RAY109

# Fundamentals of Medical Imaging

Second Edition

# Fundamentals of Medical Imaging

## Second Edition

**Paul Suetens**
*Katholieke Universiteit Leuven*

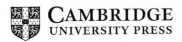

CAMBRIDGE
UNIVERSITY PRESS

CAMBRIDGE UNIVERSITY PRESS
Cambridge, New York, Melbourne, Madrid, Cape Town, Singapore, São Paulo, Delhi

Cambridge University Press
The Edinburgh Building, Cambridge CB2 8RU, UK

Published in the United States of America by Cambridge University Press, New York

www.cambridge.org
Information on this title: www.cambridge.org/suetens

First edition © Cambridge University Press 2002
Second edition © P. Suetens 2009

First published 2009

Printed in the United Kingdom at the University Press, Cambridge

*A catalog record for this publication is available from the British Library*

ISBN 978-0-521-51915-1 hardback

Additional resources for this publication at www.cambridge.org/suetens

# Contents

# Preface

This book explains the applied mathematical and physical principles of medical imaging and image processing. It gives a complete survey, accompanied by more than 300 illustrations in color, of how medical images are obtained and how they can be used for diagnosis, therapy, and surgery.

It has been written principally as a course text on medical imaging intended for graduate and final-year undergraduate students with a background in physics, mathematics, or engineering. However, I have made an effort to make the textbook readable for biomedical scientists and medical practitioners as well by deleting unnecessary mathematical details, without giving up the depth needed for physicists and engineers. Mathematical proofs are highlighted in separate paragraphs and can be skipped without hampering a fluent reading of the text.

Although a large proportion of the book covers the physical principles of imaging modalities, the emphasis is always on how the image is computed. Equipment design, clinical considerations, and diagnosis are treated in less detail. Premature techniques or topics under investigation have been omitted.

Presently, books on medical imaging fall into two groups, neither of which is suitable for this readership. The first group is the larger and comprises books directed primarily at the less numerate professions such as physicians, surgeons, and radiologic technicians. These books cover the physics and mathematics of all the major medical imaging modalities, but mostly in a superficial way. They do not allow any real understanding of these imaging modalities. The second group comprises books suitable for professional medical physicists or researchers with expertise in the field. Although these books have a numerate approach, they tend to cover the topics too deeply for the beginner and to have a narrower scope than this book.

The text reflects what I teach in class, but there is somewhat more material than I can cover in a module of 30 contact hours. This means that there is scope for the stronger student to read around the subject and also makes the book a useful purchase for those going on to do research.

In Chapter 1, an introduction to digital image processing is given. It summarizes the jargon used by the digital image community, the components defining image quality, and basic image operations used to process digital images. The theory of linear systems, described in Chapter 2 of the first edition, has been moved to an appendix. It is too high-level for the medical reader and a significant part of the engineering readers of the previous edition considered it as redundant. However, many students in physics or engineering are not familiar with linear system theory and will welcome this appendix.

Chapters 2–6 explain how medical images are obtained. The most important imaging modalities today are discussed: radiography, computed tomography, magnetic resonance imaging, nuclear medicine imaging, and ultrasonic imaging. Each chapter includes (1) a short history of the imaging modality, (2) the theory of the physics of the signal and its interaction with tissue, (3) the image formation or reconstruction process, (4) a discussion of the image quality, (5) the different types of equipment in use today, (6) examples of the clinical use of the modality, (7) a brief description of the biologic effects and safety issues, and (8) some future expectations. The imaging modalities have made an impressive evolution in a short time with respect to quality, size and applicability. This part of the book provides up-to-date information about these systems.

Chapters 7 and 8 deal with image analysis and visualization for diagnosis, therapy and surgery once images are available. Medical images can, for example, be analyzed to obtain quantitative data, or they can be displayed in three dimensions and actively used to guide a surgical intervention. Most courses separate the imaging theory from the postprocessing, but I strongly believe that they should be taken together because the topics are integrated. The interest in clinical practice today goes beyond the production and diagnosis of two-dimensional images, and the objective then is to calculate quantitative information or to use the images during patient treatment. The field of medical image analysis is in full progress and has become more mature during the last decade. This evolution has been taken into account in this second edition. The chapter on image-guided interventions of the first edition has been rewritten with a new focus. The emphasis now is on three-dimensional image visualization, not only to guide interventions, but also for diagnostic purposes.

Medical imaging and image processing can also be approached from the perspective of information and communication and the supporting technology, such as hospital information systems, the electronic patient record, and PACS (picture archiving and communication systems). However, this focus would put the emphasis on informatics, such as databases, networking, internet technology and information security, which is not the purpose of this book.

New also in this second edition is an appendix with exercises. By solving these exercises the student can test his or her insight into the matter of this book. Furthermore an ancillary website (www.cambridge. org/suetens) with three-dimensional animations has been produced which contains answers to the exercises.

In the bibliography, references to untreated topics can be found as well as more specialized works on a particular subdomain and some other generic textbooks related to the field of medical imaging and image processing.

# Acknowledgments

My colleagues of the Medical Imaging Research Center have directly and indirectly contributed to the production of this book. This facility is quite a unique place where engineers, physicists, computer scientists, and medical doctors collaborate in an interdisciplinary team. It has a central location in the University Hospital Leuven and is surrounded by the clinical departments of radiology, nuclear medicine, cardiology, and radiotherapy. Research is focused on clinically relevant questions. This then explains the emphasis in this book, which is on recent imaging technology used in clinical practice.

The following colleagues and former colleagues contributed to the first edition of the book: Bruno De Man, Jan D'hooge, Frederik Maes, Johan Michiels, Johan Nuyts, Johan Van Cleynenbreugel and Koen Vande Velde.

This second edition came about with substantial input from Hilde Bosmans (radiography), Bruno De Man (computed tomography), Stefan Sunaert (magnetic resonance imaging), Johan Nuyts (nuclear medicine), Jan D'hooge (ultrasound), Frederik Maes and Dirk Vandermeulen (image analysis), Dirk Loeckx (exercises), Christophe Deroose, Steven Dymarkowski, Guy Marchal and Luc Mortelmans (clinical use). They provided me with pieces of text, relevant clinical images and important literature; and I had indispensable discussions with them concerning content and structure.

A final reading was done by Kristof Baete, Bart De Dobbelaer, An Elen, Johannes Keustermans, Florence Kremer, Catherine Lemmens, Ronald Peeters, Janaki Rangarajan, Annemie Ribbens, Liesbet Roose, Kristien Smans, Dirk Smeets and Kevin Suetens.

I would like to express my gratitude to Walter Coudyzer for his assistance in collecting radiological data. Special thanks are due to Dominique Delaere, the information manager of the Medical Imaging Research Center, who assisted me for both this and the previous edition with the figures, illustrations and animations, consistency checking, and the webpages associated with this textbook. Thanks to his degree in biomedical engineering, he also made several improvements to the content.

# Introduction to digital image processing

## Digital images

Visible light is essentially electromagnetic radiation with wavelengths between 400 and 700 nm. Each wavelength corresponds to a different color. On the other hand, a particular color does not necessarily correspond to a single wavelength. Purple light, for example, is a combination of red and blue light. In general, a color is characterized by a spectrum of different wavelengths.

The human retina contains three types of photoreceptor cone cells that transform the incident light with different color filters. Because there are three types of cone receptors, three numbers are necessary and sufficient to describe any perceptible color. Hence, it is possible to produce an arbitrary color by superimposing appropriate amounts of three primary colors, each with its specific spectral curve. In an additive color reproduction system, such as a color monitor, these three primaries are red, green, and blue light. The color is then specified by the amounts of red, green, and blue. Equal amounts of red, green, and blue give white (see Figure 1.1(a)). Ideal white light has a flat spectrum in which all wavelengths are present. In practice, white light sources approximate this property. In a subtractive color reproduction system, such as printing or painting, these three primaries typically are

cyan, magenta, and yellow. Cyan is the color of a material, seen in white light, that absorbs red but reflects green and blue, and can thus be obtained by additive mixing of equal amounts of green and blue light. Similarly, magenta is the result of the absorption of green light and consists of equal amounts of red and blue light, and yellow is the result of the absorption of blue and consists of equal amounts of red and green light. Therefore, subtractive mixing of cyan and magenta gives blue, subtractive mixing of cyan and yellow gives green, and subtractive mixing of yellow and magenta gives red. Subtractive mixing of yellow, cyan, and magenta produces black (only absorption and no reflection) (see Figure 1.1(b)).

Note that equal distances in physical intensity are not perceived as equal distances in *brightness*. Intensity levels must be spaced logarithmically, rather than linearly, to achieve equal steps in perceived brightness. *Hue* refers to the dominant wavelength in the spectrum, and represents the different colors. *Saturation* describes the amount of white light present in the spectrum. If no white light is present, the saturation is 100%. Saturation distinguishes colorful tones from pastel tones at the same hue. In the color cone of Figure 1.2, equal distances between colors by no

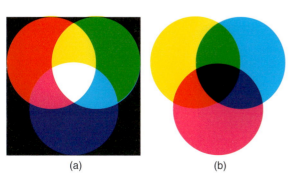

**Figure 1.1** Color mixing: **(a)** additive color mixing, **(b)** subtractive color mixing.

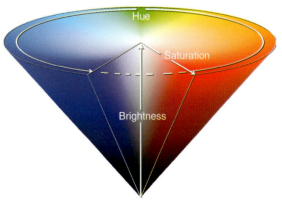

**Figure 1.2** Hue, brightness, and saturation.

means correspond to equal perceptual differences. The Commission Internationale de l'Eclairage (CIE) has defined perceptually more uniform color spaces like $L^*u^*v^*$ and $L^*a^*b^*$. A discussion of pros and cons of different color spaces is beyond the scope of this textbook.

While chromatic light needs three descriptors or numbers to characterize it, achromatic light, as produced by a black-and-white monitor, has only one descriptor, its brightness or *gray value*. Achromatic light is light with a saturation of 0%. It contains only white light.

Given a set of possible gray levels or colors and a (rectangular) grid, a *digital image* attributes a gray value (i.e., brightness) or a color (i.e., hue, saturation and brightness) to each of the grid points or *pixels*. In a digital image, the gray levels are integers. Although brightness values are continuous in real life, in a digital image we have only a limited number of gray levels at our disposal. The conversion from analog samples to discrete-valued samples is called *quantization*. Figure 1.3 shows the same image using two different quantizations. When too few gray values are used, *contouring* appears. The image is reduced to an artificial looking height map. How many gray values are needed to produce a continuous looking image? Assume that $n + 1$ gray values are displayed with corresponding physical intensities $I_0, I_1, \ldots, I_n$. $I_0$ is the lowest attainable intensity and $I_n$ the maximum intensity. The ratio $I_n/I_0$ is called the *dynamic range*. The human eye cannot distinguish subsequent intensities $I_j$ and $I_{j+1}$ if they differ less than 1%, i.e., if $I_{j+1} \leq 1.01\, I_j$. In that case $I_n \leq 1.01^n I_0$ and $n \geq \log_{1.01}(I_n/I_0)$. For a dynamic range of 100 the required number of gray values is 463 and a dynamic range of 1000 requires 694 different gray values for a continuous looking brightness. Most digital medical images today use 4096

gray values (12 bpp). The problem with too many gray values, however, is that small differences in brightness cannot be perceived on the display. This problem can be overcome for example by expanding a small gray value interval into a larger one by using a suitable gray value transformation, as discussed on p. 4 below.

In the process of digital imaging, the continuous looking world has to be captured onto the finite number of pixels of the image grid. The conversion from a continuous function to a discrete function, retaining only the values at the grid points, is called *sampling* and is discussed in detail in Appendix A, p. 228.

Much information about an image is contained in its *histogram*. The histogram $h$ of an image is a probability distribution on the set of possible gray levels. The probability of a gray value $v$ is given by its relative frequency in the image, that is,

$$h(v) = \frac{\text{number of pixels having gray value } v}{\text{total number of pixels}}. \quad (1.1)$$

## Image quality

The *resolution* of a digital image is sometimes wrongly defined as the linear pixel density (expressed in dots per inch). This is, however, only an upper bound for the resolution. Resolution is also determined by the imaging process. The more blurring, the lower is the resolution. Factors that contribute to the unsharpness of an image are (1) the characteristics of the imaging system, such as the focal spot and the amount of detector blur, (2) the scene characteristics and geometry, such as the shape of the subject, its position and motion, and (3) the viewing conditions.

Resolution can be defined as follows. When imaging a very small, bright point on a dark background, this dot will normally not appear as sharp in the image

**Figure 1.3** The same image quantized with **(a)** 8 bpp and **(b)** 4 bpp.

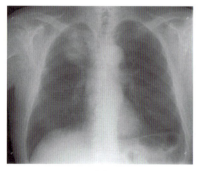

(a)

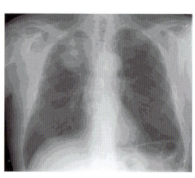

(b)

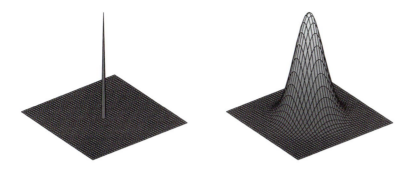

**Figure 1.4 (a)** Sharp bright spot on a dark background. **(b)** Typical image of (a). The smoothed blob is called the point spread function (PSF) of the imaging system.

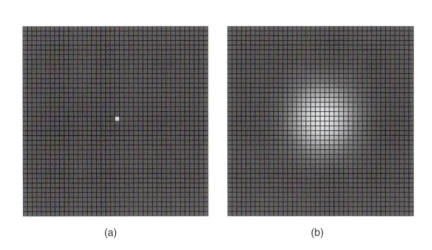

(a)         (b)

as it actually is. It will be smoothed, and the obtained blob is called the *point spread function* (PSF) (see Figure 1.4). An indicative measure of the resolution is the full width at half maximum (FWHM) of the point spread function. When two such blobs are placed at this distance or shorter from each other, they will no longer be distinguishable as two separate objects. If the resolution is the same in all directions, the *line spread function* (LSF), i.e., the actual image of a thin line, may be more practical than the PSF.

Instead of using the PSF or LSF it is also possible to use the *optical transfer function* (OTF) (see Figure 1.5). The OTF expresses the relative amplitude and phase shift of a sinusoidal target as a function of frequency. The modulation transfer function (MTF) is the amplitude (i.e. MTF = |OTF|) and the phase transfer function (PTF) is the phase component of the OTF. For small amplitudes the lines may no longer be distinguishable. An indication of the resolution is the number of line pairs per millimeter (lp/mm) at a specified small amplitude (e.g., 10%).

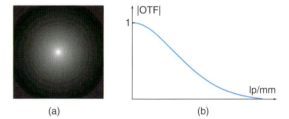

(a)         (b)

**Figure 1.5 (a)** Point spread function (PSF). **(b)** Corresponding modulation transfer function (MTF). The MTF is the amplitude of the optical transfer function (OTF), which is the Fourier transform (FT) of the PSF.

As explained in Appendix A, the OTF is the Fourier transform (FT) of the PSF or LSF.

*Contrast* is the difference in intensity of adjacent regions of the image. More accurately, it is the amplitude of the Fourier transform of the image as a function of spatial frequency. Using the Fourier transform, the image is unraveled in sinusoidal patterns with corresponding amplitude and these amplitudes represent the contrast at different spatial frequencies.

3

The contrast is defined by (1) the imaging process, such as the source intensity and the absorption efficiency or sensitivity of the capturing device, (2) the scene characteristics, such as the physical properties, size and shape of the object, and the use of contrast agents, and (3) the viewing conditions, such as the room illumination and display equipment. Because the OTF drops off for larger frequencies, the contrast of very small objects will be influenced by the resolution as well.

A third quality factor is image *noise*. The emission and detection of light and all other types of electromagnetic waves are stochastic processes. Because of the statistical nature of imaging, noise is always present. It is the random component in the image. If the noise level is high compared with the image intensity of an object, the meaningful information is lost in the noise. An important measure, obtained from signal theory, is therefore the *signal-to-noise ratio* (SNR or S/N). In the terminology of images this is the *contrast-to-noise ratio* (CNR). Both contrast and noise are frequency dependent. An estimate of the noise can be obtained by making a *flat-field* image, i.e., an image without an object between the source and the detector. The noise amplitude as a function of spatial frequency can be calculated from the square root of the so-called Wiener spectrum, which is the Fourier transform of the autocorrelation of a flat-field image.

*Artifacts* are artificial image features such as dust or scratches in photographs. Examples in medical images are metal streak artifacts in computed tomography (CT) images and geometric distortions in magnetic resonance (MR) images. Artifacts may also be introduced by digital image processing, such as edge enhancement. Because artifacts may hamper the diagnosis or yield incorrect measurements, it is important to avoid them or at least understand their origin.

In the following chapters, image resolution, noise, contrast, and artifacts will be discussed for each of the imaging modalities.

## Basic image operations

In this section a number of basic mathematical operations on images are described. They can be employed for image enhancement, analysis and visualization.

The aim of medical image enhancement is to allow the clinician to perceive better all the relevant diagnostic information present in the image. In digital radiography for example, 12-bit images with 4096 possible gray levels are available. As discussed above, it is physically impossible for the human eye to distinguish all these gray values at once in a single image. Consequently, not all the diagnostic information encoded in the image may be perceived. Meaningful details must have a sufficiently high contrast to allow the clinician to detect them easily.

The larger the number of gray values in the image, the more important this issue becomes, as lower contrast features may become available in the image data. Therefore, image enhancement will not become less important as the quality of digital image capturing systems improves. On the contrary, it will gain importance.

## Gray level transformations

Given a digital image $I$ that attributes a gray value (i.e., brightness) to each of the pixels $(i, j)$, a *gray level transformation* is a function $g$ that transforms each gray level $I(i, j)$ to another value $I'(i, j)$ independent of the position $(i, j)$. Hence, for all pixels $(i, j)$

$$I'(i, j) = g(I(i, j)). \qquad (1.2)$$

In practice, $g$ is an increasing function. Instead of transforming gray values it is also possible to operate on color (i.e., hue, saturation and brightness). In that case three of these transformations are needed to transform colors to colors.

Note that, in this textbook, the notation $I$ is used not only for the physical intensity but also for the gray value (or color), which are usually not identical. The gray value can represent brightness (logarithm of the intensity, see p. 1), relative signal intensity or any other derived quantity. Nevertheless the terms intensity and intensity image are loosely used as synonyms for gray value and gray value image.

If pixel $(i_1, j_1)$ appears brighter than pixel $(i_2, j_2)$ in the original image, this relation holds after the gray level transformation. The main use of such a gray level transformation is to increase the contrast in some regions of the image. The price to be paid is a decreased contrast in other parts of the image. Indeed, in a region containing pixels with gray values in the range where the slope of $g$ is larger than 1, the difference between these gray values increases. In regions with gray values in the range with slope smaller than 1, gray values come closer together and different values may even become identical after the transformation. Figure 1.6 shows an example of such a transformation.

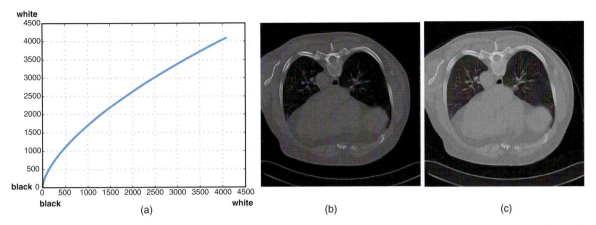

**Figure 1.6** A gray level transformation that increases the contrast in dark areas and decreases the contrast in bright regions. It can be used when the clinically relevant information is situated in the dark areas, such as the lungs in this example: **(b)** the original image, **(c)** the transformed image.

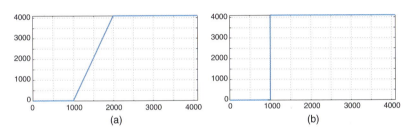

**Figure 1.7 (a)** Window/leveling with $l = 1500, w = 1000$. **(b)** Thresholding with $tr = 1000$.

A particular and popular transformation is the *window/level operation* (see Figure 1.7(a)). In this operation, an interval or window is selected, determined by the window center or level $l$, and the window width $w$. Explicitly

$$g_{l,w}(t) = \begin{cases} 0 & \text{for } t < l - \dfrac{w}{2} \\[2mm] \dfrac{M}{w}\left(t - l + \dfrac{w}{2}\right) & \text{for } l - \dfrac{w}{2} \leq t \leq l + \dfrac{w}{2} \\[2mm] M & \text{for } t > l + \dfrac{w}{2}, \end{cases} \tag{1.3}$$

where $M$ is the maximal available gray value. Contrast outside the window is lost completely, whereas the portion of the range lying inside the window is stretched to the complete gray value range.

An even simpler operation is *thresholding* (Figure 1.7(b)). Here all gray levels up to a certain threshold $tr$ are set to zero, and all gray levels above the threshold equal the maximal gray value

$$\begin{aligned} g_{\mathrm{tr}}(t) &= 0 & \text{for } t \leq tr \\ g_{\mathrm{tr}}(t) &= M & \text{for } t > tr. \end{aligned} \tag{1.4}$$

These operations can be very useful for images with a bimodal histogram (see Figure 1.8).

## Multi-image operations

A simple operation is adding or subtracting images in a pixelwise way. For two images $I_1$ and $I_2$, the sum $I_+$ and the difference $I_-$ are defined as

$$I_+(i,j) = I_1(i,j) + I_2(i,j) \tag{1.5}$$

$$I_-(i,j) = I_1(i,j) - I_2(i,j). \tag{1.6}$$

If these operations yield values outside the available gray value range, the resulting image can be brought back into that range by a linear transformation. The average of $n$ images is defined as

$$I_{\mathrm{av}}(i,j) = \frac{1}{n}(I_1(i,j) + \cdots + I_n(i,j)). \tag{1.7}$$

Averaging can be useful to decrease the noise in a sequence of images of a motionless object (Figure 1.9). The random noise averages out, whereas the object remains unchanged (if the images match perfectly).

5

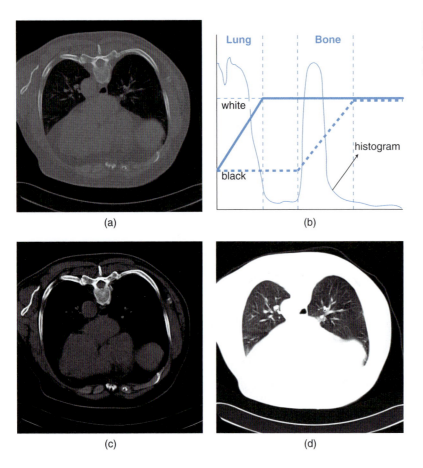

(a)

(b)

(c)

(d)

**Figure 1.8** Original CT image **(a)** with bimodal histogram **(b)**. **(c, d)** Result of window/leveling using a bone window (dashed line in (b)) and lung window (solid line in (b)), respectively.

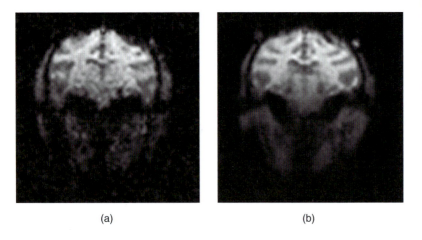

(a)

(b)

**Figure 1.9 (a)** Magnetic resonance image of a slice through the brain. This image was obtained with a $T_1$-weighted EPI sequence (see p. 82) and therefore has a low SNR. **(b)** To increase the SNR, 16 subsequent images of the same slice were acquired and averaged. (Courtesy of Professor S. Sunaert, Department of Radiology.)

This method can also be used for color images by averaging the different channels independently like gray level images. Subtraction can be used to get rid of the background in two similar images. For example, in blood vessel imaging (angiography), two images are made, one without a contrast agent and another with contrast agent injected in the blood vessels. Subtraction of these two images yields a pure image of the blood vessels because the subtraction deletes the other anatomical features. Figure 1.10 shows an example.

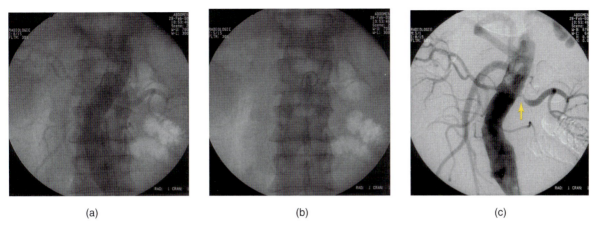

(a)               (b)               (c)

**Figure 1.10** (a) Radiographic image after injection of a contrast agent. (b) Mask image, that is, the same exposure before contrast injection. (c) Subtraction of (a) and (b), followed by contrast enhancement. (Courtesy of Professor G. Wilms, Department of Radiology.)

## Geometric operations

It is often necessary to perform elementary geometric operations on an image, such as scaling (zooming), translation, rotation, and shear. Examples are the registration of images (see p. 173) and image-to-patient registration for image-guided surgery (see p. 211). A spatial or geometric transformation assigns each point $(x, y)$ to a new location $(x', y') = S(x, y)$. The most common two-dimensional (2D) transformations can be written using homogeneous coordinates:

scaling
$$\begin{pmatrix} x' \\ y' \\ 1 \end{pmatrix} = \begin{pmatrix} s_x & 0 & 0 \\ 0 & s_y & 0 \\ 0 & 0 & 1 \end{pmatrix} \begin{pmatrix} x \\ y \\ 1 \end{pmatrix}$$

translation
$$\begin{pmatrix} x' \\ y' \\ 1 \end{pmatrix} = \begin{pmatrix} 1 & 0 & t_x \\ 0 & 1 & t_y \\ 0 & 0 & 1 \end{pmatrix} \begin{pmatrix} x \\ y \\ 1 \end{pmatrix}$$

shear
$$\begin{pmatrix} x' \\ y' \\ 1 \end{pmatrix} = \begin{pmatrix} 1 & u_x & 0 \\ u_y & 1 & 0 \\ 0 & 0 & 1 \end{pmatrix} \begin{pmatrix} x \\ y \\ 1 \end{pmatrix}$$

rotation
$$\begin{pmatrix} x' \\ y' \\ 1 \end{pmatrix} = \begin{pmatrix} \cos\theta & -\sin\theta & 0 \\ \sin\theta & \cos\theta & 0 \\ 0 & 0 & 1 \end{pmatrix} \begin{pmatrix} x \\ y \\ 1 \end{pmatrix}$$

general affine
$$\begin{pmatrix} x' \\ y' \\ 1 \end{pmatrix} = \begin{pmatrix} a_{11} & a_{12} & t_x \\ a_{21} & a_{22} & t_y \\ 0 & 0 & 1 \end{pmatrix} \begin{pmatrix} x \\ y \\ 1 \end{pmatrix}.$$

(1.8)

Composition of two such transformations amounts to multiplying the corresponding matrices.

A general affine 2D transformation depends on six parameters and includes scaling, translation, shear,

and rotation as special cases. Affine transformations preserve parallelism of lines but generally not lengths and angles. Angles and lengths are preserved by orthogonal transformations (e.g., rotations and translations)

orthogonal
$$\begin{pmatrix} x' \\ y' \\ 1 \end{pmatrix} = \begin{pmatrix} r_{11} & r_{12} & t_x \\ r_{21} & r_{22} & t_y \\ 0 & 0 & 1 \end{pmatrix} \begin{pmatrix} x \\ y \\ 1 \end{pmatrix}, \quad (1.9)$$

where the $2 \times 2$ matrix $R = \begin{pmatrix} r_{11} & r_{12} \\ r_{21} & r_{22} \end{pmatrix}$ is subject to the constraint $R^{\mathrm{T}} R = 1$.

A pixel $(x, y) = (i, j)$ of image $I(i, j)$ will be mapped onto $(x', y')$ and $x'$ and $y'$ are usually no longer integer values. To obtain a new image $I'(i', j')$ on a pixel grid, *interpolation* is used. For each $(i', j')$ the gray value $I'(i', j')$ is then calculated by simple (e.g., bilinear) interpolation between the gray values of the pixels of $I$ lying closest to the inverse transformation of $(i', j')$, i.e., $S^{-1}(i', j')$.

Today the majority of medical images are three dimensional (3D). The above matrices can easily be extended to three dimensions. For example, the general affine 3D transformation can be written as

general affine
$$\begin{pmatrix} x' \\ y' \\ z' \\ 1 \end{pmatrix} = \begin{pmatrix} a_{11} & a_{12} & a_{13} & t_x \\ a_{21} & a_{22} & a_{23} & t_y \\ a_{31} & a_{32} & a_{33} & t_z \\ 0 & 0 & 0 & 1 \end{pmatrix} \begin{pmatrix} x \\ y \\ z \\ 1 \end{pmatrix}.$$

(1.10)

While most medical images are three dimensional, interventional imaging is often still two dimensional.

7

To map the 3D image data onto the 2D image a projective transformation is needed. Assuming a pinhole camera, such as an X-ray tube, any 3D point $(x, y, z)$ is mapped onto its 2D projection point $(u, v)$ by the projective matrix (more details on p. 216)

$$\begin{pmatrix} u' \\ v' \\ w' \end{pmatrix} = \begin{pmatrix} f_x & \kappa_x & u_0 & 0 \\ \kappa_y & f_y & v_0 & 0 \\ 0 & 0 & 1 & 0 \end{pmatrix} \begin{pmatrix} x \\ y \\ z \\ 1 \end{pmatrix}$$

$$\begin{pmatrix} u \\ v \\ 1 \end{pmatrix} = \begin{pmatrix} \frac{u'}{w'} \\ \frac{v'}{w'} \\ 1 \end{pmatrix}. \qquad (1.11)$$

Using homogeneous coordinates the above geometric transformations can all be represented by matrices. In some cases, however, it might be necessary to use more flexible transformations. For example, the comparison of images at different moments, such as in follow-up studies, may be hampered due to patient movement, organ deformations, e.g., differences in bladder and rectum filling, or breathing. Another example is the geometric distortion of magnetic resonance images resulting from undesired deviations of the magnetic field (see p. 92). Geometric transformations are discussed further in Chapter 7.

## Filters

### Linear filters

From linear system theory (see Eq. (A.22)), we know that an image $I(i, j)$ can be written as follows:

$$I(i, j) = \sum_{k,l} I(k, l)\delta(i - k, j - l). \qquad (1.12)$$

For a linear shift-invariant transformation $\mathcal{L}$ (see also Eq. (A.31)),

$$\mathcal{L}(I)(i, j) = \sum_{k,l} I(k, l)\mathcal{L}(\delta)(i - k, j - l)$$

$$= \sum_{k,l} I(k, l)f(i - k, j - l)$$

$$= \sum_{k,l} f(k, l)I(i - k, j - l)$$

$$= f * I(i, j), \qquad (1.13)$$

where $f$ is called the *kernel* or *filter*, and the linear transformation on the digital image $I$ is the discrete convolution with its kernel $f = \mathcal{L}(\delta)$.

In practice, the flipped kernel $h$ defined as $h(i, j) = f(-i, -j)$ is usually used. Hence, Eq. (1.13) can be rewritten as

$$\mathcal{L}(I)(i, j) = f * I(i, j)$$

$$= \sum_{k,l} f(k, l)I(i - k, j - l)$$

$$= \sum_{k,l} h(k, l)I(i + k, j + l)$$

$$= h \bullet I(i, j), \qquad (1.14)$$

where $h \bullet I$ is the *cross-correlation* of $h$ and $I$. If the filter is symmetric, which is often the case, cross-correlation and convolution are identical.

A cross-correlation of an image $I(i, j)$ with a kernel $h$ has the following physical meaning. The kernel $h$ is used as an image *template* or *mask* that is shifted across the image. For every image pixel $(i, j)$, the template pixel $h(0, 0)$, which typically lies in the center of the mask, is superimposed onto this pixel $(i, j)$, and the values of the template and image that correspond to the same positions are multiplied. Next, all these values are summed. A cross-correlation emphasizes patterns in the image similar to the template.

Often local filters with only a few pixels in diameter are used. A simple example is the $3 \times 3$ mask with values $1/9$ at each position (Figure 1.11). This filter performs an averaging on the image, making it smoother and removing some noise. The filter gives the same weight to the center pixel as to its neighbors. A softer way of smoothing the image is to give a high weight to the center pixel and less weight to pixels further away from the central pixel. A suitable filter for

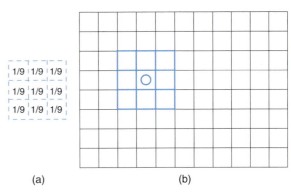

(a)                    (b)

**Figure 1.11 (a)** $3 \times 3$ averaging filter. **(b)** The filter as floating image template or mask.

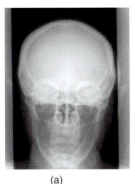 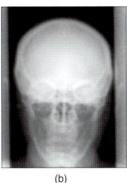 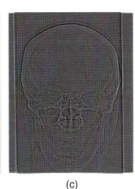

(a)    (b)    (c)

**Figure 1.12** (a) Radiography of the skull. (b) Low-pass filtered image with a Gaussian filter (20 × 20 pixels, $\sigma = 15$). (c) High-pass filtered image obtained by subtracting (b) from (a).

this operation is the discretized Gaussian function

$$g(\vec{r}) = \frac{1}{2\pi\sigma^2}\, e^{(-r^2/2\sigma^2)} \qquad \vec{r} = (i,j). \qquad (1.15)$$

Small values are put to zero in order to produce a local filter. The Fourier transform of the Gaussian is again Gaussian. In the Fourier domain, convolution with a filter becomes multiplication. Taking this into account, it is clear that a Gaussian filter attenuates the high frequencies in the image. These averaging filters are therefore also called *low-pass* filters. In contrast, filters that emphasize high frequencies are called *high-pass* filters. A high-pass filter can be constructed simply from a low-pass one by subtracting the low-pass filter $g$ from the identity filter $\delta$. A high-pass filter enhances small-scale variations in the image. It extracts edges and fine textures. An example of low-pass and high-pass filtering is shown in Figure 1.12.

Other types of linear filters are differential operators such as the gradient and the Laplacian. However, these operations are not defined on discrete images. Because derivatives are defined on differentiable functions, the computation is performed by first fitting a differentiable function through the discrete data set. This can be obtained by convolving the discrete image with a continuous function $f$. The derivative of this result is evaluated at the points $(i,j)$ of the original sampling grid. For the 1D partial derivative this sequence of operations can be written as follows:

$$\frac{\partial}{\partial x} I(i,j) \approx \left[ \frac{\partial}{\partial x} \left( \sum_{k,l} I(k,l) f(x-k, y-l) \right) \right]_{x=i, y=j}$$

$$= \left[ \sum_{k,l} \frac{\partial f}{\partial x}(i-k, j-l) I(k,l) \right]. \qquad (1.16)$$

Hence, the derivative is approximated by a convolution with a filter that is the sampled derivative of some differentiable function $f(\vec{r})$. This procedure can now be used further to approximate the gradient and the Laplacian of a digital image:

$$\nabla I = \nabla f * I$$
$$\nabla^2 I = \nabla^2 f * I, \qquad (1.17)$$

where it is understood that we use the discrete convolution. If $f$ is a Gaussian $g$, the following differential convolution operators are obtained:

$$\nabla g(\vec{r}) = -\frac{1}{\sigma^2} g(\vec{r}) \cdot \vec{r}$$
$$\nabla^2 g(\vec{r}) = \frac{1}{\sigma^4}(r^2 - 2\sigma^2) \cdot g(\vec{r}). \qquad (1.18)$$

For $\sigma = 0.5$, this procedure yields approximately the following $3 \times 3$ filters (see Figure 1.13):

Gaussian

| 0.01 | 0.08 | 0.01 |
|------|------|------|
| 0.08 | 0.64 | 0.08 |
| 0.01 | 0.08 | 0.01 |

$\dfrac{\partial}{\partial x}$

| 0.05 | 0 | −0.05 |
|------|---|-------|
| 0.34 | 0 | −0.34 |
| 0.05 | 0 | −0.05 |

$\dfrac{\partial}{\partial y}$

| 0.05 | 0.34 | 0.05 |
|------|------|------|
| 0 | 0 | 0 |
| −0.05 | −0.34 | −0.05 |

$\nabla^2$

| 0.3 | 0.7 | 0.3 |
|-----|-----|-----|
| 0.7 | −4 | 0.7 |
| 0.3 | 0.7 | 0.3 |

$$(1.19)$$

**9**

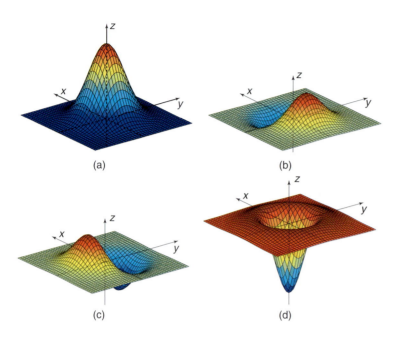

(a)

(b)

(c)

(d)

**Figure 1.13** **(a)** A Gaussian function. **(b)** Derivative of the Gaussian in the $x$-direction. **(c)** Derivative of the Gaussian in the $y$-direction. **(d)** Laplacian of the Gaussian.

Note that integration of a Gaussian over the whole spatial domain must be 1, and for the gradient and Laplacian this must be 0. To satisfy this condition, the numbers in the templates above, which are spatially limited, were adapted.

The Laplacian of a Gaussian is sometimes approximated by a difference of Gaussians with different values of $\sigma$. This can be derived from Eq. (1.18). Rewriting it as

$$\left(\frac{r^2}{\sigma^4} + \frac{2}{\sigma^2}\right) g(\vec{r}) - \frac{4}{\sigma^2} g(\vec{r}) \qquad (1.20)$$

shows us that the second term is proportional to the original Gaussian $g$, while the first term drops off more slowly because of the $r^2$ and acts as if it were a Gaussian with a larger value of $\sigma$ (the $2/\sigma^2$ added to the $r^2/\sigma^4$ makes it a monotonically decreasing function in the radial direction).

Popular derivative filters are the Sobel operator for the first derivative, and the average - $\delta$ for the Laplacian, which use integer filter elements:

Sobel

| 1 | 0 | $-1$ |
|---|---|---|
| 2 | 0 | $-2$ |
| 1 | 0 | $-1$ |

average - $\delta$

| 1 | 1 | 1 |
|---|---|---|
| 1 | $-8$ | 1 |
| 1 | 1 | 1 |

$$(1.21)$$

Note that, if we compute the convolution of an image with a filter, it is necessary to extend the image at its boundaries because pixels lying outside the image will be addressed by the convolution algorithm. This is best done in a smooth way, for example by repeating the boundary pixels. If not, artifacts appear at the boundaries after the convolution.

As an application of linear filtering, let us discuss edge enhancement using *unsharp masking*. Figure 1.14 shows an example. As already mentioned, a low-pass filter $g$ can be used to split an image $I$ into two parts: a smooth part $g * I$, and the remaining high-frequency part $I - g * I$ containing the edges in the image or image details. Hence

$$I = g * I + (I - g * I). \qquad (1.22)$$

Note that $I - g * I$ is a crude approximation of the Laplacian of $I$. Unsharp masking enhances the image details by emphasizing the high-frequency part and assigning it a higher weight. For some $\alpha > 0$, the output image $I'$ is then given by

$$\begin{aligned} I' &= g * I + (1 + \alpha)(I - g * I) \\ &= I + \alpha(I - g * I) \\ &= (1 + \alpha)I - \alpha \, g * I. \end{aligned} \qquad (1.23)$$

The parameter $\alpha$ controls the strength of the enhancement, and the parameter $\sigma$ is responsible for the size

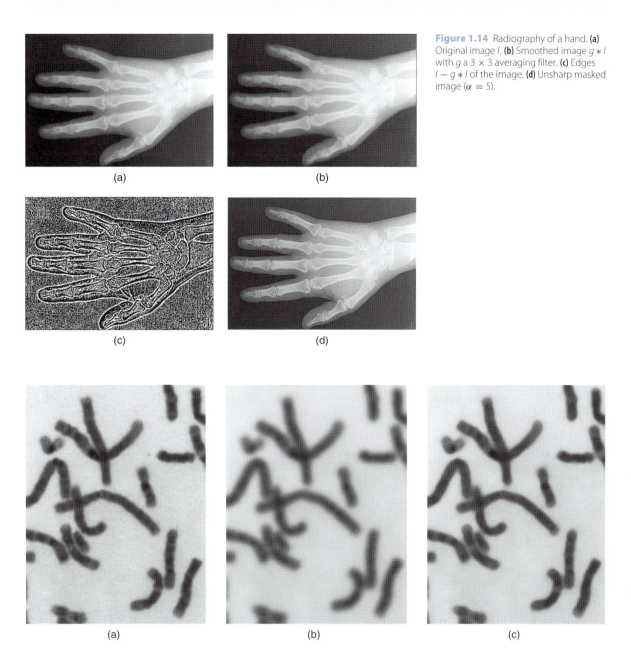

**Figure 1.14** Radiography of a hand. **(a)** Original image $I$. **(b)** Smoothed image $g * I$ with $g$ a $3 \times 3$ averaging filter. **(c)** Edges $I - g * I$ of the image. **(d)** Unsharp masked image ($\alpha = 5$).

(a)

(b)

(c)

(d)

(a)

(b)

(c)

**Figure 1.15** **(a)** Original karyotype (chromosome image). **(b)** Image smoothed with a Gaussian filter. **(c)** Image filtered with a median filter.

of the frequency band that is enhanced. The smaller the value of $\sigma$, the more unsharp masking focuses on the finest details.

### Nonlinear filters

Not every goal can be achieved by using linear filters. Many problems are better solved with nonlinear methods. Consider, for example, the denoising problem. As explained above, the averaging filter removes noise in the image. The output image is, however, much smoother than the input image. In particular, edges are smeared out and may even disappear. To avoid smoothing, it can therefore be better to calculate the median instead of the mean value in a small window around each pixel. This procedure better preserves the edges (check this with paper and pencil on a step edge). Figure 1.15 shows an example on a chromosome image.

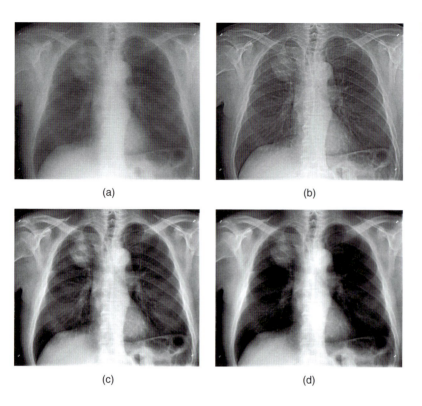

(a)

(b)

(c)

(d)

**Figure 1.16** The effect of the filter size in unsharp masking. **(a)** Original image (1024 × 1248 pixels). Unsharp masking with filter size **(b)** 10, **(c)** 60, and **(d)** 125. Image (b) shows enhanced fine details but an overall reduction of the contrast. In image (d), large-scale variations, which correspond to the lungs and the mediastinum, are enhanced, and most of the small details are suppressed. Image (c) shows a case somewhere between (b) and (d).

## Multiscale image processing

In the previous sections a number of basic image operations have been described that can be employed for image enhancement and analysis (see for example Figures 1.6 and 1.14).

Gray value transformations (Figure 1.6), such as the widespread window/level operation, increase the contrast in a subpart of the gray value scale. They are quite useful for low-contrast objects situated in the enhanced gray value band. Unfortunately, features outside this gray value interval are attenuated instead of enhanced. In addition, gray value transformations do not make use of the spatial relationship among object pixels and therefore equally enhance meaningful and meaningless features such as noise.

Spatial operations overcome this problem. Differential operations, such as unsharp masking (Figure 1.14), enhance gray value variations or edges, whereas other operations, such as spatial averaging and median filtering, reduce the noise. However, they focus on features of a particular size because of the fixed size of the mask, which is a parameter that must be chosen. Figure 1.16 shows the effect of the filter size for unsharp masking. Using a low-pass filter, the image is split into a low-pass and a remaining high-pass part. Next, the high-pass part is emphasized, both parts are added again (Eq. (1.23)), and the result is normalized to the available gray value range. If the filter size is small, this procedure emphasizes small-scale features and suppresses gray value variations that extend over larger areas in the image. With a large-size filter, large image features are enhanced at the expense of the small details. With this method, the following problems are encountered.

- The image operation is tuned to a particular frequency band that is predetermined by the choice of the filter size. However, diagnostic information is available at all scales in the image and is not limited to a particular frequency band.

- Gray value variations in the selected frequency band are intensified equally. This is desired for low-contrast features but unnecessary for high-contrast features that are easily perceivable.

It is clear that a method is needed that is independent of the spatial extent or scale of the image features and emphasizes the amplitude of only the low-contrast features. Multiscale image processing has been studied extensively, not only by computer scientists but also by neurophysiologists. It is well known that the human visual system makes use of a multiscale approach. However, this theory is beyond the scope of this textbook. More about multiscale image analysis can be found, for example, in [1].

[1] B. M. ter Haar Romeny. *Front-End Vision and Multi-Scale Image Analysis: Multi-Scale Computer Vision Theory and Applications written in Mathematica*, Volume 27 of *Computational Imaging and Vision*. Springer, 2003.

# Chapter 2

# Radiography

## Introduction

X-rays were discovered by Wilhelm Konrad Röntgen in 1895 while he was experimenting with cathode tubes. In these experiments, he used fluorescent screens, which start glowing when struck by light emitted from the tube. To Röntgen's surprise, this effect persisted even when the tube was placed in a carton box. He soon realized that the tube was emitting not only light, but also a new kind of radiation, which he called X-rays because of their mysterious nature. This new kind of radiation could not only travel through the box. Röntgen found out that it was attenuated in a different way by various kinds of materials and that it could, like light, be captured on a photographic plate. This opened up the way for its use in medicine. The first "Röntgen picture" of a hand was made soon after the discovery of X-rays. No more than a few months later, radiographs were already used in clinical practice. The nature of X-rays as short-wave electromagnetic radiation was established by Max von Laue in 1912.

## X-rays

X-rays are electromagnetic waves. Electromagnetic radiation consists of photons. The energy $E$ of a photon with frequency $f$ and wavelength $\lambda$ is

$$E = hf = \frac{hc}{\lambda}, \qquad (2.1)$$

where $h$ is Planck's constant and $c$ is the speed of light in vacuum; $hc = 1.2397 \times 10^{-6}$ eV m. The electromagnetic spectrum (see Figure 2.1) can be divided into several bands, starting with very long radio waves, used in magnetic resonance imaging (MRI) (see Chapter 4), extending over microwaves, infrared, visible and ultraviolet light, X-rays, used in radiography, up to the ultrashort-wave, high energetic $\gamma$-rays, used in nuclear imaging (see Chapter 5). The wavelength for X-rays is on the order of Angstrøms ($10^{-10}$ m) and,

consequently, the corresponding photon energies are on the order of keV (1 eV $= 1.602 \times 10^{-19}$ J).

X-rays are generated in an *X-ray tube*, which consists of a vacuum tube with a *cathode* and an *anode* (Figure 2.2(a)). The cathode current $J$ releases electrons at the cathode by thermal excitation. These electrons are accelerated toward the anode by a voltage $U$ between the cathode and the anode. The electrons hit the anode and release their energy, partly in the form of X-rays, i.e., as *bremsstrahlung* and *characteristic radiation*. Bremsstrahlung yields a continuous X-ray spectrum while characteristic radiation yields characteristic peaks superimposed onto the continuous spectrum (Figure 2.2(b)).

### Brehmsstrahlung

The energy (expressed in eV) and wavelength of the bremsstrahlung photons are bounded by

$$E \leq E_{max} = qU, \qquad \lambda \geq \lambda_{min} = \frac{hc}{qU}, \qquad (2.2)$$

where $q$ is the electric charge of an electron. For example, if $U = 100$ kV, then $E_{max} = 100$ keV.

### Characteristic radiation

The energy of the electrons at the cathode can release an orbital electron from a shell (e.g., the K-shell), leaving a hole. This hole can be refilled when an electron of higher energy (e.g., from the L-shell or the M-shell) drops into the hole while emitting photons of a very specific energy. The energy of the photon is the difference between the energies of the two electron states; for example, when an electron from the L-shell (with energy $E_L$) drops into the K-shell (getting energy $E_K$) a photon of energy

$$E = E_L - E_K \qquad (2.3)$$

is emitted. Such transitions therefore yield characteristic peaks in the X-ray spectrum.

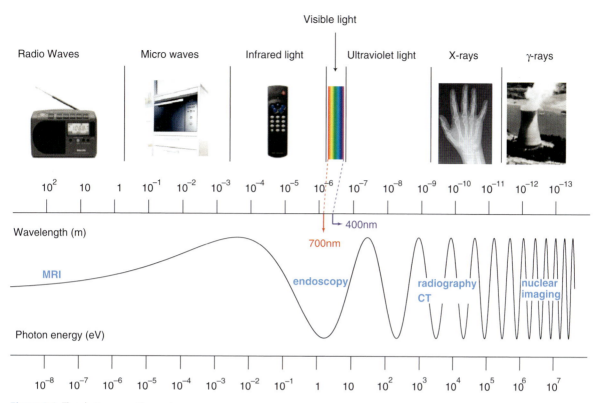

**Figure 2.1** The electromagnetic spectrum.

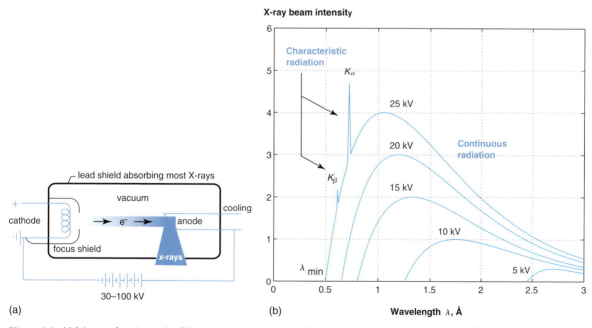

**Figure 2.2** (a) Scheme of an X-ray tube. (b) Intensity distribution in the Röntgen spectrum of molybdenum for different voltages. The excitation potential of the K-series is 20.1 kV. This series appears as characteristic peaks in the 25 kV curve. The peaks $K_\alpha$ and $K_\beta$ are due to L-shell and M-shell drops respectively.

The important parameters of an X-ray source are the following.

- The amount of electrons hitting the anode and, consequently, the amount of emitted photons controlled by the cathode current multiplied by the time the current is on (typically expressed in mA s). Typical values range from 1 to 100 mA s.
- The energy of the electrons hitting the anodes and, consequently, the energy of the emitted photons (typically expressed in keV), controlled by the voltage between cathode and anode (typically expressed in kV). For most examinations the values vary from 50 to 125 kV. For mammography the voltage is 22–34 kV. The energy of the atom defines the upper limit of the photon energy.
- The total incident energy (typically expressed in joules, $1\,J = 1\,kV\,mA\,s$) at the anode, defined by the product of the voltage, the cathode current and the time the current is on. Note that almost all of this energy is degraded to heat within the tube. Less than 1% is transmitted into X-rays.

## Interaction with matter
## Interaction of photons with matter

X-rays and $\gamma$-rays are ionizing waves. Such photons are able to ionize an atom, i.e., to release an electron from the atom. Photons with energy less than 13.6 eV are nonionizing. These photons cannot eject an electron from its atom, but are only able to raise it to a higher energy shell, a process called *excitation*. Ionizing photons can interact with matter in different ways.

- The energy of X-ray photons can be absorbed by an atom and immediately released again in the form of a new photon with the same energy but traveling in a different direction. This nonionizing process is called *Rayleigh scattering* or *coherent scattering* and occurs mainly at low energies (<30 keV). The lower the energy the higher is the scattering angle. In most radiological examinations it does not play a major role because the voltage used is typically in the range from 50 to 125 kV. For mammography, however, the voltage is lower (22–34 kV) and Rayleigh scatter cannot be neglected.
- A photon can be absorbed by an atom while its energy excites an electron. The electron then escapes from its nucleus in the same direction as

the incoming photon was traveling. This mechanism is called *photoelectric absorption*.

- A second possibility is that the photon transfers only part of its energy to eject an electron with a certain kinetic energy. In that case, a photon of the remaining lower energy is emitted and its direction deviates from the direction of the incoming photon. The electron then escapes in another direction. This process is called *Compton scattering*.
- A third mechanism is *pair production*. If the energy of a photon is at least 1.02 MeV, the photon can be transformed into an electron and a positron (electron–positron pair). A positron is the antiparticle of an electron, with equal mass but opposite charge. Soon after its formation, however, the positron will meet another electron, and they will annihilate each other while creating two photons of energy 511 keV that fly off in opposite directions. This process finds its application in nuclear medicine.
- At still higher energies, photons may cause nuclear reactions. These interactions are not used for medical applications.

## Interaction of an X-ray beam with tissue

Consider an X-ray beam and a material of thickness $d = x_{out} - x_{in}$ (see Figure 2.3(a)). Inside the material, the beam is attenuated by the different types of interaction explained above. Although the individual interactions are of statistical nature, the macroscopic intensity of the beam follows a deterministic exponential law: The intensity of the outgoing beam $I_{out}$ is related to the intensity of the incoming beam $I_{in}$ by

$$I_{out} = I_{in}\, e^{-\mu\, d}, \tag{2.4}$$

where $\mu$ is called the *linear attenuation coefficient* (typically expressed in $cm^{-1}$). This simple law is only valid when the material is homogeneous and the beam consists of photons of a single energy. Actually, $\mu$ is a function of both the photon energy and the material, that is, $\mu = \mu(E, \text{material})$, for example:

$$\mu(10\,keV, H_2O) = 5\,cm^{-1}$$
$$\mu(100\,keV, H_2O) = 0.17\,cm^{-1}$$
$$\mu(10\,keV, Ca) = 144\,cm^{-1}$$
$$\mu(100\,keV, Ca) = 0.40\,cm^{-1}. \tag{2.5}$$

Equation (2.4) can be generalized as follows.

(a)

(b)

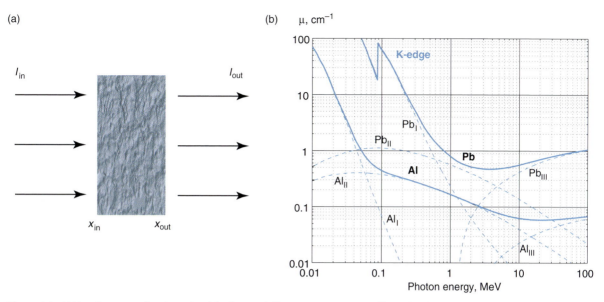

**Figure 2.3** **(a)** X-ray beam traveling through a slab of material. **(b)** Linear attenuation coefficient for photons in aluminum and lead. The solid curves represent the total linear attenuation coefficient. The dashed lines show the partial linear attenuation coefficient for each of the three effects: I for photoelectric absorption, dominant at low energies; II for Compton scattering, dominant at higher energies; III for pair production, dominant at very high energies.

- When a beam of single-energy photons travels through a nonhomogeneous medium, $I_{out}$ is related to $I_{in}$ by

$$I_{out} = I_{in}\, e^{-\int_{x_{in}}^{x_{out}} \mu(x)\,dx}. \qquad (2.6)$$

- A real X-ray beam does not contain a single photon energy but a whole spectrum of energies. Making the intensity distribution of the incoming beam a function of the energy, that is, $I_{in} = \int_0^\infty \sigma(E)\,dE$, the intensity of the outgoing beam is equal to

$$I_{out} = \int_0^\infty \sigma(E)\, e^{-\int_{x_{in}}^{x_{out}} \mu(E,x)\,dx}\,dE. \qquad (2.7)$$

Figure 2.3(b) shows that at low energies photoelectric absorption is most prominent while at intermediate energies the Compton scattering dominates. Pair production exists only at very high energies. Photoelectric absorption occurs at photon energies higher than the binding energy of K-shell electrons. Hence, the attenuation coefficient suddenly increases at this energy, known as the *K-edge*. Figure 2.3(b) also shows that with increasing energy, photoelectric absorption decreases more rapidly than Compton scattering. Note also that the linear attenuation coefficient increases with the atomic number $Z$. With increasing $Z$, photoelectric absorption increases more rapidly than Compton scattering.

Often the *mass attenuation coefficient* ($\mu_m$) is used instead of the linear attenuation coefficient:

$$\mu_m = \mu/\rho, \qquad (2.8)$$

where $\rho$ is the mass density of the attenuating medium. For example, for water $\rho = 1\,g/cm^3$ and for calcium $\rho = 1.55\,g/cm^3$. Hence,

$$\mu_m(10\text{ keV}, H_2O) = 5\,cm^2/g$$
$$\mu_m(100\text{ keV}, H_2O) = 0.17\,cm^2/g$$
$$\mu_m(10\text{ keV}, Ca) = 93\,cm^2/g \qquad (2.9)$$
$$\mu_m(100\text{ keV}, Ca) = 0.258\,cm^2/g.$$

## X-ray detectors

To produce an image from the attenuated X-ray beam, the X-rays need to be captured and converted to image information. Some detectors for digital radiography are relatively recent developments. Older but still in use are the screen–film detector and the image intensifier.

**17**

# Screen–film detector

## Screen

Photographic film is very inefficient for capturing X-rays. Only 2% of the incoming X-ray photons contribute to the output image on a film. This percentage of contributing photons corresponds to the probability that an X-ray photon (quantum) is absorbed by the detector. It is known as the *absorption efficiency*. The low sensitivity of film for X-rays would yield prohibitively large patient doses. Therefore, an intensifying screen is used in front of the film. This type of screen contains a heavy chemical element that absorbs most of the X-ray photons. When an X-ray photon is absorbed, the kinetic energy of the released electron raises many other electrons to a higher energy state. When returning to their initial state they produce a flash of visible light, called a *scintillation*. Note that these light photons are scattered in all directions. Consequently, two intensifying screens can be used, i.e., one in front and one behind the film, to increase the absorption efficiency further. The portion of the light that is directed toward the film contributes to the exposure of the film. In this way, the absorption efficiency can be increased to more than 50% instead of the 2% for film. Because the light is emitted in all directions, a smooth light spot (the PSF, see p. 3) instead of a sharp peak hits the film and causes image blurring.

X-ray intensifying screens consist of scintillating substances that exhibit luminescence. *Luminescence* is the ability of a material to emit light after excitation, either immediately or delayed.

- *Fluorescence* is the prompt emission of light when excited by X-rays and is used in intensifying screens. A material is said to fluoresce when light emission begins simultaneously with the exciting radiation and light emission stops immediately after the exciting radiation has stopped. Initially, calcium tungstate ($CaWO_4$) was most commonly used for intensifying screens. Advances in technology have now resulted in the use of rare earth compounds, such as gadolinium oxysulfide ($Gd_2O_2S$). A more recent scintillator material is thallium-doped cesium iodide (CsI:Tl), which has not only an excellent absorption efficiency but also a good resolution because of the needle-shaped or pillarlike crystal structure, which limits lateral light diffusion.

- *Phosphorescence* or afterglow is the continuation of light emission after the exciting radiation has stopped. If the delay to reach peak emission is longer than $10^{-8}$ seconds or if the material continues to emit light after this period, it is said to phosphoresce. Phosphorescence in screens is an undesirable effect, because it causes ghost images and occasionally film fogging.

## Film

The film contains an emulsion with silver halide crystals (e.g., AgBr). When exposed to light, the silver halide grains absorb optical energy and undergo a complex physical change. Each grain that absorbs a sufficient amount of photons contains dark, tiny patches of metallic silver called development centers. It is important to note that the amount of photons required is independent of the grain size. When the film is developed, the development centers precipitate the change of the entire grain to metallic silver. The more light reaching a given area of the film, the more grains are involved and the darker the area after development. In this way a negative is formed. After development, the film is fixed by chemically removing the remaining silver halide crystals.

In radiography, the negative image is the final output image. In photography, the same procedure has to be repeated to produce a positive image. The negative is then projected onto a sensitive paper carrying silver halide emulsion similar to that used in the photographic film.

Typical characteristics of a film are its *graininess*, *speed*, and *contrast*.

- *Graininess* The image derived from the silver crystals is not continuous but grainy. This effect is most prominent in fast films. Indeed, because the amount of photons needed to change a grain into metallic silver upon development is independent of the grain size, the larger the grains, the faster the film becomes dark.

- *Speed* The speed of a film is inversely proportional to the amount of light needed to produce a given amount of metallic silver on development. The speed is mainly determined by the silver halide grain size. The larger the grain size the higher the speed because the number of photons needed to change the grain into metallic silver upon development is independent of the grain size. Speed is expressed in ASA (American Standards Association) or in ISO (International Standards Organization). These units are the same.

For X-ray imaging with a screen–film combination, it makes more sense to speak about the speed of the screen–film combination: how many X-ray photons are needed to produce a certain density on the film. The speed then depends on the properties of the intensifying screen and the film, but also on the quality of film–screen contact, and on a good match between the emission spectrum of the screen and the spectral sensitivity of the film used.

Because light is emitted in all directions, a significant proportion, about 50%, of that light is not directed toward the film. A reflective layer behind the screen–film–screen redirects it toward the film, ensuring that it contributes to exposure. This has the advantage of increasing the speed of the screen–film–screen combination with a corresponding reduction in patient dose.

- *Contrast* The most widely used description of the photosensitive properties of a film is the plot of the *optical density* $D$ versus the logarithm of the *exposure* $E$. This curve is called the *sensitometric curve*. The exposure is the product of incident light intensity and its duration. The optical density is defined by

$$D = \log \frac{I_{\text{in}}}{I_{\text{out}}}, \qquad (2.10)$$

where $I_{\text{in}}$ and $I_{\text{out}}$ are the incoming and outgoing light intensity when exposing the developed film with a light source. Note that $I_{\text{in}}$ and $I_{\text{out}}$ are different from the incident light intensity in the definition of the exposure $E$, in which it refers to the light emitted by the intensifying screen during X-ray irradiation.

Figure 2.4 shows a typical sensitometric curve. It is S-shaped. In low- and high-density areas, contrast is low and there is little information. Only the linear part is really useful and its slope characterizes the film contrast. The maximal slope of the curve is known as the *gamma* of the film. Note that a larger slope implies a higher contrast at the cost of a smaller useful exposure range.*

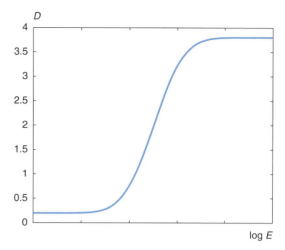

**Figure 2.4** Typical sensitometric curve for radiographic film. $D$ is the optical density and $E$ the exposure.

# Image intensifier

An *image intensifier* works as follows (see Figure 2.5). A fluorescent screen converts the X-rays into visible light. The emitted light hits a photocathode, and the energy of the photons releases electrons from this cathode. A large potential difference between the cathode and the output accelerates the ejected electrons. The resulting electron beam is directed onto a small fluorescent screen by electrostatic or magnetic focusing and converted to light photons again. This focusing makes the system suitable to be coupled to a camera without any loss of light. The main advantage of an image intensifier system is that it is capable of producing dynamic image sequences in real time at video rate, a process known as *fluoroscopy*. However, when compared with film–screen systems, the images are degraded in three ways.

- The spatial resolution will generally be less than that of a film–screen system because of the limited camera resolution.
- Because of the additional conversions (light → electrons → light), the noise increases slightly.
- Geometric distortion occurs, called *pin-cushion distortion*, particularly toward the borders of the image.

# Detectors for digital radiography
## Storage phosphors

A special case of phosphorescence is when part of the absorbed energy is not released immediately in

---

* Double contrast films also exist. Their sensitometric curve contains two linear parts with a different slope, i.e., a high-contrast part as usual, continued by a low-contrast part at high optical densities. This increases the perceptibility in hyperdense regions, such as in mammography at the border of the breast.

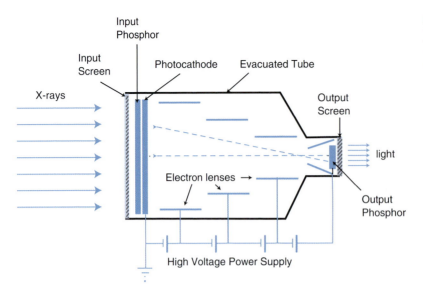

Figure 2.5 Scheme of an image intensifier. The camera is placed against the output screen to minimize light loss. (Reprinted with permission of Kieran Maher.)

the form of light. The temporarily stored energy can be released upon stimulation by other forms of energy such as laser light. This phenomenon is called *photostimulated luminescence* and is used in digital radiography. This type of scintillator is called a *storage phosphor* or *photostimulable phosphor*. The screen–film combination is then replaced by a screen coated with such a scintillator. When X-rays are absorbed by the phosphor, electrons are pumped up from the valence band to the conduction band. In a classical scintillator plate such an electron falls back to the valence band while releasing its energy in the form of a light photon. In a storage phosphor, however, these electrons are trapped by *electron traps*, which are impurities in the scintillator. In this way, the incident X-ray energy is converted into stored energy. After exposure a latent image is trapped in the scintillator. The latent image can be stored in the phosphor plate for a considerable period after exposure. It takes 8 hours to decrease the stored energy by about 25%. The stored energy can be extracted by pixelwise scanning with a laser beam. This way the trapped electrons receive a new energy shot that allows them to escape from their trap and fall back into the valence band. The latent image information is thereby released as visible light, which is captured by an optic array and transmitted to a photomultiplier. The photomultiplier converts the detected light into an analog electrical signal. This analog signal is then converted in an A/D converter to a digital bit stream. The residual information on the scintillator screen is erased by a strong light source, after which the screen can be reused for new X-ray

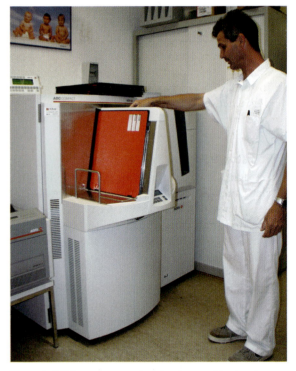

Figure 2.6 This system scans the latent image with a laser beam and erases the residual image on the storage phosphor after which the screen can be reused for new X-ray exposure.

exposure. As soon as the radiologic technician puts the cassette into the scanner (Figure 2.6), this whole laser scanning and cleaning process is done automatically.

Storage phosphor screens provide a much wider useful exposure range than conventional film–screen systems. Moreover, the storage phosphor is a linear detector. This means there is no contrast reduction in the low- and high-density areas of the image, as is the case with the S-shaped sensitometric curve. Consequently, the system is much more tolerant to over-exposure and underexposure, and retakes caused by suboptimal exposure settings (mA s, kV) are reduced. In theory, a reduction of the radiation dose per image is also possible because of the available contrast at low exposure. However, dose reduction adversely affects the SNR of the resulting image. Therefore, reducing the dose per examination must be considered in relationship to the diagnostic information required. Often, the greed for diagnostic detail slightly increases the dose rather than reducing it.

A second advantage of digital radiography is that the image is available for computer postprocessing such as image enhancement and quantification. Moreover, the image can easily be stored and transported in digital form, making the images more accessible and making large film archives unnecessary. Today, digital *picture archiving and communication systems* (PACS) are part of hospital information systems, making the medical images immediately available through the digital network in the same way as the other patient information.

### Active matrix flat panel detectors

Newer detector technologies for digital radiography are flat panel detectors with fast-imaging capability. These systems produce nearly real time images, as opposed to storage phosphor systems which require a readout scan on the order of a minute and a workflow similar to that for screen–film systems.

Traditional electronic capturing devices, including CCDs (charge-coupled devices), are almost exclusively based upon Si-crystal technology, and for manufacturing reasons this restricts the devices to small areas. This is because it is difficult and expensive to create a large defect-free semiconductor crystal. A flat, large-area integrated circuit, called an *active matrix array*, can easily be made by depositing a 2D array of identical semiconductor elements onto an amorphous material, such as hydrogenated amorphous silicon (a-Si:H).

A light-sensitive active matrix array can be produced by depositing an array of photodiodes onto the a-Si:H substrate. By coupling it to a fluorescent plate it functions as a large and fast flat panel X-ray detector.

In spite of the technological progress in scintillator materials, the conversion of X-ray radiation into light photons negatively influences the PSF because of the light distribution in different directions. A more recent technique eliminates the need for a scintillator by using a photoconductor, such as amorphous selenium (a-Se) or cadmium telluride (CdTe), instead of a phosphor. When exposed to radiation, the photoconductor converts the energy of the X-ray photons directly into an electrical conductivity proportional to the intensity of the radiation. To scan this latent image, the photoconductor layer is placed upon an active matrix array that consists of a 2D array of capacitors (instead of photodiodes) deposited onto the amorphous substrate. These capacitors store the electric charge produced by detected X-ray photons until it is read out by the electronic circuit of the active matrix array. This technology is known as *direct radiography* as against the indirect approach where light is produced by a scintillator as an intermediate step in the transformation of X-rays to a measurable signal.

Active matrix flat panel detectors have become an accepted technology for mammography because of their overall performance (see p. 24 below on DQE).*

## Dual-energy imaging

By taking two radiographic images, each capturing a different energy spectrum, the image of substances with a high atomic number (e.g., bone, calcifications, stents) can be separated from that of the soft tissue by proper image processing. This way two different selective images are obtained, for example, a soft-tissue image and a bone image. Several methods have been proposed to calculate tissue selective images. The method explained here is also used in computed tomography (p. 48).

Two system configurations have been used. The first captures two radiographic images in a short time interval (e.g., 200 ms) and at different X-ray tube voltages (e.g., peaks at 110–150 kV and at 60–80 kV). The second configuration contains two layers of scintillator detectors and acquires the images in a single exposure. The top layer detects and filters most low-energy photons, while the bottom layer detects primarily high-energy photons. A third configuration is promising but immature. It uses photon counting detectors

---

* Commercial mammography systems exist that are able to count the individual X-ray photons with a very high absorption efficiency. To obtain their unsurpassed DQE they make use of crystalline silicon strip detectors in combination with a slit-scanning technology.

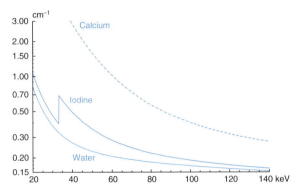

**Figure 2.7** Linear attenuation coefficient as a function of the energy for calcium (Ca), water and the contrast agent iodine (I) in water (10 mg/ml). Note the K-edge discontinuity of I at 33.2 keV.

that count and measure the energy of the photons. This *multi-energy* technique has an improved spectral sensitivity, needs only one radiographic image and is insensitive to patient motion.

Dual-energy imaging relies on the dependence of the attenuation coefficient $\mu$ on the energy $E$ (Figure 2.7). In the absence of K-edge discontinuities in the used energy range $[E_{min}, E_{max}]$ the linear attenuation coefficient can be approximated as

$$\mu(E) \approx \mu_p(E) + \mu_C(E)$$

$$\approx a_p \frac{1}{E^m} + a_C f_{KN}(E). \qquad (2.11)$$

The two components express the attenuation due to photoelectric interaction and Compton scatter respectively. The exponent $m$ is an empirically defined parameter (e.g., $m = 3$ [2]). $f_{KN}(E)$ is the so-called Klein–Nishina function. The tissue-dependent coefficients $a_p$ and $a_C$ are related to the physical material properties:

$$a_p \approx K_p \frac{\rho}{A} Z^n, \qquad n \approx 4$$

$$a_C \approx K_C \frac{\rho}{A} Z \qquad (2.12)$$

where $K_p$ and $K_C$ are constants, $\rho$ is the mass density, $A$ the mass number and $Z$ the atomic number of the attenuating medium [2].

Using Eq. (2.11) it can easily be shown that the attenuation coefficient of an arbitrary substance $S$ can

[2] R. E. Alvarez and A. Macovski. Energy-selective reconstructions in x-ray computerized tomography. *Physics in Medicine and Biology*, 21(5): 733–744, 1976.

be written as a linear combination of the attenuation coefficient of two selected materials, provided that the attenuation properties of both basis materials are sufficiently different (e.g., bone and soft tissue)

$$\mu_S(E) = a_1 \cdot \mu_1(E) + a_2 \cdot \mu_2(E). \qquad (2.13)$$

Substituting Eq. (2.13) in Eq. (2.7) for a spectrum with energy range $[E_{min}, E_{max}]$ yields

$$I(x, y) = \int_{E_{min}}^{E_{max}} \sigma(E)\, e^{-\int_{L_{x,y}} \mu(E,s)\, ds}\, dE$$

$$= \int_{E_{min}}^{E_{max}} \sigma(E)\, e^{-\int_{L_{x,y}} (a_1(s)\cdot\mu_1(E) + a_2(s)\cdot\mu_2(E))\, ds}\, dE, \qquad (2.14)$$

where $L_{x,y}$ is the projection line arriving at pixel $(x, y)$ of the radiographic image. When taking images, the tissue-dependent coefficients $a_1$ and $a_2$ are unknown. Defining

$$A_1(x, y) = \int_{L_{x,y}} a_1(s)\, ds$$

$$A_2(x, y) = \int_{L_{x,y}} a_2(s)\, ds, \qquad (2.15)$$

Eq. (2.14) can be written as

$$I(x, y)$$
$$= \int_{E_{min}}^{E_{max}} \sigma(E)\, e^{-(A_1(x,y)\cdot\mu_1(E) + A_2(x,y)\cdot\mu_2(E))}\, dE. \qquad (2.16)$$

$A_1(x, y)$ and $A_2(x, y)$ represent the equivalent thickness of the basis materials along ray $L_{x,y}$. In this equation $A_1(x, y)$ and $A_2(x, y)$ are unknown, but they can be retrieved. Indeed, if two radiographic images are acquired, each at a different energy with corresponding spectra $\sigma_{LE}$ and $\sigma_{HE}$, the following system of two nonlinear equations must be solved to calculate $A_1(x, y)$ and $A_2(x, y)$ in pixel $(x, y)$

$$I_{HE}(x, y)$$
$$= \int_{E_{min}}^{E_{max}} \sigma_{LE}(E)\, e^{-(A_1(x,y)\cdot\mu_1(E) + A_2(x,y)\cdot\mu_2(E))\, ds}\, dE$$

$$I_{LE}(x, y)$$
$$= \int_{E_{min}}^{E_{max}} \sigma_{HE}(E)\, e^{-(A_1(x,y)\cdot\mu_1(E) + A_2(x,y)\cdot\mu_2(E))\, ds}\, dE. \qquad (2.17)$$

In case of a single exposure with spectrum $\sigma_{LE}$ and two detector layers, the second spectrum $\sigma_{HE}$ is defined as

$$\sigma_{HE}(E) = \sigma_{LE}(E)\, e^{-\mu_f(E)\, t_f}, \qquad (2.18)$$

where $\mu_f(E)$ and $t_f$ are the known attenuation coefficient and thickness of the filtering top detector layer.

Various approaches exist to solve Eqs. (2.17). For example, the inverse relationship can be modeled by a second- or third-order polynomial. If more than two measurements and corresponding equations are available, an optimization strategy is required to solve the overdetermined system. This is for example the case when photon-counting detectors can be used. More information on numerical optimization can be found in [3].

Using the obtained values of $A_1(x, y)$ and $A_2(x, y)$ the original radiographic image can be separated into two material equivalent images (e.g., bone and soft tissue). Note that the above theory needs some modification in the presence of a substance with an observable K-edge in the energy range $[E_{min}, E_{max}]$. In that case Eqs. (2.11) and (2.13) have to be extended with a third component and corresponding coefficients $a_K$ and $a_3$ respectively. This yields a third unknown $A_3$ in Eq. (2.16) and, hence, requires a multi-energy approach with at least three different measurements [4]. The original image is then separated into three instead of two basis images, the third being an image of the substance with K-edge. The strength of *K-edge imaging* is that the energy dependence of a material with K-edge is very different around its K-edge, resulting in a high sensitivity for multi-energy imaging. K-edge imaging is immature but offers opportunities for target-specific contrast agents and drugs, particularly in multi-energy CT (see p. 48).

# Image quality
## Resolution
The image resolution of a radiographic system depends on several factors.

[3] J. Nocedal and S. Wright. *Numerical Optimization*, Volume XXII of *Springer Series in Operations Research and Financial Engineering*. Springer, second edition, 2006.
[4] E. Roessl and R. Proksa. K-edge imaging in x-ray computed tomography using multi-bin photon counting detectors. *Physics in Medicine and Biology*, 52: 4679–4696, 2007.

- The size of the focal spot. The anode tip should make a large angle with the electron beam to produce a nicely focused X-ray beam.

- The patient. Thicker patients cause more X-ray scattering, deteriorating the image resolution. Patient scatter can be reduced by placing a collimator grid in front of the screen (see p. 24). The grid allows only the photons with low incidence angle to reach the screen.

- The light scattering properties of the fluorescent screen.

- The film resolution, which is mainly determined by its grain size.

- For image intensifier systems and digital radiography, the sampling step at the end of the imaging chain is an important factor.

The resolving power (i.e., the frequency where the MTF is 10%) of clinical screen–film combinations varies from 5 up to 15 lp/mm. In most cases, spatial resolution is not a limiting factor in reader performance with film. For images with storage phosphors, a resolving power of 2.5 up to 5 lp/mm (at 10% contrast) is obtained. This corresponds to a pixel size of 200 to 100 $\mu$m, which is mostly sufficient except for mammography, for which more recent detector technology (see active matrix flat panel detectors, p. 21) is needed. Depending on the size of the object, it is clear that images with 2000 by 2000 pixels and even more are needed to obtain an acceptable resolution.

## Contrast
The contrast is the intensity difference in adjacent regions of the image. According to Eq. (2.7) the image intensity depends on the attenuation coefficients $\mu(E, x)$ and thicknesses of the different tissue layers encountered along the projection line. Because the attenuation coefficient depends on the energy of the X-rays, the spectrum of the beam has an important influence on the contrast. Soft radiation, as used in mammography, yields a higher contrast than hard radiation.

Another important factor that influences the contrast is the absorption efficiency of the detector, which is the fraction of the total radiation hitting the detector that is actually absorbed by it. A higher absorption efficiency yields a higher contrast.

In systems with film, the contrast is strongly determined by the contrast of the photographic film. The higher the contrast, the lower the useful exposure range. In digital radiography, contrast can be adapted after the image formation by using a suitable gray value transformation (see p. 4). Note however that such a transformation also influences the noise, thus keeping the CNR unchanged.

## Noise

Quantum noise, which is due to the statistical nature of X-rays, is typically the dominant noise factor. A photon-detecting process is essentially a Poisson process (the variance is equal to the mean). Therefore, the noise amplitude (standard deviation) is proportional to the square root of the signal amplitude, and the SNR also behaves as the square root of the signal amplitude. This explains why the dose cannot be decreased unpunished. Doing so would reduce the SNR to an unacceptable level. Further conversions during the imaging process, such as photon–electron conversions, will add noise and further decrease the SNR.

To quantify the quality of an image detector the measure *detective quantum efficiency* (DQE) is often used. The image detector is one element in the imaging chain and to quantify its contribution to the SNR, the DQE is used, which expresses the signal-to-noise transfer through the detector. The DQE can be calculated by taking the ratio of the squared SNR at the detector output to the squared SNR of the input signal as a function of spatial frequency:

$$DQE = \frac{SNR_{out}^2(f)}{SNR_{in}^2(f)}. \qquad (2.19)$$

It is a measure of how the available signal-to-noise ratio is degraded by the detector. Several factors influence the DQE, particularly the absorption efficiency of the detector, the point spread function of the detector and the noise introduced by the detector. Figure 2.8 shows an example of the DQE as a function of frequency for three different detector technologies.

## Artifacts

Although other modalities suffer more from severe artifacts than radiography, X-ray images are generally not artifact free. Scratches in the detector, dead pixels, unread scan lines, inhomogeneous X-ray beam intensity (heel effect), afterglow, etc., are not uncommon and deteriorate the image quality.

## Equipment

Let us now take a look at the complete radiographic imaging chain, which is illustrated schematically in Figure 2.9. It consists of the following elements.

- The X-ray source.
- An aluminum filter, often complemented by a copper filter. This filter removes low-energy photons, thus increasing the mean energy of the photon beam. Low-energy photons deliver doses to the patient but are useless for the imaging process because they do not have enough energy to travel through the patient and never reach the detector. Because low-energy photons are called soft radiation and high-energy photons hard radiation, this removal of low-energy photons from the beam is called *beam hardening*.
- A collimator to limit the patient area to be irradiated.

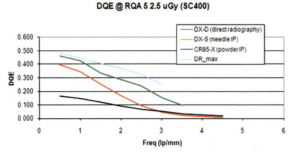

**Figure 2.8** DQE of four digital X-ray detection systems, obtained under standardized measurement conditions. The DQE curve is cut off at a frequency close to the Nyquist frequency, i.e., half of the sampling frequency. (Courtesy of Agfa HealthCare.)

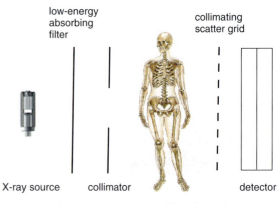

**Figure 2.9** Schematic representation of the radiographic imaging chain.

- The patient, who attenuates the X-ray beam and produces scatter.

- A collimating scatter grid. This is a collimator that absorbs scatter photons. It stops photons with large incidence angle, whereas photons with small incidence angle can pass right through the grid. The grid can be made of lead, for example. Note that a scatter grid is not always used in paediatrics because in small children the scatter is limited.

- The detector. This can be a screen–film combination in which a film is sandwiched between two screens (see p. 18), an image intensifier coupled to a camera (see p. 19), a cassette containing a storage-phosphor plate (see p. 19), or an active matrix flat panel detector (see p. 21) or dual-layer detector (see p. 21).

Figure 2.10 shows a general purpose radiographic room. The table can be tilted in any orientation, from the horizontal to the vertical position. The X-ray system contains a tray for a conventional film-based or a storage phosphor cassette, as well as an image intensifier beneath the table. More recent X-ray systems contain an active matrix flat panel detector with fast-imaging capability, which replaces the cassette and image intensifier (Figure 2.11).

Figure 2.12 shows a 3D rotational angiography system (3DRA). Images of the blood vessels can be made from any orientation by rotating the C-arm on which the X-ray tube and image detector are mounted at both ends. By continuously rotating the C-arm over a large angle (180° and more), sufficient projection images are obtained to reconstruct the blood vessels in three dimensions (3D) (Figure 2.13). The mathematical procedure used to calculate a 3D image from its projections is also used in computed tomography (CT) and is explained in Chapter 3.

## Clinical use

Today, the majority of the radiographic examinations in a modern hospital are performed digitally. X-ray images can be static or dynamic. Static or still images

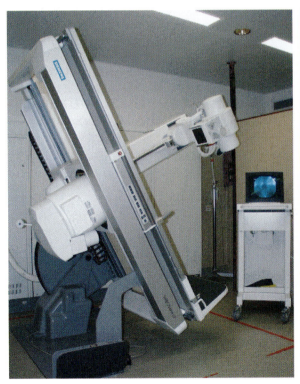

(a)

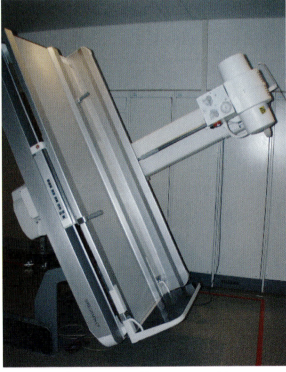

(b)

**Figure 2.10** Multipurpose radiographic room. The table can be tilted in any orientation. Both an image intensifier and a storage phosphor are available.

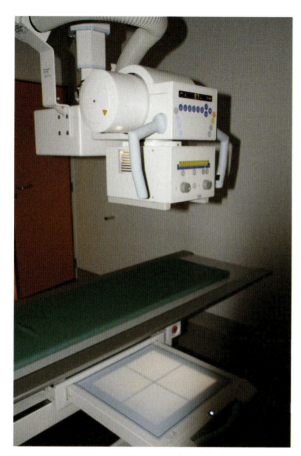

**Figure 2.11** In more recent X-ray systems the cassette and image intensifier are replaced by an active matrix flat panel detector. This picture shows a Siemens system with large-area amorphous silicon detector coupled to a CsI scintillator plate.

*Radiographic images*

These are made of all parts of the human body. They are still responsible for the majority of radiological examinations. The most common investigations include the following.

- skeletal X-rays (see Figure 2.14),
- chest images (radiographs of the thoracic cavity and heart, see Figure 2.15),
- mammography (images of the breasts, see Figure 2.16),
- dental X-rays (images of the teeth and jaw).

*Fluoroscopic images*

These are image sequences produced in real time. Consequently, their application field focuses on investigations in which motion or the instant availability of the images, or both, are crucial. This application field is obviously narrower than that of radiographic examinations, which explains why the number of fluoroscopic guided examinations is an order of magnitude lower. The most typical applications, in decreasing order of occurrence, include the following.

- Interventional fluoroscopy (see Figure 2.17). This application is responsible for the majority of fluoroscopic sequences. Typically, the images are used to guide and quickly verify surgical actions, particularly in bone surgery, such as for osteosynthesis (traumatology, orthopedics).

- Angiography (see Figure 2.18), which takes images of blood vessels through the injection of an iodine-containing fluid into the arteries or veins. Usually, subtraction images are made by mathematically subtracting postcontrast and precontrast images followed by a simple gray level transformation to increase the image contrast of the vessels. The result is an image in which the blood vessels appear as contrasting line patterns on a homogeneous background. Obviously, it is essential that the patient does not move during the imaging procedure, to avoid motion blurring and subtraction artifacts in the images. Traditionally, angiography has been used for diagnosis of conditions such as heart ischemiae caused by plaque buildup. However, today radiologists, cardiologists, and vascular surgeons also use the X-ray angiography procedure to guide minimally invasive interventions of the blood vessels, such as for vascular repermeabilization (Figure 2.12).

are made with a film–screen combination or with digital radiography, whereas dynamic images are obtained with an image intensifier or an active matrix flat panel detector and viewed in real time on a TV monitor or computer screen. Dynamic image sequences are commonly known as fluoroscopic images as against radiographic images, which refer to static images.

In X-ray images, the attenuation differences of various nonbony matter are usually too small to distinguish them. A contrast agent or dye (i.e., a substance with a high attenuation coefficient) may overcome this problem. It is especially useful for intravascular (blood vessels, heart cavities) and intracavitary (kidney, bladder, etc.) purposes.

Following are a number of typical examples of frequently used examinations. They are subdivided into radiographic images and fluoroscopic images.

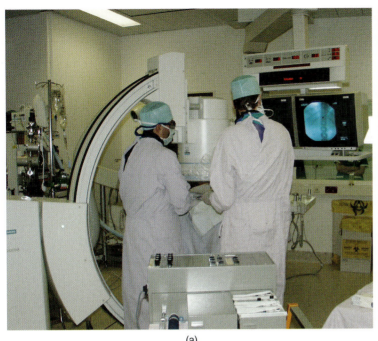
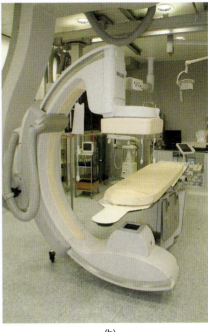

(a)                                                        (b)

**Figure 2.12** 3D rotational angiography (3DRA). **(a)** C-arm with X-ray tube and image intensifier at both ends. **(b)** More recent system in which the image intensifier has been replaced by an active matrix flat panel detector with an acquisition frame rate of up to six 2048 × 2048 images (12 bbp) per second. By rotating the C-arm on a circular arc (e.g., 240° in 4 s) around the patient, a series of projection images are acquired that can be used to compute a 3D image of the blood vessels. (Courtesy of Professor G. Wilms, Department of Radiology.)

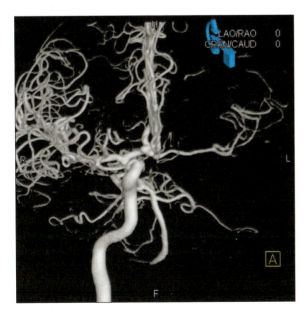

**Figure 2.13** 3D image of the cerebral blood vessels reconstructed from a series of 2D projection images around the patient, obtained with the 3DRA system shown in Figure 2.12(b). Selective injection of the right internal carotid artery in a patient with a subarachnoid hemorrhage showing an aneurysm of the anterior communicating artery. (Courtesy of Professor G. Wilms, Department of Radiology.)

- Barium fluoroscopy of the gastrointestinal tract after the patient swallows barium contrast solution and/or where the contrast is instilled via the rectum (see Figure 2.19).
- Urography (image of the kidneys and bladder) using an iodine-containing contrast fluid.

## Biologic effects and safety

Even at very low X-ray doses the energy deposited by ionizing radiation, such as X-rays, may be sufficient to damage or destroy cells. Although this generally has no negative consequence, the probability always exists that modifications in single cells could lead to malignancy (cancer) or genetic changes. There is no evidence of a threshold dose below which the probability would be zero. If the X-ray dose increases, the frequency of cell damage and the occurrence of cancer increases, but not the severity of the cancer.

Malignant disease and heritable effects, for which the probability but not the severity is proportional to the dose, without any threshold, are *stochastic effects* of radiation. *Deterministic effects* of radiation also exist.

27

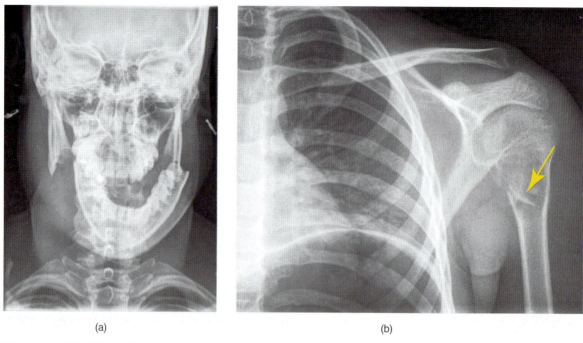

(a)

(b)

**Figure 2.14** **(a)** Double mandibular fracture with strong displacement to the left. **(b)** Solitary humeral bone cyst known as "fallen leaf sign". (Courtesy of Dr. L. Lateur, Department of Radiology.)

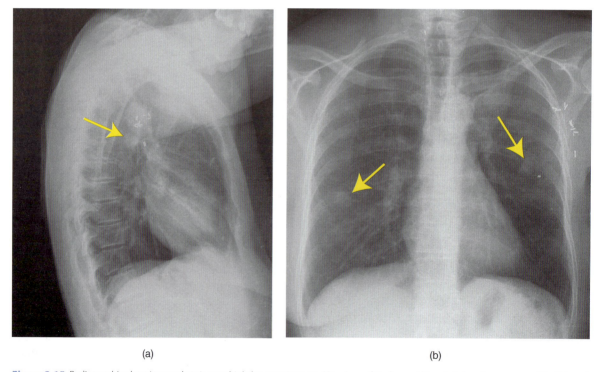

(a)

(b)

**Figure 2.15** Radiographic chest image showing multiple lung metastases. (Courtesy of Professor J. Verschakelen, Department of Radiology.)

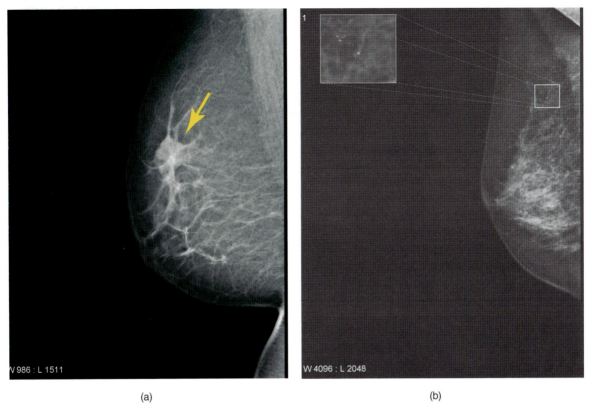

(a)                                                                              (b)

**Figure 2.16** **(a)** Dense opacity with spicular border in the cranial part of the right breast; histological proven invasive ductal carcinoma. **(b)** Cluster of irregular microcalcifications suggesting a low differentiated carcinoma. (Courtesy of Dr. Van Ongeval, Department. of Radiology.)

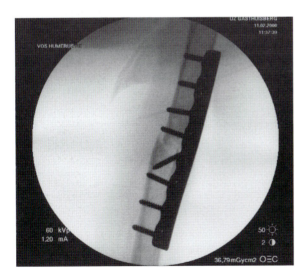

**Figure 2.17** Postoperative fluoroscopic control of bone fixation with plate and screws after a complete fracture of the humerus. (Courtesy of Dr. L. Lateur, Department of Radiology.)

They are injuries to a large population of cells where repair mechanisms fail and the complete tissue is damaged. Deterministic effects are characterized by a threshold dose and an increase in the severity of the tissue reaction with increasing dose.

The SI unit of *absorbed dose*, $D$, is the *gray (Gy)*. One Gy is one joule per kilogram of irradiated material. If the average absorbed dose, $D_T$, in organ or tissue $T$ is known, it is, for example, possible to predict the onset of *deterministic effects*. Tables of threshold values can be found in the literature. For example, a dose of 5 Gy in a single exposure at the level of the eye lens can cause visual impairment due to cataract. In clinical practice deterministic effects are rare.

The probability of stochastic effects from radiation depends heavily on the type of radiation. Some types of radiation are more detrimental per unit of absorbed dose than others. To assess the risk of the *stochastic effects* of radiation in a particular organ or tissue $T$,

**29**

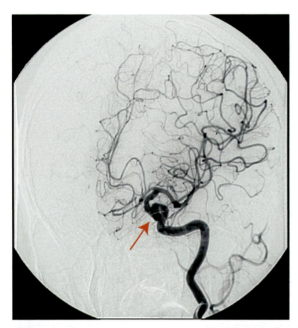

**Figure 2.18** Cerebral angiogram showing an aneurysm or saccular dilation of a cerebral artery. (Courtesy of Professor G. Wilms, Department of Radiology.)

the *equivalent dose*, $H_T$, is used:

$$H_T = \Sigma_R (w_R \cdot D_{T,R}), \qquad (2.20)$$

where $D_{T,R}$ is the average absorbed dose from radiation of type $R$ in tissue or organ $T$ and $w_R$ is the radiation weighted factor, which is a measure of its relative biological impact per unit of absorbed dose. The SI unit of equivalent dose is the *sievert (Sv)*. The radiation weighting factor for X-rays, electrons and muons is 1, for protons and charged pions it is 2, and for heavier particles 20. For neutrons there is no single value but the weighting factor is a function of the neutron energy. In most medical imaging applications only X-rays are involved and $w_R$ is simply 1. In the literature, factors can be found that relate the equivalent organ or tissue dose to the risk of stochastic effects. For example, lung cancer occurs on average in 114 cases per 10 000 persons per sievert, yielding a so-called *nominal risk coefficient** of lung cancer induction of 1.14%/Sv.

* "Nominal risk coefficients are derived by averaging sex and age-at-exposure lifetime risk estimates in representative populations" (*Annals of the ICRP*, publication 103, 2007).

To assess the overall *radiation detriment*[†] from stochastic effects, the *effective dose*,[††] also expressed in sieverts (Sv), is used. The effective dose is the tissue weighted sum of equivalent doses in all irradiated tissues or organs of the body, that is,

$$E = \Sigma_T (w_T \cdot H_T), \qquad (2.21)$$

where $H_T$ is the equivalent dose in tissue or organ $T$ and $w_T$ the *tissue weighting factor*. The weights $w_T$ represent the (rounded) relative radiation detriments of the individual organs and tissues. The sum of all weights equals 1:

$$\Sigma_T w_T = 1. \qquad (2.22)$$

For example, the nominal risk coefficient, expressed in cases per 10 000 persons per sievert, for the liver is 30. The detriment, i.e., the radiation detriment adjusted nominal risk coefficient, is 26.6. Given a total detriment for all organs and tissues of 574, the relative detriment is 0.046 (rounded: $w_{liver} = 0.04$).

Tissue weighting factors can be found in the "2007 Recommendations of the International Commission on Radiological Protection" (*Annals of the ICRP*, publication 103). They are averaged over all ages and both sexes and therefore do not apply to particular individuals. Red bone marrow, colon, lung, stomach and breast have a tissue weighting factor of 0.12. Gonads have 0.08; bladder, oesophagus, liver and thyroid have 0.04; bone surface, brain, salivary glands and skin have 0.01. Thirteen remainder tissues have been defined, i.e., adrenals, extrathoracic region, gall bladder, heart, kidneys, lymphatic nodes, muscle, oral mucosa, pancreas, prostate (male), small intestine, spleen, thymus and uterus/cervix (female). Because the sum of all

[†] "Radiation detriment is a concept used to quantify the harmful effects of radiation exposure in different parts of the body. It is determined from nominal risk coefficients, taking into account the severity of the disease in terms of lethality and years of life lost. Total detriment is the sum of the detriment for each part of the body (tissues and/or organs)" (*Annals of the ICRP*, publication 103, 2007).

[††] "The concept of "effective dose" associated with a given exposure involves weighting individual organs and tissues of interest by the relative detriments for these parts of the body. In such a system, the weighted sum of the tissue-specific dose equivalents, called the effective dose, should be proportional to the total estimated detriment from the exposure, whatever the distribution of equivalent dose within the body. The components of detriment are essentially the same for cancer and heritable disease and, if desired, these detriments may be combined" (*Annals of the ICRP*, publication 103, 2007).

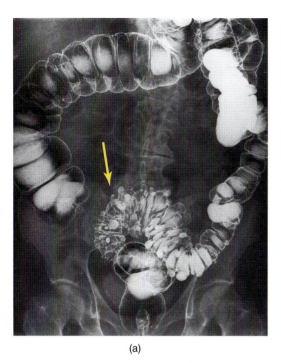

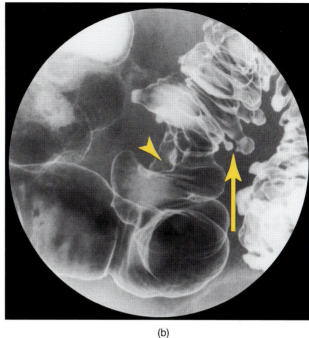

(a)  (b)

**Figure 2.19** **(a)** Double contrast (barium + gas insufflation) enema with multiple diverticula in the sigmoid colon (arrows). **(b)** Polypoid mass proliferating intraluminally (arrowhead on the spotview). (Courtesy of Professor E. Ponette, Department of Radiology.)

weights equals 1, the weight for the remainder tissues is 0.12. It must be applied to the arithmetic mean dose of the 13 organs and tissues.

Effective dose is a valuable measure to compare different examinations. Examples of effective doses for some typical radiographic examinations are: dental 0.005–0.02 mSv; chest 0.01–0.05 mSv; skull 0.1–0.2 mSv; pelvis 0.7–1.4 mSv; lumbar spine 0.5–1.5 mSv. Note that many examinations require more than one or a continuous X-ray exposure, which increases the dose. The use of fluoroscopy for diagnostic and therapeutic reasons may yield doses around 5 mSv. Examples are intravenous urography (3 mSv), barium enema (8 mSv) and endoscopic retrograde cholangiopancreatography (4 mSv). Interventional procedures, such as performed in the angiography room or in the catheterization lab, may have much higher doses, and occasionally even skin doses that reach the thresholds for deterministic effects. Relatively low doses are seen with cerebral angiography (5 mSv) and much higher doses for transjugular intrahepatic portosystemic shunt procedures (TIPS) (70 mSv). Compare this to the dose equivalent due to natural sources, which is 2–3 mSv per year.

According to the International Commission on Radiological Protection (ICRP) the relative radiation detriment adjusted nominal risk coefficient for cancer is 5.5%/Sv and for heritable effects up to the second generation is 0.2%/Sv. For adults (18 to 64 years), these risk factors are a little lower, i.e., 4.1%/Sv and 0.1%/Sv respectively.

Because of the potential risk of medical irradiation, the ICRP recommends keeping the magnitude of individual examination doses as low as reasonably achievable (ALARA principle). There are no dose limits for patients, but every exposure should be justified. This is, to a large extent, a medical decision. The physician should have as much knowledge as possible about previous examinations of the patient and about the patient's condition. Pregnancy, for example, is a state where risks are increased. Most countries have now introduced diagnostic reference levels and can verify in this way whether the X-ray doses for typical examinations in medical centers are too high or too low. Particular attention is given to screening examinations because they are performed on asymptomatic people. In this regard, there is a lot of experience in breast cancer screening programs, where

European Guidelines are widely applied. Special attention should also be given to children and to high-dose imaging, such as interventional radiology.

Furthermore, the ICRP recommends limiting all exposed workers from regulated radiation practices to 20 mSv per year when averaged over five years and the public to 1 mSv per year. In particular, physicians may receive a significant exposure when doing procedures under fluoroscopy, but they too must not exceed 20 mSv per year. There are strict protection protocols they have to follow, among which is the protection of the body and the thyroid gland with a lead apron and collar. A dosimeter, which is a small device clipped to the personnel's clothing, measures the cumulative absorbed dose.

## Future expectations

Today, other imaging modalities, such as ultrasound, CT, and MRI, have largely replaced a number of X-ray examinations. Examples are arthrography (joints), myelography (spinal cord), cholangiography (bile ducts), cholecystography (gall bladder), and pyelography (urinary tract). Although radiography will remain an important imaging modality, this evolution can be expected to continue.

Flat panel detectors for a large field of view and with a fast readout capability will become available for 3D imaging. Hence, 2D projective imaging will further be augmented by 3D volumetric imaging (see also Chapter 3).

It can also be expected that the DQE of the detectors will continue to improve, yielding reduced radiation doses or images with enhanced contrast-to-noise ratio. Furthermore, *photon counting* detectors, which count the number of photons and measure their energy, will become commercially available by employing direct radiography with very fast readout capability.

Currently all medical images can be fully integrated into the hospital information system. The images can be interpreted on screen by the radiologist and electronically transmitted to the referring physician. It can be expected that manual interventions during the image acquisition process, such as cassette handling and parameter setting, will be further reduced. This will have a strong impact on the work flow in a medical imaging department. Furthermore, the computer will behave as an intelligent assistant for the radiologist and will improve his/her performance. Computer aided diagnosis (CAD) is discussed in more detail in Chapter 7.

# Chapter 3

# X-ray computed tomography

## Introduction

*X-ray computed tomography* or *CT* (Figure 3.1) is an imaging modality that produces cross-sectional images representing the X-ray attenuation properties of the body. The word tomography originates from the Greek words $\tau o \mu o \varsigma$ (slice) and $\gamma \rho \alpha \phi \epsilon \iota \nu$ (to write). Image formation of a cross-section is based on the following procedure. X-rays are produced by an X-ray tube, attenuated by the patient and measured by an X-ray detector. Using thin X-ray beams, a set of lines is scanned covering the entire field of view (Figure 3.2(a) shows a parallel-beam geometry and Figure 3.2(b) shows a fan-beam geometry). This process is repeated for a large number of angles (Figure 3.2(c) and (d)), yielding line attenuation measurements for all possible angles and for all possible distances from the center. Based on all these measurements, the actual attenuation at each point of the scanned slice can be *reconstructed*. Although the imaging modalities of Chapters 4 and 5 (MR, PET, and SPECT) also represent a kind of computed tomography, the term CT (originally CAT) is allocated for X-ray comput(eriz)ed (axial) tomography. The physics of X-rays, their production, and interactions with tissue have already been discussed in Chapter 2.

The history of CT began in 1895, when Wilhelm Konrad Röntgen reported the discovery of what he called "a new kind of rays." Röntgen received the first Nobel Prize in Physics in 1901. Reconstruction of a function from its projections was first formulated by Johann Radon in 1917. Before the invention of computed tomography, other kinds of tomography existed.

- **Linear tomography** (Figure 3.3(a)) The X-ray source and film move at constant speed in opposite directions. Under these circumstances, one section of the patient (plane $P_1$–$P_2$) is always projected at the same position on the film, whereas the rest of the body is averaged out. In addition to linear tube and detector movement, curved paths (circular, elliptical, hypocycloidal, ...) have been used as well.

- **Axial transverse tomography** (Figure 3.3(b)) The film is positioned horizontally in front of the patient and slightly below the focal plane. Both the patient

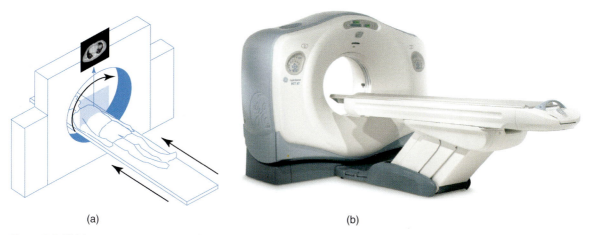

(a)                                        (b)

**Figure 3.1** **(a)** Schematic representation, and **(b)** photograph of a CT scanner. (Courtesy of GE Healthcare.)

and the film rotate at the same fixed speed around a vertical axis while the X-ray source remains stationary. Under these circumstances, the focal plane in the patient remains in sharp focus throughout the rotation, whereas all other planes are averaged out.

The first CT scanner (the EMI scanner) was developed by Godfrey N. Hounsfield in 1972. His work was based on mathematical and experimental methods developed by A. M. Cormack a decade earlier. Hounsfield and Cormack shared the Nobel Prize in Physiology or Medicine in 1979. The first whole-body CT scanner (the ACTA scanner) was developed by

Robert S. Ledley in 1974. Since the introduction of helical and multi-slice CT (respectively in 1989 and 1998), CT has opened the way to 3D images of the heart and has brought dynamic (4D) studies within reach.

In modern CT scanners, the images consist of $512 \times 512$ pixels representing the *CT number*, which is expressed in *Hounsfield units* (HU). The CT number is defined as

$$\text{CT number (in HU)} = \frac{\mu - \mu_{H_2O}}{\mu_{H_2O}} \cdot 1000, \quad (3.1)$$

where $\mu$ is the linear attenuation coefficient. With this definition, air and water have a CT number of, respectively, $-1000$ HU and $0$ HU. Bone falls on the positive side of the scale, but has no unique CT number. This value ranges from several hundreds to over 1000 HU. The reason is that $\mu$ of bone (and all other tissues) depends on its composition and structure, e.g., cortical or trabecular, as well as on the energy of the absorbed X-rays (see Figure 2.3).

Some clinical applications look at air–tissue or tissue–bone contrasts on the order of 1000 HU, but other clinical exams focus on small soft tissue contrasts of a few HU. An optimal perception requires a suitable gray level transformation. In clinical practice, this is done by a real time window/level operation. The window and level respectively define the width and center of the displayed gray level interval. Figure 3.4 shows an example of a CT image of the chest with two different window/level settings, the first to visualize the lungs (a), and the second to emphasize the soft tissues (b).

## X-ray detectors in CT
### Energy integrating detectors
Most recent commercial CT detectors consist of a scintillator crystal ($CdWO_4$, $Y_2O_3$, CsI, $Gd_2O_2S$) in combination with a photodiode. The scintillator

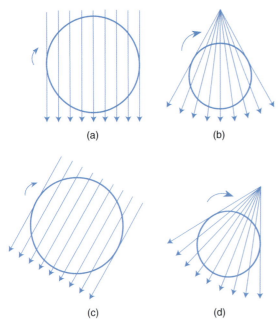

**Figure 3.2** Basic scanning procedure in CT. A set of lines is scanned covering the entire field of view: **(a)** parallel-beam geometry and **(b)** fan-beam geometry. This process is repeated for a large number of angles (**c** and **d**).

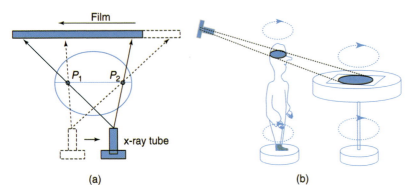

**Figure 3.3 (a)** Linear tomography. The X-ray source and film move at constant speed in opposite directions. **(b)** Axial transverse tomography. The film is positioned horizontally in front of the patient and slightly below the focal plane. Both the patient and the film rotate at the same fixed speed around a vertical axis while the X-ray source remains stationary.

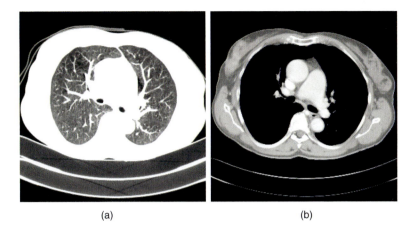

**Figure 3.4** CT image of the chest with different window/level settings: **(a)** for the lungs (window 1500 and level −500), and **(b)** for the soft tissues (window 350 and level 50).

(a)  (b)

material converts X-rays into visible light (scintillations), which then hits the photodiode, causing it to produce an electric current. Individual scintillator pieces are assembled into a reflector matrix in order to define the detector cells. The scintillators are produced with high optical quality so that the few millimeters thickness necessary to have a very high absorption efficiency (96%) also has good transfer of light to the photodiode. Recent scintillators also offer a very fast response time (on the order of microseconds). Due to the finite thickness of the septa in the antiscatter grid, the absorption efficiency of the detector is limited by the area fill fraction, typically on the order of 80%. The multichannel readout electronics or data acquisition system (DAS) connects to the photodiode. The DAS integrates the photocurrent from the diode and converts the electric charge signal to voltage using a transimpedance amplifier. The DAS also performs the analog to digital conversion with typical sample rates on the order of a couple of kilohertz. One limitation of these detectors is the susceptibility to electronic noise introduced by the transimpedance amplifier. For detectors using scintillator/photodiodes, electronic noise dominates the quantum noise at low signal levels, leading to noise streaks (see p. 50) in the images.

## Photon counting detectors

Recently photon counting detectors are receiving increased attention for CT. They are based on direct conversion (see *direct radiography*, p. 21). A direct conversion material such as cadmium telluride (CdTe) or cadmium-zinc-telluride (CZT) converts an X-ray photon into a certain electronic charge proportional to its energy. The charge produced in direct conversion is about ten times that produced by the scintillator/

photodiode combination and the electronic noise no longer dominates the signal from individual X-rays. This difference allows an electronic circuit to detect these charge packages and count the number of photons. The fact that these detectors count the number of photons instead of integrating their energy improves the CNR by 10 to 20%. First, carefully defining a detection threshold eliminates the impact of electronic noise. Second, the difference in attenuation between two tissues is generally larger for low-energy X-rays. Hence, the total CNR can be increased by assigning a higher weight to the detected low-energy X-ray photons.

Yet, the main reason to consider photon counting detectors is their ability to measure the amount of charge, and hence the energy, of the corresponding X-ray. The energy resolution can be much better than for example that of dual layer scintillator detectors, or even dual kV methods for dual-energy imaging (see p. 21). Remaining challenges for commercial introduction of direct conversion detectors for CT applications include stability and the count rate limits, and therefore it will be several years before scintillator-based detectors will be replaced on commercial CT scanners.

## Imaging

## Data acquisition

### Projection and Radon transform

Consider the 2D parallel-beam geometry in Figure 3.5(a) in which $\mu(x, y)$ represents the distribution of the linear attenuation coefficient in the $xy$-plane. It is assumed that the patient lies along the $z$-axis and that $\mu(x, y)$ is zero outside a circular *field of view* with diameter FOV. The X-ray beams make an angle

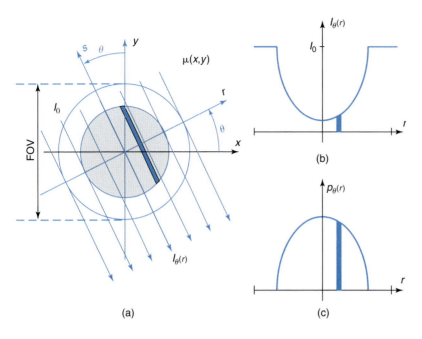

**Figure 3.5** **(a)** Parallel-beam geometry with coordinate systems. The X-ray beams make an angle $\theta$ with the $y$-axis and are at distance $r$ from the origin. **(b)** An intensity profile $I_\theta(r)$ is measured for every view (defined by an angle $\theta$). $I_0$ is the unattenuated intensity. **(c)** The attenuation profiles $p_\theta(r)$, obtained by log-converting the intensity profiles $I_\theta(r)$, are the projections of the function $\mu(x,y)$ along the angle $\theta$.

$\theta$ with the $y$-axis. The unattenuated intensity of the X-ray beams is $I_0$. A new coordinate system $(r, s)$ is defined by rotating $(x, y)$ over the angle $\theta$. This gives the following transformation formulas:

$$
\begin{bmatrix} r \\ s \end{bmatrix} = \begin{bmatrix} \cos\theta & \sin\theta \\ -\sin\theta & \cos\theta \end{bmatrix} \begin{bmatrix} x \\ y \end{bmatrix}
$$
$$
\begin{bmatrix} x \\ y \end{bmatrix} = \begin{bmatrix} \cos\theta & -\sin\theta \\ \sin\theta & \cos\theta \end{bmatrix} \begin{bmatrix} r \\ s \end{bmatrix}.
\tag{3.2}
$$

For a fixed angle $\theta$, the measured intensity profile as a function of $r$ is shown in Figure 3.5(b) and is given by

$$
I_\theta(r) = I_0 \cdot e^{-\int_{L_{r,\theta}} \mu(x,y)\,ds}
$$
$$
= I_0 \cdot e^{-\int_{L_{r,\theta}} \mu(r\cdot\cos\theta - s\cdot\sin\theta, r\cdot\sin\theta + s\cdot\cos\theta)\,ds},
\tag{3.3}
$$

where $L_{r,\theta}$ is the line that makes an angle $\theta$ with the $y$-axis at distance $r$ from the origin. Actually, the spectrum of the X-ray tube and the attenuation depend on the energy, yielding (see Eq. (2.7))

$$
I_\theta(r)
$$
$$
= \int_0^\infty \sigma(E) \cdot e^{-\int_{L_{r,\theta}} \mu(E, r\cdot\cos\theta - s\cdot\sin\theta, r\cdot\sin\theta + s\cdot\cos\theta)\,ds}\,dE.
\tag{3.4}
$$

However, in practice it is typically assumed that the X-rays are monochromatic, and Eq. (3.3) is used as an approximation.*

Each intensity profile is transformed into an attenuation profile:

$$
p_\theta(r) = -\ln\frac{I_\theta(r)}{I_0}
$$
$$
= \int_{L_{r,\theta}} \mu(r\cdot\cos\theta - s\cdot\sin\theta, r\cdot\sin\theta + s\cdot\cos\theta)\,ds,
\tag{3.5}
$$

where $p_\theta(r)$ is the *projection* of the function $\mu(x,y)$ along the angle $\theta$ (Figure 3.5(c)). Note that $p_\theta(r)$ is zero for $|r| \geq \text{FOV}/2$.

$p_\theta(r)$ can be measured for $\theta$ ranging from 0 to $2\pi$. Because concurrent beams coming from opposite sides theoretically yield identical measurements, attenuation profiles acquired at opposite sides contain redundant information. Therefore, as far as parallel-beam geometry is concerned, it is sufficient to measure $p_\theta(r)$ for $\theta$ ranging from 0 to $\pi$.

Stacking all these projections $p_\theta(r)$ results in a 2D dataset $p(r, \theta)$ called a *sinogram* (see Figure 3.6). Assume a distribution $\mu(x,y)$ containing a single dot, as in Figure 3.7(a) and (b). The corresponding

---

* Dual-energy CT is a recent development and is introduced on p. 48.

projection function $p(r, \theta)$ (Figure 3.7(c)) has a sinusoidal shape, which explains the origin of the name sinogram. In mathematics, the transformation of any function $f(x, y)$ into its sinogram $p(r, \theta)$ is called the *Radon transform*:

$$p(r, \theta) = \mathcal{R}\{f(x, y)\}$$

$$= \int_{-\infty}^{\infty} f(r \cdot \cos\theta - s \cdot \sin\theta, r \cdot \sin\theta + s \cdot \cos\theta)\, ds.$$

$$(3.6)$$

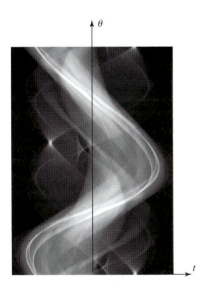

**Figure 3.6** A sinogram is a 2D dataset $p(r, \theta)$ obtained by stacking the 1D projections $p_\theta(r)$.

## Sampling

Until now, we have assumed that data are available for all possible angles $\theta$ and distances $r$. In practice, we have a limited number $M$ of projections or views and a limited number $N$ of detector samples. Hence, the discrete sinogram $p(n\Delta r, m\Delta\theta)$ can be represented as a matrix with $M$ rows and $N$ columns; $\Delta r$ is the detector sampling distance, and $\Delta\theta$ is the rotation interval between subsequent views. Taking into account that $p(r, \theta)$ becomes zero for $|r| \geq \text{FOV}/2$, and assuming a beam width $\Delta s$, the minimum number of detector samples can be calculated.

Figure 3.8 shows a projection (a) and its Fourier transform (FT) (b). Assuming a block-shaped beam aperture (c), the projection is convolved with this block, resulting in a smoothed projection (e). Correspondingly, the FT (b) is multiplied with a sinc function (d), resulting in an FT (f) with strongly reduced high-frequency content. The discrete nature of the measurements resulting from the limited number of detector samples is modeled by multiplying the convolved data (e) with a pulse train (g), yielding the sampled signal (i). This corresponds to convolving the FT (f) with a reciprocal pulse train (h). The resulting spectrum (j) is obtained by shifting and adding spectrum (f). A certain amount of aliasing is unavoidable.

To limit aliasing, the contributions of (f) in (j) must be separated as far as possible or at least far enough to let the first zero-crossings coincide. Let $\Delta s$ be the

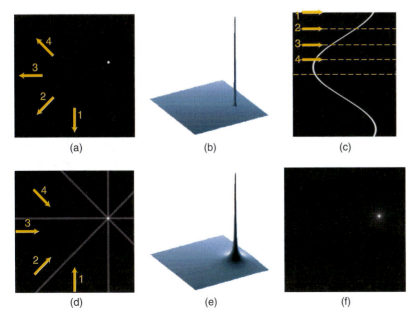

(a)  (b)  (c)

**Figure 3.7** (a and b) Image and surface plot of a distribution $\mu(x, y)$ containing one single dot. The arrows indicate four arbitrary projection directions.
(c) 360°-sinogram obtained by projecting $\mu(x, y)$. The arrows indicate the views that correspond to the four projection directions in (a). (d) Backprojection (see p. 38) of the four views chosen in (a). (e and f) Surface plot and image of the straightforward backprojection of the entire sinogram in (c).

(d)  (e)  (f)

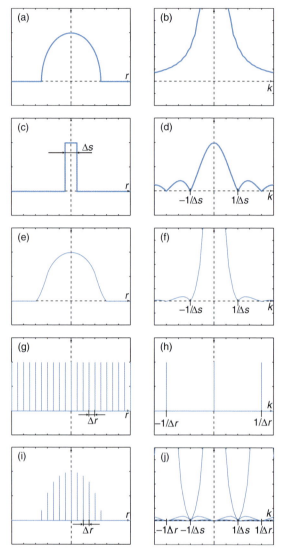

**Figure 3.8** Illustration of required detector sampling: **(a)** projection, **(c)** beam aperture, **(e)** smoothed projection, **(g)** pulse train, **(i)** sampled signal; **(b, d, f, h, j)** corresponding FTs.

beam width (see (c)); then, the width of the main lobe in (d) and in (f) is $2/\Delta s$. This means that the distance between the pulses in (h), which is $1/\Delta r$, must be at least equal to $2/\Delta s$

$$\frac{1}{\Delta r} \geq \frac{2}{\Delta s} \qquad (3.7)$$

or

$$\Delta r \leq \frac{\Delta s}{2}, \qquad (3.8)$$

that is, the sampling distance $\Delta r$ must not exceed $\Delta s/2$, or at least two samples per beam width are

required. Equation (3.8) also follows from the *Nyquist criterion*, which is explained in Appendix A, p. 228. For example, a field of view of 50 cm and a beam width of 1 mm requires about 1000 detector channels.

A rigorous determination of the minimum number of views is less straightforward [5]. Typically the number of views per 360° is on the order of the number of detector channels. For example, GE scanners with 888 detector channels acquire 984 views per rotation and Siemens scanners with 768 detector cells use 1056 views per 360°.

Means to improve sampling include quarter detector offset and in-plane focal spot wobble or deflection.

## 2D image reconstruction

### Backprojection

Given the sinogram $p(r, \theta)$, the question is how to reconstruct the distribution $\mu(x, y)$ (or, generically, the function $f(x, y)$). Intuitively, one could think of the following procedure. For a particular line $(r, \theta)$, assign the value $p(r, \theta)$ to all points $(x, y)$ along that line. Repeat this (i.e., integrate) for $\theta$ ranging from 0 to $\pi$. This procedure is called *backprojection* and is given by

$$b(x, y) = \mathcal{B}\{p(r, \theta)\}$$
$$= \int_0^\pi p(x \cdot \cos\theta + y \cdot \sin\theta, \theta) \, d\theta. \qquad (3.9)$$

Figure 3.7(d–f) illustrates backprojection for a dot. By backprojecting only a few projections, the image in Figure 3.7(d) is obtained. The backprojection of all the projections is shown in Figure 3.7(e) and (f). The image is blurred when compared to the original. The narrow peak of the original dot has a conelike shape after reconstruction. From this example, it is clear that a simple backprojection is unsatisfactory.

The discrete version of the backprojection becomes

$$b(x_i, y_j) = \mathcal{B}\{p(r_n, \theta_m)\}$$
$$= \sum_{m=1}^{M} p(x_i \cos\theta_m + y_j \sin\theta_m, \theta_m) \, \Delta\theta. \qquad (3.10)$$

Note, however, that the values $(x_i \cos\theta_m + y_j \sin\theta_m)$ generally do not coincide with the discrete positions $r_n$.

[5] P. M. Joseph and R. A. Schulz. View sampling requirements in fan beam computed tomography. *Medical Physics*, 7(6): 692–702, November 1980.

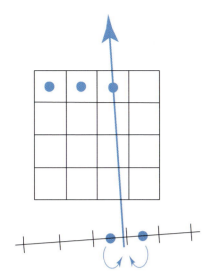

**Figure 3.9**
Discrete
backprojection with
interpolation. For
each view, a
projection line
through each pixel
is drawn. The
intersection of this
line with the
detector array is
computed and the
corresponding
projection value is
calculated by
interpolation
between its
neighboring
measured values.

Interpolation is therefore required. Figure 3.9 illustrates this. For each view, a projection line through each pixel is drawn. The intersection of this line with the detector array is then computed, and the corresponding projection value is calculated by inter-polation between its neighboring measured values. This is called pixel-driven or voxel-driven backpro-jection with linear interpolation. In 3D, the principle is the same, but the interpolation becomes bilinear.

## Projection theorem

We need a mathematical instead of an intuitive answer to the question "given the sinogram $p(r, \theta)$, what is the original function $f(x, y)$?" This means that we need a mathematical expression for the inverse Radon transform

$$f(x, y) = \mathcal{R}^{-1}\{p(r, \theta)\}. \qquad (3.11)$$

The *projection theorem*, also called the *central slice the-orem*, gives an answer to this question. Let $F(k_x, k_y)$ be the 2D FT of $f(x, y)$

$$F(k_x, k_y) = \iint_{-\infty}^{\infty} f(x, y)\, e^{-2\pi i(k_x x + k_y y)}\, dx\, dy \qquad (3.12)$$

and $P_\theta(k)$ the 1D FT of $p_\theta(r)$

$$P_\theta(k) = \int_{-\infty}^{\infty} p_\theta(r)\, e^{-2\pi i(k\cdot r)}\, dr. \qquad (3.13)$$

Let $\theta$ be variable. Then $P_\theta(k)$ becomes a 2D function $P(k, \theta)$. The projection theorem now states that

$$P(k, \theta) = F(k_x, k_y) \qquad (3.14)$$

$$\text{with} \quad \begin{cases} k_x = k \cdot \cos\theta \\ k_y = k \cdot \sin\theta \\ k = \sqrt{k_x^2 + k_y^2}, \end{cases} \qquad (3.15)$$

that is, the 1D FT with respect to variable $r$ of the Radon transform of a 2D function is the 2D FT of that function. Hence, it is possible to calculate $f(x, y)$ for each point $(x, y)$ based on all its projections $p_\theta(r)$, $\theta$ varying between 0 and $\pi$.

*Proof of Eq. (3.14)*
By definition, the 2D FT of $f(x, y)$ is

$$F(k_x, k_y) = \iint_{-\infty}^{\infty} f(x, y)\, e^{-2\pi i(k_x x + k_y y)}\, dx\, dy. \qquad (3.16)$$

Using Eq. (3.15) this becomes

$$F(k_x, k_y) = \iint_{-\infty}^{\infty} f(x, y)\, e^{-2\pi i(k\cdot\cos\theta\cdot x + k\cdot\sin\theta\cdot y)}\, dx\, dy. \qquad (3.17)$$

For any choice of $\theta$ we can define a change in coordi-nates using Eq. (3.2) and the Jacobian determinant

$$J = \begin{vmatrix} \cos\theta & -\sin\theta \\ \sin\theta & \cos\theta \end{vmatrix} = 1, \qquad (3.18)$$

to transform the Cartesian coordinates $x$ and $y$ to the polar coordinates $r$ and $s$:

$$F(k_x, k_y) = \iint_{-\infty}^{\infty} f(r \cdot \cos\theta - s \cdot \sin\theta, s \cdot \cos\theta + r \cdot \sin\theta)$$
$$\cdot e^{-2\pi i(k\cdot\cos\theta(r\cdot\cos\theta - s\cdot\sin\theta) + k\cdot\sin\theta(s\cdot\cos\theta + r\cdot\sin\theta))}\, ds\, dr. \qquad (3.19)$$

Because $\cos^2\theta + \sin^2\theta = 1$, this can be reduced to

$$F(k_x, k_y) = \iint_{-\infty}^{\infty} f(r \cdot \cos\theta - s \cdot \sin\theta, s \cdot \cos\theta + r \cdot \sin\theta)$$
$$\cdot e^{-2\pi i(k\cdot r)}\, ds\, dr. \qquad (3.20)$$

The function $e^{-2\pi i(k \cdot r)}$ is independent of $s$ and can be placed outside the inner integral:

$$F(k_x, k_y) = \int_{-\infty}^{\infty} \left[ \int_{-\infty}^{\infty} f(r \cdot \cos\theta - s \cdot \sin\theta, s \cdot \cos\theta \right.$$

$$\left. + r \cdot \sin\theta) \, ds \right] e^{-2\pi i(k \cdot r)} \, dr. \tag{3.21}$$

From Eq. (3.6) it is clear that the inner integral is the projection $p(r, \theta)$:

$$F(k_x, k_y) = \int_{-\infty}^{\infty} p(r, \theta) \, e^{-2\pi i(k \cdot r)} \, dr. \tag{3.22}$$

By definition the right-hand side is the 1D FT of $p(k, \theta)$, that is, $P(k, \theta)$.

### Direct Fourier reconstruction

Based on the projection theorem, we can use the following algorithm to calculate $f(x, y)$.

1.  Calculate the 1D FT $\mathcal{F}_1$ of all the projections $p_\theta(r)$:

$$\mathcal{F}_1\{p_\theta(r)\} = P_\theta(k). \tag{3.23}$$

2.  Put all the values of the 1D function $P_\theta(k)$ on a polar grid to obtain the 2D function $P(k, \theta)$ (Figure 3.10(a)). The data samples need to be interpolated to a Cartesian grid (Figure 3.10(b)) in order to obtain $F(k_x, k_y)$.

3.  Calculate the 2D IFT $\mathcal{F}_2^{-1}$ of $F(k_x, k_y)$:

$$\mathcal{F}_2^{-1}\{F(k_x, k_y)\} = f(x, y). \tag{3.24}$$

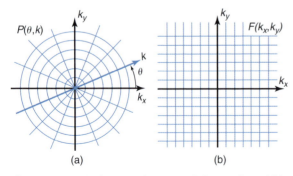

(a)　　　　　(b)

**Figure 3.10** (a) The function $P(k, \theta)$ is sampled on a polar grid. (b) Samples of the function $F(k_x, k_y)$ on a Cartesian grid are required for direct Fourier reconstruction.

The interpolation in step 2 can cause artifacts, making direct Fourier reconstruction less popular than reconstruction by filtered backprojection, which is discussed below.

### Filtered backprojection (FBP)

To avoid interpolation, the polar version of the 2D inverse FT (Eq. (A.74)) can be used:

$$f(x, y) = \int_0^\pi \int_{-\infty}^{\infty} P(k, \theta) \, |k| \, e^{i2\pi kr} \, dk \, d\theta, \tag{3.25}$$

with $r = x \cos\theta + y \sin\theta$. Defining

$$P^*(k, \theta) = P(k, \theta) \cdot |k| \tag{3.26}$$

and

$$p^*(r, \theta) = \int_{-\infty}^{+\infty} P^*(k, \theta) \, e^{i2\pi kr} \, dk, \tag{3.27}$$

Eq. (3.25) becomes

$$f(x, y) = \int_0^\pi p^*(r, \theta) \, d\theta. \tag{3.28}$$

Hence, the function $f(x, y)$ can be reconstructed by backprojecting $p^*(r, \theta)$, which is the inverse 1D FT with respect to $k$ of $P^*(k, \theta)$. The function $P^*(k, \theta)$ is obtained by multiplying $P(k, \theta)$ by the *ramp filter* $|k|$. This explains the name *filtered backprojection*. Because a multiplication in the Fourier domain can be written as a convolution in the spatial domain, $p^*(r, \theta)$ can also be written as

$$p^*(r, \theta) = \int_{-\infty}^{+\infty} p(r', \theta) \, q(r - r') \, dr' \tag{3.29}$$

with

$$q(r) = \mathcal{F}^{-1}\{|k|\}$$

$$= \int_{-\infty}^{+\infty} |k| \, e^{i2\pi kr} \, dk. \tag{3.30}$$

The function $q(r)$ is called the convolution kernel. This yields the following reconstruction scheme.

1.  Filter the sinogram $p(r, \theta)$:

$$\forall \theta \quad p_\theta^*(r) = p_\theta(r) * q(r), \text{ or}$$

$$P_\theta^*(k) = P_\theta(k) \cdot |k|. \tag{3.31}$$

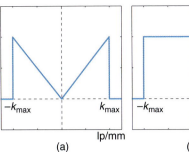

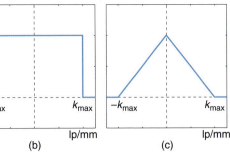

**Figure 3.11** **(a)** For a discrete implementation, the ramp filter $|k|$ is cut off at frequency $k_{max}$. The resulting filter is the difference of a block function **(b)** and a triangular function **(c)**.

(a)  (b)  (c)

lp/mm    lp/mm    lp/mm

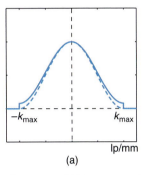

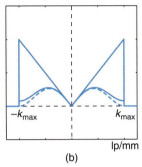

(a)  (b)

lp/mm    lp/mm

**Figure 3.12** **(a)** Hamming window with $\alpha = 0.54$ and Hanning window (dashed line) with $\alpha = 0.5$. **(b)** Ramp filter and its products with a Hamming window and a Hanning window (dashed line).

a smoothing window (Hanning, Hamming, Shepp-Logan, Butterworth) suppresses the highest spatial frequencies and reduces these artifacts. For example, the window

$$
H(k) = \begin{cases} \alpha + (1 - \alpha) \cos\left( \dfrac{\pi k}{k_{max}} \right) & \text{for } |k| < k_{max} \\ 0 & \text{for } |k| \geq k_{max} \end{cases}
$$

$$(3.34)$$

with $\alpha = 0.54$ is the Hamming window, and with $\alpha = 0.5$ the Hanning window (Figure 3.12(a)).

Figure 3.12(b) shows the products of a ramp filter and a Hamming–Hanning window.

### Fan-beam FBP

The previous reconstruction algorithms are all based on the assumption that the data have been acquired in a parallel-beam geometry. In third and fourth generation CT scanners, the acquired data are not ordered in parallel subsets but in fans (Figure 3.2). Figure 3.13(a) shows the coordinates $(r, \theta)$ used in parallel-beam geometries together with the coordinates $(\gamma, \beta)$ used in fan-beam geometries with the detectors placed along a circular arc; $\beta$ is the angle between the source and the $y$-axis, and $\gamma$ is the angle between the ray through $(x, y)$ and the center line of the associated fan. The *fan-angle* is the angle formed by the fan. As can be seen in Figure 3.13(b), measurements for $\beta$ ranging from 0 to $\pi$ do not include all possible line measurements in the case of a fan-beam geometry. For example, if the X-ray tube starts above the patient ($\beta = 0$) and rotates clockwise over 180°, the vertical line with accompanying question mark in Figure 3.13(b) is not measured. Actually, a range from 0 to $(\pi + \text{fan-angle})$ is required in order to include

2. Backproject the filtered sinogram $p^*(r, \theta)$:

$$
f(x, y) = \int_0^\pi p^*(x \cos\theta + y \sin\theta, \theta) \, d\theta. \quad (3.32)
$$

Because of its divergent nature, the continuous filter $|k|$ is not useful in practice. However, from Figure 3.8(j) it follows that for discrete projection data, the useful Fourier content is limited to frequencies smaller than $k_{max} = 1/\Delta s = 1/2\Delta r$. Therefore, the ramp filter $|k|$ can be limited to these frequencies and is cut off at $k_{max}$ (Figure 3.11(a)). This filter, called the Ram–Lak filter after its inventors Ramachandran and Lakshiminarayanan, can be written as the difference of a block and a triangle (Figure 3.11(b) and (c)). Their inverse FTs yield

$$
q(r) = \frac{k_{max} \sin(2\pi k_{max} r)}{\pi r} - \frac{1 - \cos(2\pi k_{max} r)}{2\pi^2 r^2}.
$$

$$(3.33)$$

Usually, frequencies slightly below $k_{max}$ are unreliable because of aliasing and noise. Application of

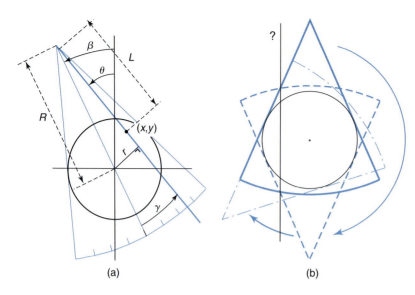

(a)

(b)

**Figure 3.13** **(a)** Fan-beam geometry with detectors placed on a circular arc: $\beta$ is the angle between the center line of the fan and the $y$-axis, $\gamma$ is the angle between the center line and the ray through point $(x, y)$. $L$ is the distance from the source to $(x, y)$. **(b)** With the fan-beam geometry a measurement range from $\beta = 0$ to $(\pi + \text{fan-angle})$ is required to acquire all the projection lines.

all line measurements. For simplicity, we will assume that data for $\beta$ ranging from 0 to $2\pi$ are available (360° acquisition). Two possible reconstruction approaches exist.

- Rebinning involves the reordering of the data into parallel data and requires interpolation.
- An adapted equation for filtered backprojection can be used.

Substituting Eq. (3.29) in Eq. (3.28) and limiting $r'$ in the integration to $[-\text{FOV}/2, \text{FOV}/2]$ yields

$$f(x, y) = \frac{1}{2} \int_0^{2\pi} \int_{-\text{FOV}/2}^{+\text{FOV}/2} p(r', \theta)$$

$$\cdot\, q(x \cos \theta + y \sin \theta - r')\, dr'\, d\theta. \quad (3.35)$$

The factor $1/2$ compensates for the modification of the integration limits from 0 to $2\pi$. Using the coordinates $(\gamma, \beta)$ for a fan-beam geometry (Figure 3.13(a)), the following coordinate transformations can be derived:

$$\theta = \gamma + \beta$$
$$r = R \sin \gamma, \quad (3.36)$$

where $R$ is the distance from the top of the fan, i.e. the position of the source, to the center of the FOV.

Introducing these new coordinates in Eq. (3.35) yields

$$f(x, y) = \frac{1}{2} \int_0^{2\pi} \int_{-\frac{\text{fan-angle}}{2}}^{+\frac{\text{fan-angle}}{2}} p(\gamma', \beta)$$

$$\cdot\, q(x \cos(\gamma + \beta) + y \sin(\gamma + \beta) - R \sin \gamma')$$

$$\cdot\, R \cos \gamma'\, d\gamma'\, d\beta. \quad (3.37)$$

After a few calculations [6] the following fan-beam reconstruction formula can be derived:

$$f(x, y) = \int_0^{2\pi} \frac{1}{L^2} \int_{-\frac{\text{fan-angle}}{2}}^{+\frac{\text{fan-angle}}{2}} [R \cos \gamma' \cdot p(\gamma', \beta)]$$

$$\cdot\, \frac{1}{2} \left( \frac{\gamma - \gamma'}{\sin(\gamma - \gamma')} \right)^2 q(\gamma - \gamma')\, d\gamma'\, d\beta, \quad (3.38)$$

where $L$ is the distance from the image point $(x, y)$ to the top of the fan. Note that this expression is a modified FBP weighted with $1/L^2$. The inner integral is a convolution of $p(\gamma, \beta)$, weighted with $R \cos \gamma$, with a modified filter kernel $\frac{1}{2} (\gamma / \sin \gamma)^2 q(\gamma)$.

A similar equation can be derived for the case that the detectors lie on a straight line perpendicular to the center line of the fan. In this configuration the coordinates $(t, \beta)$ are used (Figure 3.14); $t$ is the distance from the origin to the ray through $(x, y)$ measured

[6] A. C. Kak and M. Slaney. *Principles of Computerized Tomographic Imaging.* New York: IEEE Press, 1987.

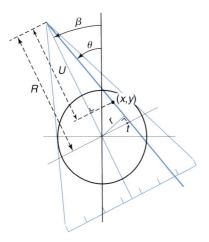

**Figure 3.14** Fan-beam geometry with collinear detectors: $\beta$ is the angle between the center line of the fan and the y-axis. $t$ is the distance from the origin to the ray through point $(x, y)$ measured in the direction parallel to the detector array. $U$ is the projection of the source-to-point distance onto the central fan ray.

parallel to the detector array. It can be shown [6] that the weighted FBP can now be written as

$$f(x, y) = \int_0^{2\pi} \frac{1}{(U/R)^2} \int_{-\infty}^{+\infty} \left[ \frac{R}{\sqrt{R^2 + t'^2}} \cdot p(t', \beta) \right]$$
$$\cdot \frac{1}{2} q(t - t') \, dt' \, d\beta, \qquad (3.39)$$

where $U$ is the projection of the source-to-point distance onto the central ray of the fan.

In dynamic applications, such as cardiac CT, discussed below, it is important to keep the scan segment as short as possible, to minimize motion blur. Since Eqs. (3.38) and (3.39) are based on 360° worth of data, a different reconstruction formula is desired for cardiac imaging. A widespread (approximate) method is the so-called Parker weighting, which uses 180° plus fan-angle worth of data and applies a weighting term to downweight projection lines that are measured twice [7].

# Imaging in three dimensions
## Single-slice CT
### Circular CT
The most straightforward way to image an entire volume is to scan a number of consecutive slices by circular tube–detector rotations alternated with small

[7] D. L. Parker. Optimal short scan convolution reconstruction for fan beam CT. *Medical Physics*, 9(2): 254–257, March 1982.

table shifts. This is also known as axial scanning. To acquire a complete 3D data set and not lose any resolution by this axial sampling, the Nyquist criterion should be satisfied (see p. 38 and Figure 3.8). The maximum distance between consecutive slices depends on the effective slice thickness, which is typically represented by the full width at half maximum (FWHM) of the slice sensitivity profile (SSP) at the center of the field of view (FOV). If we assume a rectangular SSP of width $\Delta z$, the data are to be convolved with a block function with width $\Delta z$. The maximum distance between two slices is then $\Delta z/2$, that is, at least two slices per slice thickness must be acquired in order to minimize aliasing from axial sampling (cf. Eq. (3.8)).

### Helical CT
A technique that is widely used nowadays is *helical CT*. The X-ray tube rotates continuously around the patient, just as in 2D CT. At the same time, the patient is slowly translated through the gantry. Hence, the tube describes a helical orbit (like a screw) with respect to the patient. This explains the origin of the term *helical CT*. While the term *helical CT* is mathematically more accurate, *spiral CT* is also in common use as a synonym.

The *table feed* (TF) is the axial distance over which the table translates during a complete tube rotation of 360°. The pitch ratio – or simply *pitch* – is the ratio between the table feed and the slice thickness.

Figure 3.15 compares circular and helical CT; $\beta$ is the angular position of the X-ray tube and $z$ its axial position relative to the patient. In circular CT (Figure 3.15(a)) the data are acquired for discrete axial positions $\{z_1, z_2, \ldots\}$ and for angular tube positions $\beta$ ranging from 0 to $2\pi$. In helical CT (Figure 3.15(b) and (c)) the data are acquired while $\beta$ and $z$ increase simultaneously.

Assume we want to reconstruct a slice at a particular axial position $z_1$. Data for $\beta$ ranging from 0 to $\pi$ (plus fan-angle) are needed at this position, while only one view at angle $\beta^*$ is available. This problem is solved by interpolation from measurements at adjacent axial positions. The dots in Figure 3.15(b) illustrate this for 360° linear interpolation.

Now consider only the views at angle $\beta_i$. The axial sampling distance for such views is TF. As in circular CT, the real data are convolved with the axial SSP. Assuming a rectangular SSP of width $\Delta z$ and following the same reasoning as for circular CT, we come to the conclusion that the maximum sampling distance is

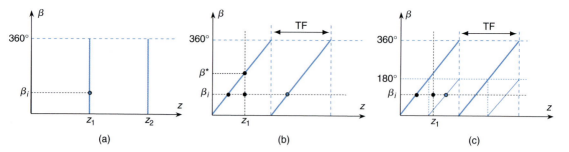

Figure 3.15 (a) In circular CT, data are acquired at discrete axial positions $\{z_1, z_2, \ldots\}$ and for angular tube positions $\beta$ ranging from 0 to $2\pi$. (b and c) In helical CT, data are acquired while $\beta$ and $z$ increase simultaneously. In (b) 360° linear interpolation is used and in (c) 180° linear interpolation is used to obtain a complete dataset at one particular axial position $z_1$.

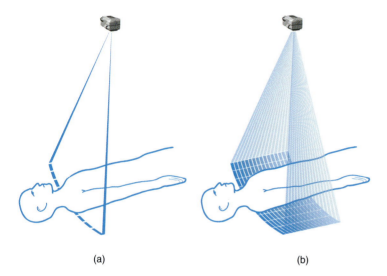

Figure 3.16 (a) Single-slice CT versus (b) multi-slice CT: a multi-slice CT scanner can acquire multiple slices simultaneously by using multiple adjacent detector arrays. (Reprinted with permission of RSNA.)

$\Delta z/2$. Hence, for a slice thickness $\Delta z$, the maximum table feed is TF $= \Delta z/2$ (pitch $= 0.5$).

Taking into account that concurrent but opposite rays yield identical measurements (Figure 3.15(c)), the axial sampling density can be doubled by using 180° interpolation. The sampling distance then becomes TF/2, and the maximum table feed TF $= \Delta z$ (pitch $= 1.0$). Increasing the pitch to a value above one reduces the scan time, however, at the cost of image quality.* Note that with a fan-beam geometry, opposite rays are not separated exactly by TF/2, and the axial distance from a particular ray to an opposite ray depends on its position within the fan.

## Multi-slice CT

In modern CT scanners, the detector array consists of multiple detector rows, in order to measure several

slices per rotation of the X-ray tube (Figure (3.16)). The number of slices can also be boosted by combining multiple detector rows with longitudinal focal spot wobble, providing interlaced slices. This way, for example, a 32-row CT scanner is marketed as a 64-slice scanner.

The pitch can be defined here as the ratio of the table feed to the total X-ray beam thickness, i.e., the thickness of the complete stack of slices. Using the same pitch values as in single-slice CT yields a reduction of the scan time by the number of detector rows, resulting in reduced motion artifacts.[†] Using,

---

* Theoretically, the patient dose would reduce as the pitch increases, but in practice the dose is often kept constant by increasing the mA s to maintain the CNR.

[†] For multi-slice CT scanners, the maximum pitch can be determined intuitively as follows. In order to reconstruct any single slice, the minimum required view angle range is 180° plus the fan-angle. Simplistically this can be used to define the time during which the patient can translate by an amount equal to the longitudinal coverage of the beam at isocenter. The pitch by definition equals the translation for 360° of rotation, so the pitch cannot be larger than 360/(180 + fan-angle) or about 1.5. Note that this calculation

for example, a 64-row system with 0.5 mm detectors (referred to the isocenter), a pitch of 1.0 and a 0.33 second rotation, it is possible to obtain a CT of the lungs (e.g., 40 cm) in about 4 seconds.

If the distance between the X-ray tube and the detector array is large, or the axial width of the detectors is limited, or both, all the projection lines can be assumed to be parallel to the central plane. In this case, the problem reduces to the reconstruction of a series of 2D images. This is the case, for example, if there are only four adjacent detector rows. For 16-slice scanners, however, this assumption does not hold anymore. An approximate solution then consists of tilting each image plane to minimize its mean $z$-distance to the X-ray source positions involved in the reconstruction of that plane. After 2D reconstruction of the tilted image planes, axial slices are achieved by interpolation. This technique is called *tilted plane reconstruction*.

As the number of detector rows increases (64 and higher), artifacts become more visible. Fully 3D reconstruction methods are then recommended (discussed below).

Note that with a multi-slice CT scanner, the operator is able to specify slices thicker than the detector width. Thicker slices have a higher SNR. They can be obtained by convolving the measured projection values along the $z$-axis with a smoothing filter. This is called *z-filtering*. Reconstruction of thick slices using thinner detector arrays has the advantage that the nonlinear partial volume effect is reduced (see p. 51).

## Volumetric CT

An increased number of detector rows is good for reduced scan time and cardiac imaging in particular. An entire volume may even be acquired in one single orbit of the X-ray tube. However, it also comes with an increased cone angle. Unfortunately, except for the central plane, the in-plane data required for 2D reconstruction are not measured and true 3D reconstruction is required.

In three dimensions, the projection theorem states that the 3D Fourier transform of a function in the direction of $\vec{k}$ equals the 1D Fourier transform along the same direction of the *plane* integrals perpendicular to that direction. From this the 3D inverse Radon transform can be derived. The connection between

cone-beam measurements and planar integrals was made by Grangeat [8].

The projection theorem provides a mathematical solution to true 3D reconstruction in cases where source trajectories are sufficient to provide all Radon plane integrals and where there is no truncation on the detector. However, axial truncation cannot be avoided in clinical CT where patients are much larger than the longitudinal extent of the detector. Furthermore, the number of scan configurations is limited for practical reasons. Typically used in clinical routine are circular and helical scanning.

### Circular cone-beam reconstruction

For circular trajectories the source and detector make a circular orbit around the patient (Figure 3.17). For this configuration stable exact reconstruction is theoretically impossible except for voxels on the midplane. There is simply not sufficient information in the measurements. So we have to rely on an approximate reconstruction algorithm. The most famous algorithm is the so-called FDK algorithm proposed in 1984 by Feldkamp *et al.* [9]. It essentially extends the 2D weighted FBP (Eq. (3.39)) to three dimensions, that is,

$$f(x, y, z)$$
$$= \int_0^{2\pi} \frac{1}{(U/R)^2} \int_{-\infty}^{+\infty} \left[ \frac{R}{\sqrt{R^2 + t'^2 + \zeta^2}} \cdot p(t', \zeta, \beta) \right]$$
$$\cdot \frac{1}{2} q(t - t') \, dt' \, d\beta, \tag{3.40}$$

where $\zeta$ is the height of the tilted fan above the rotation center of the source and $U$ is the projection of the source-to-point distance onto the central ray of the untilted fan (see Figure 3.17).

Because the algorithm offers only an approximate solution, cone-beam artifacts are unavoidable. They can become severe for larger cone angles and challenging phantoms.

[8] P. Grangeat. Mathematical framework of cone beam 3d reconstruction via the first derivative of the radon transform. In G. T. Herman, A. K. Louis, and F. Natterer, editors, *Mathematical Methods in Tomography*, Number 1497 of *Lecture Notes in Mathematics*, pages 66–97, Berlin: Springer–Verlag, 1990.
[9] L. A. Feldkamp, L. C. Davis, and J. W. Kress. Practical cone-beam algorithm. *Journal of the Optical Society of America A*, 1(6): 612–619, 1984.

does not take the Nyquist criterion for optimal $z$-resolution into consideration and yields only an upper bound for the pitch.

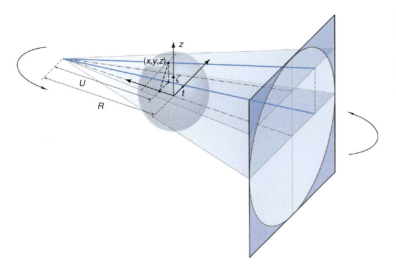

**Figure 3.17** Circular cone-beam geometry. This is a 3D extension of the 2D fan-beam geometry shown in Figure 3.14. The source and detector make a circular orbit around the z-axis. The tilted fan through point $(x, y, z)$ intersects the z-axis at height $\zeta$. $t$ is defined as in the 2D case. $U$ is the projection of the source-to-point distance onto the central ray of the untilted fan.

### Helical cone-beam reconstruction

Unlike for circular scanning, a helical cone-beam acquisition results in a complete data set, provided the helical pitch is not too large ($\leq 1.3$). The first exact FBP algorithm for helical cone beam was proposed by Katsevich [10]. Other exact FBP-type algorithms have also been developed including the derivative back-projection (DBP) approach. The DBP approach can provide accurate reconstruction in some cases even in the presence of axial truncation.

Despite the existence of exact helical cone-beam reconstruction algorithms, most manufacturers use approximate algorithms, like FDK based approaches, because they are preferable in terms of noise, noise uniformity and other quality characteristics.

### Iterative reconstruction

Although widely used in nuclear medicine (PET and SPECT), iterative reconstruction has only recently been introduced in commercial CT scanners. There are several reasons for this. First, the data sets in CT are much larger than in nuclear medicine and iterative reconstruction then becomes computationally very intensive. Second, many iterative algorithms have a statistical basis. Count rates have been much lower in nuclear medicine, resulting in increased noise. This explains the stronger need for a statistical approach in nuclear medicine. However, CT has evolved towards lower dose and volumetric acquisition. Iterative methods can cope with noisy data, which is more prominent

in low-dose CT, and they are directly applicable to 3D reconstruction. Furthermore, the ever-increasing computer capacity brings iterative reconstruction within reach. Iterative reconstruction is discussed in more detail in Chapter 5 on nuclear medicine.

## Cardiac CT

The full heart can be imaged in a few seconds by performing a low-pitch helical scan or by combining a limited number of large-coverage circular scans, also known as axial scanning. A particular cardiac phase is reconstructed by collecting its projection data from subsequent heart cycles, which requires a synchronization with the ECG signal. Dynamic 3D images (often called 4D images) of the heart can be obtained by subdividing the cardiac cycle into different phases.

Axial scanning is the most straightforward acquisition mode. Contiguous volume slabs at a selected phase of the cardiac cycle are scanned and reconstructed in subsequent heart beats at one slab per heart beat. This acquisition mode is also known as the step-and-shoot method. Note that systems that acquire data of the complete heart in less than a single rotation (180° plus fan-angle) are also commercially available. For example, a 320-row scanner with a detector size of 0.5 mm is able to scan a volume of 16 cm. If the X-ray beam coverage is large enough to measure an entire organ in one rotation, axial scanning eliminates the dose due to helical overscan, and it also enables dynamic phenomena to be imaged for one single organ (perfusion, cardiac cine). A drawback of circular cone-beam scanning, however, is the

[10] A. Katsevich. Analysis of an exact inversion algorithm for spiral cone-beam ct. *Physics in Medicine and Biology*, 47: 2583–2597, 2002.

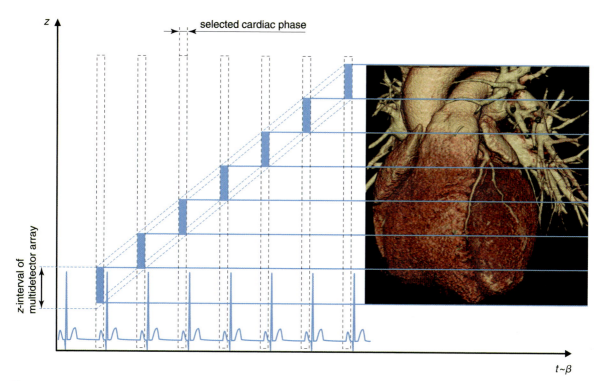

**Figure 3.18** Principle of data acquisition for helical cardiac CT. The oblique lines represent the $z$-interval of the multidetector array as a function of time or angular tube position $\beta$.

fundamental incompleteness of the data, leading to cone-beam artifacts.

Figure 3.18 shows the acquisition principle for helical scanning. A particular phase of the heart cycle is selected in the ECG signal. To guarantee the reconstruction of contiguous volume slabs and avoid gaps in the $z$-direction, care has to be taken to collect sufficient projection data for each $z$-value. This can only be obtained by decreasing the slope of the oblique lines, which corresponds to a pitch reduction. If the projection data needed for each particular $z$-value can be collected during one heart cycle, the shaded regions must be contiguous in the $z$-direction. Using, for example, a 128-row system with 0.5 mm detectors (referred to the isocenter) and a 0.33 second rotation time, a heart rate of 60 bpm requires a reduced pitch of 0.25, and a coronary angiogram with a scan length around 20 cm is obtained in about 4 seconds.

To avoid motion artifacts the heart should be scanned during its short quiescent intervals, say during one fourth of the heart cycle. During this time, projection data spread around 180° plus fan-angle must be collected. For example, a rotation time of 0.33 seconds and a fan-angle of 50° results in a scan

time of 0.21 seconds per slab. Hence, one fourth of the heart cycle should take at least 0.21 seconds.* This corresponds to a maximum heart rate of 71 bpm. Ultrashort scan algorithms add the fan-angle of only the cardiac region, i.e., about 30°. This reduces the scan time to 0.19 seconds per slab and increases the maximum heart rate slightly to 78 bpm. A dual-source CT scanner, with two X-ray tubes positioned 90° apart, relaxes this limitation. For this configuration the half-scan interval is 90° plus 30°, giving a scan time of only 0.11 seconds per slab and a maximum heart rate of 136 bpm.

The importance of a good selection of the quiescent phase is clear knowing that some coronary arteries can reach speeds well over 40 mm per second, so even in the dual source example the motion blur could rise to 4.4 mm and more without ECG synchronization. Unfortunately, different parts of the heart have different optimal phases, and the motion is never completely zero. Hence, strategies for further improving temporal resolution are desired and

---

* Beta-blockers are often used to reduce the heart rate.

47

algorithmic motion correction approaches are being widely researched.

# Dual-energy CT

Dual-energy imaging [2] (see also p. (21)) opens the way to tissue characterization. It requires that two energy spectra are captured. Different spectra can be obtained in several different ways.

- A conventional CT scanner can perform two consecutive rotations at different kV.

- The kV can be quickly modulated between low and high kV while a single circular or helical acquisition is performed. This requires a special high-voltage generator and a very fast detector.

- The dual-source CT scanner has two X-ray tubes that are positioned 90° apart, which can be operated at different kV.

- A detector with two separate layers of scintillators acquires two different spectra since the top layer will absorb most low-energy photons, and the bottom layer will detect more high-energy photons.

- A photon-counting detector counts the X-ray photons in different energy bins, by comparing the signal with certain energy thresholds. This multi-energy approach also offers the possibility of using and visualizing substances with K-edge (see p. 23, K-edge imaging).

The method is similar to that described in Chapter 2 for dual-energy radiography. It starts from the knowledge that the attenuation coefficient of an arbitrary substance can be written as a linear combination of the attenuation coefficient of two selected materials (e.g., water and iodine*) in the absence of K-edge discontinuities in the used energy range $[E_{min}, E_{max}]$. Hence

$$\mu(E, x, y) = a_1(x, y) \cdot \mu_1(E) + a_2(x, y) \cdot \mu_2(E). \tag{3.41}$$

[2] R. E. Alvarez and A. Macovski. Energy-selective reconstructions in x-ray computerized tomography. *Physics in Medicine and Biology*, 21(5): 733–744, 1976.
* Iodine has a relatively low K-edge energy of 33.2 keV, which is too low to play a role in general purpose CT. For dedicated CT operating at lower kV, such as breast CT or small animal CT, it cannot be neglected.

Substituting Eq. (3.41) in Eq. (3.4) for a spectrum with energy range $[E_{min}, E_{max}]$ yields

$$\begin{aligned}
I_\theta(r) &= \int_{E_{min}}^{E_{max}} \sigma(E) \, e^{-\int_{L_{r,\theta}} \mu(E, x, y) \, ds} \, dE \\
&= \int_{E_{min}}^{E_{max}} \sigma(E) \, e^{-\int_{L_{r,\theta}} (a_1(x,y) \cdot \mu_1(E) + a_2(x,y) \cdot \mu_2(E)) \, ds} \, dE,
\end{aligned} \tag{3.42}$$

where $L_{r,\theta}$ is the projection line. In dual-energy CT the unknown tissue-dependent coefficients $a_1(x, y)$ and $a_2(x, y)$ can be reconstructed from $A_1(r, \theta)$ and $A_2(r, \theta)$, which are defined as

$$A_1(r, \theta) = \int_{L_{r,\theta}} a_1(x, y) \, ds$$

$$A_2(r, \theta) = \int_{L_{r,\theta}} a_2(x, y) \, ds. \tag{3.43}$$

Reconstruction can be performed by, for example, filtered backprojection. Although $A_1$ and $A_2$ are unknown, they can be retrieved in a similar way as in dual-energy radiography: Eq. (3.42) is rewritten as

$$I_\theta(r) = \int_{E_{min}}^{E_{max}} \sigma(E) \, e^{-(A_1(r,\theta) \cdot \mu_1(E) + A_2(r,\theta) \cdot \mu_2(E))} \, dE. \tag{3.44}$$

Two different spectra $\sigma_{LE}$ and $\sigma_{HE}$ yield a system of two nonlinear equations (see Eq. (2.17)) from which $A_1$ and $A_2$ can be solved.

The basis material decomposition process described above is performed in the projection domain, but it can be done in the image domain as well, i.e., after the image reconstruction. The coefficients $A_1(r, \theta)$ and $A_2(r, \theta)$ in Eq. (3.44) must simply be replaced by $a_1(x, y)$ and $a_2(x, y)$. The main advantage of the projection domain approach is that it eliminates beam hardening artifacts. Beam hardening causes a shift in average energy and corresponding attenuation coefficient along the X-ray path as it penetrates tissue (see p. 51).

It is important to notice that dual-energy CT does not just yield equivalent thicknesses ($A_1$ and $A_2$) of two basis materials as in dual-energy radiography, but the tissue-specific coefficients $a_1(x, y)$ and $a_2(x, y)$ are obtained for each pixel (Figure 3.19). From these values monochromatic images at any energy or single-substance images can be calculated. Applications of dual-energy CT include:

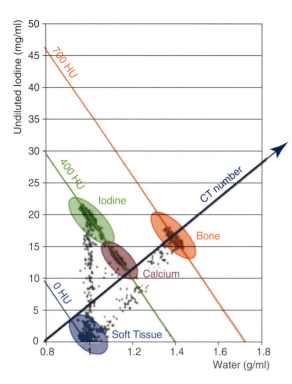

**Figure 3.19** Using multi-energy imaging each pixel can be represented as a linear combination of the attenuation coefficient of two basis materials. In conventional CT, different materials with the same average attenuation cannot be distinguished. In dual-energy imaging the material dependence of each tissue is characterized and therefore true tissue characterization can be performed. (Courtesy of GE Healthcare.)

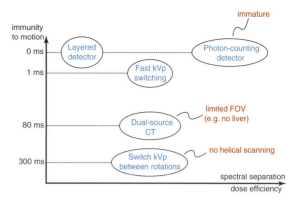

**Figure 3.20** Multi-energy: comparison of different implementations. Photon-counting detectors have the best performance. (Courtesy of GE Healthcare.)

approach is the most favorable, but the technology is still under development (Figure 3.20). For dynamic imaging, it is important that two measurements of the same projection line at different energies occur simultaneously. In this respect, the detector-based methods and the fast switching method are the most favorable, while the rotate–rotate method and the dual-source method simply do not allow projection-based decomposition for dynamic imaging (Figure 3.20). Furthermore, the dual-source method may be limited to a reduced field of view if the second detector is smaller.

## Image quality
### Resolution

The spatial resolution in a CT image depends on a variety of factors.

- The size of the focal spot. The focal spot is the area on which the electrons hit the anode and where the X-rays originate. It is usually positioned at a small angle relative to the imaging plane so that the thermal length (physical) can be much larger than the optical length (projected) in order to spread the heat production over a larger thermal area.

- The size of the detector channels, as well as the amount of channel-to-channel crosstalk.

- The X-ray beam width is a combination of the above two factors. For locations closer to the focal spot, the focal spot size dominates the beam width. For locations closer to the detector, the detector cell size dominates the beam width.

- elimination of beam hardening artifacts,

- automatic segmentation, for example automatic bone removal,

- retrospective generation of (virtual) monochromatic images at any possible energy,

- tissue characterization,

- virtual unenhanced images. Dual kV examination with contrast agent allows an image to be produced as if there were no contrast agent. This eliminates the need for two scans, i.e., a precontrast (unenhanced) and a contrast scan.

Two important criteria for dual-energy CT are the energy separation and the co-registration. The measurements need to occur at very different effective energies in order to do an effective material decomposition. If the effective energies are too similar, the noise will be amplified. In this respect, the dual-layer solution is the least favorable and the photon-counting

- The continuous rotation of the tube–detector introduces a certain amount of azimuthal blur, which increases linearly with distance from the center of rotation. Hence, azimuthal blur can be significant at the periphery of the field of view.

- The reconstruction kernel or convolution filter, which can be tuned to enhance high frequencies for the sharpest images or to suppress high frequencies for reduction of noise and aliasing.

- The interpolation process inherent to backprojection. This depends on the available sample density, which in turn depends on the channel size, the helical pitch, the detector quarter offset and focal spot wobble or deflection.

- The voxel size. Normally, the voxel size is chosen smaller than the spatial resolution of the system, as defined by the above factors. Only if the voxel size is chosen larger, for example to save computation time, does it become the bottleneck and determine the spatial resolution.

The in-plane spatial resolution in CT is typically defined as the value at which the MTF reaches a given percentage of its maximum. Current clinical CT scanners have an in-plane spatial resolution between 5 lp/cm and 15 lp/cm (at 10% MTF), depending on the reconstruction kernel. The effective slice thickness (FWHM of the SSP at the center of the field of view) can be as low as 0.5 mm.

## Noise

Three types of noise can be distinguished in CT: quantum noise or statistical noise, electronic noise, and round-off or quantization noise that results from the limited dynamic range of the detector. The main contribution is from quantum noise, which is due to the statistical nature of X-rays. It can be represented as a Poisson distribution: the variance is equal to the mean and the probability of measuring $n$ photons when $\lambda$ photons are expected is $P(n \mid \lambda) = (e^{-\lambda} \cdot \lambda^n)/n!$. The amount of noise depends on the following.

- The total exposure. Increasing the mA s increases the SNR, thus reducing the relative quantum noise at the expense, however, of patient dose and tube load.

- The reconstruction algorithm. Both the applied filters and the interpolation methods influence the image noise.

Typically, the standard deviation because of noise is a few HU. In high-contrast applications higher noise levels (lower dose) can be tolerated.

The reconstruction algorithm transforms measured signal noise into structured image noise. In the presence of metal objects, this results in alternating dark and bright thin streaks radiating from the metal objects. A phantom simulation illustrates this. Figure 3.21(a) shows an artifact-free reconstructed section of a water bowl with an iron rod. Adding Poisson noise to the simulated intensities results in streak artifacts, as shown in Figure 3.21(b).

## Contrast

The contrast between an object and its background depends primarily on the respective attenuation properties, but also on a variety of physical factors such as the spectrum of the X-ray tube, the amount of beam hardening and scatter, and the detection nonlinearity. Because the images are digital, the displayed contrast is modulated by the gray level transformation (e.g., window/level) after the image formation. This makes noise the main limitation on the perception of low-contrast details. Note that the ability to detect low-contrast details is much higher in CT than in radiography. The main reason is that radiography delivers projection images in which multiple structures are superimposed into the image, while CT scans are images of thin body slices.

## Image artifacts
### Undersampling

As discussed on p. 37, a minimum number of detector samples and views are required. Taking too few samples results in the following phenomena.

- If the number of detector samples is too small, aliasing occurs. In particular, a sharp edge in a projection will be badly approximated, resulting in a high-frequency damped oscillation around the edge. During reconstruction, this error is backprojected along the line tangent to the edge in the image. This results in several types of artifacts, as illustrated by the phantom simulation in Figure 3.21(c). Aliasing artifacts can be prevented by increasing the number of detector samples, by increasing the beam width (at the expense of spatial resolution), or by giving an offset of $\Delta r/4$ ($\Delta r$ is the sampling distance) to the detectors in order

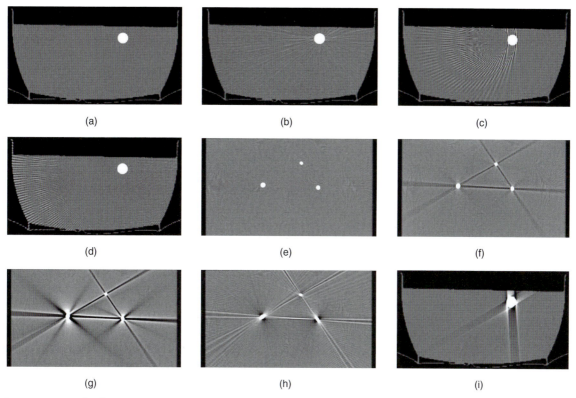

**Figure 3.21** **(a)** Artifact-free reconstruction of a simulated water bowl with iron rod. **(b)** Same slice reconstructed after noise was added to the simulated sinogram. **(c)** Aliasing artifacts occur when the number of detector samples is too small. **(d)** Peripheral streaks occur when the number of views is too small. **(e)** Artifact-free reconstruction of a plexiglass plate with three amalgam fillings. **(f)** Beam hardening artifacts occur when a polychromatic spectrum is simulated. **(g)** Same section after the addition of scatter. **(h)** Strong gradients in the image result in partial volume artifacts. This effect was artificially eliminated in all the other images. **(i)** Motion artifacts caused by a short movement of the iron rod.

to obtain two interleaved sets of detector samples separated by 180°.

- If the number of views is too small, alternating dark and bright streaks occur in the peripheral image region where the sampling density is smallest. This is illustrated in Figure 3.21(d).

### Beam hardening

Low-energy photons are preferentially absorbed. Therefore, an X-ray beam *hardens* as it passes through tissue. The harder a beam, the less it is further attenuated. All beams passing through a particular pixel follow different paths and therefore experience a different degree of beam hardening. Hence, they perceive different attenuation values in that pixel. This phenomenon causes beam hardening artifacts such as a reduced attenuation toward the center of an object (cupping) and streaks that connect objects with strong attenuation. Figure 3.21(e) shows an artifact-free section of a phantom that consists of a plexiglass

(polymethyl methacrylate) plate and three amalgam fillings. Simulating the same section using a polychromatic spectrum results in beam hardening artifacts shown in Figure 3.21(f).

### Scatter

Not all photons that arrive at the detector follow a straight path from the X-ray tube. Typically, up to 30% of the detected radiation is due to scatter. The contribution of scatter to the measured intensity profile is very smooth. Because of the scattered photons, the attenuation of a particular beam is underestimated. The larger the integrated attenuation along a particular projection line, the smaller is the theoretical intensity and thus the larger the relative error resulting from scatter. Scatter yields streak artifacts, as shown in Figure 3.21(g).

### Nonlinear partial volume effect

Because of the finite beam width, every measurement represents an intensity averaged over this beam width.

51

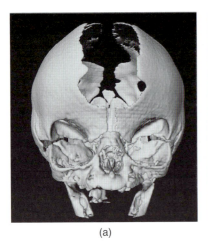
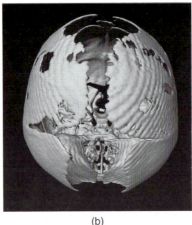

(a)                          (b)

**Figure 3.22** The stairstep artifact is visible in 3D images as a helical winding along inclined surfaces. (Courtesy of Professor M. H. Smet, Department of Radiology and Professor J. Van Cleynenbreugel, Lab. Medical Image Computing.)

Afterwards, this measured intensity is log-converted to calculate the integrated linear attenuation along the beam (Eq. (3.5)). However, it can be shown that this value is always an underestimation of the integrated averaged attenuation. The larger the attenuation differences across the beam width, the larger this underestimation. This results in the streaks tangent to edges shown in Figure 3.21(h).

### Motion

A short movement of an object during the acquisition results in inconsistent measurements and causes two streaks, that is, a streak that connects the object and the position of the X-ray tube at the moment the object moves, and a streak that connects the object and the X-ray tube at its start–stop position. The simulation in Figure 3.21(i) shows the streak artifacts that result from a short movement of the iron rod. More gradual movement, such as cardiac motion, may also cause streak artifacts but will result primarily in a blurred representation of the moving parts.

### Stairstep artifact

In helical CT, the representation of a 3D surface involves longitudinal interpolation in the reconstruction step as well as in the surface rendering step. Stairstep artifacts occur when the helical pitch is too large or when the reconstruction interval is too small. This artifact is visible in longitudinal reslices as regular stairstep disruptions along inclined edges and in 3D images as a black or white helical winding along inclined surfaces, such as the skull (Figure 3.22), dense ribs and contrast filled coronaries.

**Figure 3.23** The windmill artifact, also called the bearclaw artifact, is visible as a pattern of black and white spokes originating from positions with a high $z$-gradient. (Courtesy of GE Healthcare.)

### Windmill artifact

The windmill artifact (also called bearclaw artifact) is a $z$-aliasing artifact that occurs primarily in helical cone-beam CT. The helical cone-beam reconstruction process involves interpolation between detector rows. The amount of blur introduced by this interpolation process changes as a function of view angle due to the helical motion. This results in a typical pattern of black and white spokes originating from a strong $z$-gradient (Figure 3.23).

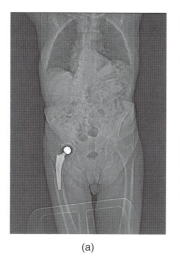

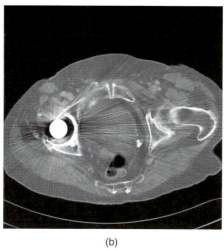

(a)　　　　　　　　(b)

**Figure 3.24** CT scan of a patient with a prosthetic hip implant, obtained with a multi-slice CT scanner. **(a)** Topogram, that is, an image of the projections $p_\theta(r)$ for a particular angle $\theta$ and varying depth $z$. This image looks like a radiograph. It is typically used as an overview image to define the region for subsequent scanning. **(b)** CT image of a slice through the prosthesis showing streak artifacts due to the metallic implant. (Courtesy of Professor G. Marchal, Department of Radiology.)

## Other artifacts

A variety of other artifacts is due to poor calibration or system failure such as detector failure, noisy calibration, a change of the detector efficiency between the calibration and the actual measurement, irregular table translation, and mechanical instability of the tube–detector unit.

Figure 3.24 shows a practical example of the *metal streak artifact* caused by a hip prosthesis. Metal artifacts are due to a combination of beam hardening, scatter, nonlinear partial volume effect, and noise.

The *blooming artifact* is a very common artifact that typically occurs when imaging calcified plaque. It is caused by a combination of beam hardening and limited spatial resolution and leads to an overestimation of the plaque size and an underestimation of the vessel lumen.

A more detailed overview of CT image artifacts is given in [11].

## Equipment
## Tomosynthesis

Radiography and CT can be seen as two ends of a spectrum: radiography gives one projection image without depth information; CT uses a thousand projection images to image an entire volume, voxel by voxel, i.e., with perfect depth information. Tomosynthesis can be seen as a compromise between radiography

and CT: a low number (typically tens) of projection images are combined to compute 3D images with limited depth information. Tomosynthesis reconstruction techniques include simple backprojection (also called shift-and-add), which is intrinsically the principle used in linear tomography (Figure 3.3(a)), filtered backprojection, and iterative reconstruction.

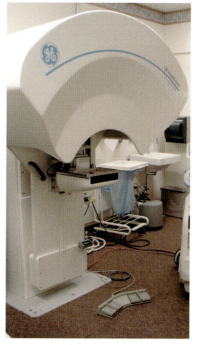

**Figure 3.25** Second generation Digital Breast Tomosynthesis prototype installed at the University of Michigan for clinical research. (Courtesy of GE Healthcare.)

[11] J. Hsieh. *Computed Tomography: Principles, Design, Artifacts, and Recent Advances.* Cambridge: Cambridge University Press, SPIE Publications, SPIE Monograph, Volume PM114, 2003.

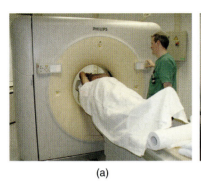 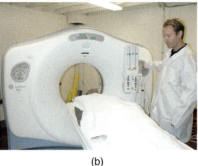

(a)                                         (b)

**Figure 3.26** The external design of a multi-slice scanner is not significantly different from that of a single-slice scanner. **(a)** Philips Brilliance CT 64-channel with 64 detector rows. **(b)** GE Lightspeed VCT with 64 detector rows.

In nonmedical applications, tomosynthesis is usually called laminography. The most prominent medical applications of tomosynthesis are in chest imaging and mammography. Tomosynthesis was enabled by the introduction of digital flat panel detector technologies; chest tomosynthesis became commercially available in 2004. The first Digital Breast Tomosynthesis research prototype was completed in 1999 by GE Global Research in collaboration with Massachusetts General Hospital. Figure 3.25 shows a second generation Digital Breast Tomosynthesis prototype installed at the University of Michigan for clinical research.

## General purpose scanners

General purpose scanners (Figure 3.26) typically contain multiple detector rows. Because of their large FOV ($\geq$ 50 cm) and high rotation speed (up to 3 rotations per second) active matrix flat panel detectors are typically not useful. Although large size flat panel detectors exist (p. 21), their frame rate is still too low for most radiological examinations, including cardiac and dynamic studies.

Multi-slice CT with helical acquisition was introduced in 1998. Initially these scanners contained only four detector rows, but rapidly this number increased to 16, 64, 128, 256, and even 320. With a 320-row scanner and a detector size of 0.5 mm referred to the isocenter, for example, a total volume of 16 cm is covered, making this system suitable for operation in the axial scan mode and for performing a cardiac scan in one single rotation (0.35 s). Until recently all manufacturers were competing to have the largest number of detector rows, also referred to as the slice wars. Today, most manufacturers believe this comes with too many image quality tradeoffs and prefer to focus on other performance improvements.

The basic geometry is shown in Figure 3.27(a) and (b). In front of the X-ray tube is a collimator (Figure 3.27(a) and (c)), which limits the transmitted X-rays to the detector and prevents useless irradiation of the patient. A post-patient collimator or antiscatter grid consisting of many small attenuating plates between the detector cells (Figure 3.27(a) and (d)) is used to limit the detected scattered radiation. The circle inscribed by the tube–detector fan determines the field of view (FOV). Data and power are transmitted from and to the rotating tube–detector unit through *slip rings* (not shown). The power is transmitted through a brush slip ring and the data are transmitted via an RF or optical slip ring. Slip rings eliminate the mechanical problems that would be implied by cables connecting fixed and rotating parts. The gantry (this is the part of the CT scanner that contains the rotating parts) can be tilted over a limited angle for imaging oblique slices (Figure 3.28).

## Dedicated scanners

Today several special purpose CT scanners exist. They are typically cheaper and smaller than general purpose systems. They make use of the principle of circular cone-beam scanning and acquire volumetric data in a single orbit of the X-ray tube. In many applications the field of view can be limited and/or the scan time is not critical. This opens the way to use flat panel digital X-ray detectors (FPDs) yielding high spatial resolution images. Current commercial systems acquire the data in seconds to tens of seconds. Below are some examples.

### Oral and maxillofacial CT

A variety of in-office scanners for the maxillofacial area are commercially available today. Figure 3.29 shows two of them with an open design. The patient

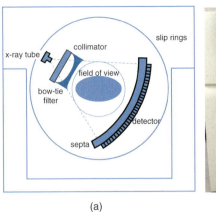

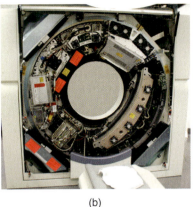

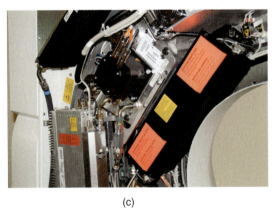

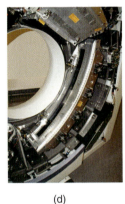

(a)

(b)

**Figure 3.27** (a) and (b) The basic internal geometry of a multi-slice helical CT scanner. Collimators are placed in front of the X-ray tube and the detectors. Because the patient's body attenuates primarily the X-rays of the interior part of the beam, a bow-tie shaped filter compensates for this by mainly attenuating the exterior X-rays, this way ensuring a more uniform signal at the detectors. (c) X-ray tube with adjustable collimating split. This particular scanner has no bow-tie filter. (d) Detector array with post-patient collimator.

(c)

(d)

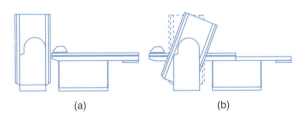

(a)                    (b)

**Figure 3.28** Schematic views of a helical CT scanner showing gantry tilt and table translation.

sits comfortably on a chair and the tube–detector frame rotates in a horizontal plane. This technology has been the onset of new diagnostic and interventional procedures such as oral implant surgery planning (see, for example, Figure 8.42 in Chapter 8), orthodontic treatment planning, and quantitative analysis of bone and joint morphology and function.

## Interventional CT

Modern C-arm systems for interventional fluoroscopy and angiography with flat panel detector, such as the

3DRA system shown in Figure 2.12, are able to reconstruct a 3D image from the acquired projection data. Figure 3.30 shows a mobile scanner dedicated to spine and orthopedic surgery. The system can be used in combination with an intraoperative navigation system (Chapter 8, p. 208) to navigate accurately through the CT images with the surgical instruments. Figure 3.31 shows a portable system dedicated to intraoperative imaging of sinuses, skull base, and temporal bones.

## Breast CT

A few research groups [12] have developed dedicated breast CT scanners. The patient is typically placed in the prone position, and the gantry is positioned horizontally underneath the patient (Figure 3.32). The X-ray tube and flat panel detector system then rotate around the pendant breast, acquiring the cone-beam

[12] K. K. Lindfors, J. M. Boone, T. R. Nelson, K. Yang, A. L. C. Kwan, and D. F. Miller. Dedicated breast CT: initial clinical experience. *Radiology*, 246(3): 725–733, 2008.

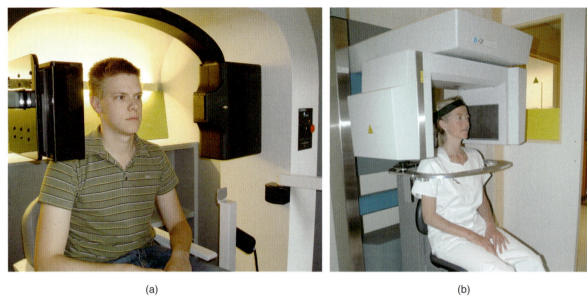

**Figure 3.29** Cone-beam CT scanners for the oral and maxillofacial area. **(a)** Iluma CT (Imtec). (Courtesy of Dr. G. Swennen, AZ Sint-Jan, Brugge.) **(b)** i-CAT CT (Imaging Sciences International). (Courtesy of Dr. N. Nadjmi, Eeuwfeestkliniek, Antwerpen.)

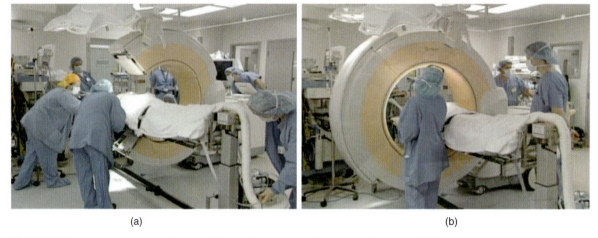

**Figure 3.30** O-arm imaging system (Medtronic). **(a)** A mobile gantry enables lateral patient access. **(b)** Once in place the gantry closes around the patient into an "O"-shaped gantry that can be tilted in any orientation.

projections which allow reconstruction of the 3D volume data set of the breast. The principal benefit of this approach is that the 3D data set allows the radiologist to avoid overlapping anatomy, and the hope is that more breast cancers will be detected using this 3D technique, compared to 2D mammography. One of the main challenges is to image the complete breast, and not miss any portion due to the proximity to the chest wall or into the axillary tail. Even if breast CT is not found to be useful for breast cancer screening, it is likely that it will have a role to play as a secondary imaging device during the diagnostic breast examination. In this role, it can rule out so-called summation artifacts and be used for image guided robotic biopsy guidance.

## Electron beam tomography

In electron beam tomography (EBT), sometimes called ultrafast CT or cardiovascular CT, the X-ray

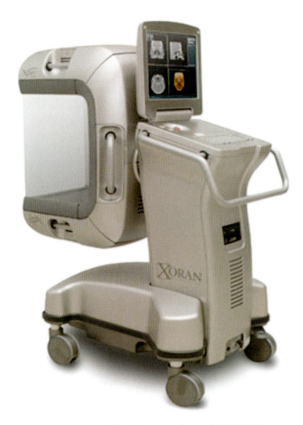

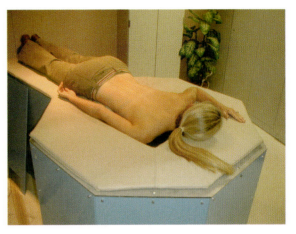

**Figure 3.32** Breast CT prototype by John Boone *et al*. The patient is placed in prone position and the X-ray tube and detector rotate around the pendant breast. (Courtesy of UC Davis Health Systems.)

**Figure 3.31** Portable CT with an open design (xCAT ENT, Xoran Technologies), dedicated to head and neck imaging (sinuses, skull base and temporal bones).

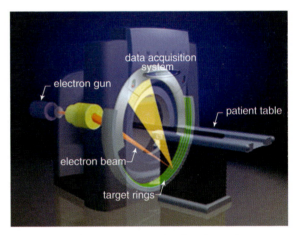

**Figure 3.33** Schematic representation of an electron beam tomographic scanner. The impact of electrons on the target rings produces X-rays that are collimated and directed onto the detectors. (Courtesy of GE Healthcare.)

tube – formerly a compact unit – has become an integrated part of the system (Figure 3.33). Electrons, produced by an electron gun, pass through an electromagnetic focusing coil and are bent electromagnetically onto one of four tungsten target rings lying in the gantry below the patient. The impact of electrons on the target rings produces X-rays that are directed onto a double ring of cadmium tungstate detector elements located in the gantry above the patient. The X-rays are tightly collimated before passing through the patient. Each sweep of a target ring requires 50 ms, and there is an 8 ms delay to reset the beam. This provides a temporal resolution of 17 frames per second. Each frame consists of two slices, one for each detector ring. The images produced by the EBT scanner have a resolution of 0.25–0.5 mm in the imaging plane. The axial resolution is 1.5–10.0 mm, depending on the collimation selected by the operator. These features make the EBT scanner useful to produce images of the beating heart. However, at this moment, the number of installed EBT scanners around the world is rather limited.

## Multiple X-ray tubes

Most commercial clinical scanners are based on the so-called third generation architecture. A single X-ray tube and a single detector assembly are positioned face-to-face and rotated jointly around the patient. Berninger and Redington presented the idea of replicating the source and detector, as illustrated in Figure 3.34.

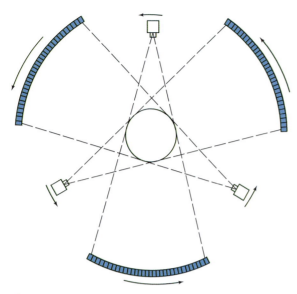

**Figure 3.34** CT architecture with three sources and three detectors. Berninger and Redington first proposed replicating the X-ray tube and detector assembly.

The dynamic spatial reconstructor (DSR) (Figure 3.35(a)) may have been the first real multi-source prototype. It is a unique experimental 4D X-ray CT scanner developed at the Mayo Clinic by Richard Robb *et al.* [13]. It allows simultaneous scanning of up to 240 cross-sections at a maximum frame rate of 60 Hz (60 volumes per second). The DSR consists of 14 X-ray tubes and 14 2D detectors (Figure 3.35(b)). The X-ray tubes are placed on a 160° circular arc with very large diameter and are pulsed sequentially over a period of 11 ms (hence 60 Hz). The detectors are located diametrically opposed to the X-ray tubes. Each detector consists of an image intensifier and a high-definition television camera. Because of the large diameter, the X-rays in different slices can be considered to be parallel, and the 3D reconstruction problem reduces to the 2D reconstruction of a series of 2D slices.

About 25 years later, Siemens developed the first commercial two-tube scanner, also known as dual-source CT. The main advantage of this architecture is its improved temporal resolution. In today's state-of-the-art CT scanners, the gantry rotation time is reduced to about 0.35 s, but it is mechanically challenging to reduce that time even further, which justifies the

renewed interest in multi-source architectures. The dual-source CT system almost doubles the temporal resolution. However, the cross-scatter from the second source into the first detector is reported to result in a scatter-to-primary ratio as high as 100% for obese patients, corresponding to a severe dose penalty. Therefore, more research will be needed on both hardware (scatter rejection) and software (scatter correction) methods for dual-source CT.

## X-rays tubes with multiple spots

Almost all modern CT architectures are based on one or more single-spot X-ray tubes possibly with focal spot wobble.

Another class of X-ray sources has multiple spots distributed along the longitudinal axis in the $z$-direction. It has been shown that the combined information from the multiple spots in the $z$-direction effectively eliminates cone-beam artifacts.

Another example of a distributed X-ray source with a deflected electron beam is the transmission X-ray source developed by NovaRay, formerly known as Cardiac Mariners, and Nexray, Palo Alto, California, USA, with thousands of focal spots. This area source was first used to demonstrate the concept of inverse-geometry CT. In addition to eliminating cone-beam artifacts, this architecture has the benefit of a small photon-counting detector and very good absorption efficiency.

A related architecture is based on discrete electron emitters, resulting in a 2D array source with tens of focal spots (see Figure 3.36). This source architecture is more compact than the above and perhaps more compatible with the concept of a virtual bow-tie, where the operation of each spot is modulated in real time to optimize image quality and minimize dose, depending on the patient anatomy.

In recent decades, advances in detector technologies defined the so-called "slice wars." We expect that in the next decade dramatic advances in distributed X-ray sources may define a new revolution in CT and give birth to a wide class of new multi-source CT architectures, including line sources, inverse-geometry CT, and ultimately a rebirth of stationary CT, which means that neither the source nor the detector is in motion during the data acquisition process.

## Clinical use

The main virtue of X-ray computed tomography is its ability to produce a series of cross-sectional images

[13] R. A. Robb. The dynamic spatial reconstructor: an x-ray video-fluoroscopic ct scanner for dynamic volume imaging of moving organs. *IEEE Transactions on Medical Imaging*, 1(1): 22–33, July 1982.

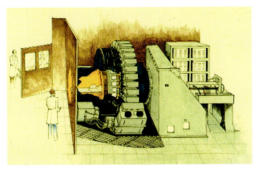

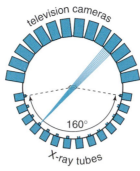

**Figure 3.35** Schematic view of the dynamic spatial reconstructor (DSR). 14 X-ray tubes are placed on a 160° circular arc and 14 television cameras are located diametrically opposite to the X-ray tubes. Image provided courtesy of Richard A. Robb, Ph.D., Biomedical Imaging Resource, Mayo Clinic.

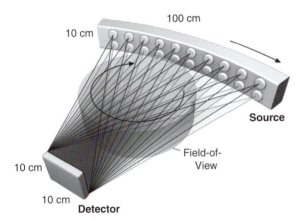

**Figure 3.36** An inverse-geometry architecture with tens of spots combining the benefits of a line source in $z$, a small photon-counting detector, and a virtual bow tie. Reproduced with permission from Bruno De Man and SPIE.

of the human body. As compared with the projection images in radiography, true 3D images and a better contrast between different tissues are obtained.

CT is applied to obtain anatomical images of all parts of the human body. The most common investigations include the following:

- head and neck (brain, maxillofacial structures, inner ear, soft tissues of the neck (Figure 3.37)),

- thorax (lungs, chest wall and mediastinum, heart and great vessels (Figure 3.38)),

- urogenital tract (kidneys, adrenals, urinary bladder, prostate, female genital organs, retroperitoneal cavity (Figure 3.39)),

- abdomen (gastrointestinal tract, liver, pancreas, peritoneal cavity, spleen (Figure 3.40)),

- musculoskeleton system (bone fractures, calcium studies, soft tissue tumors, muscle tissue (Figure 3.41)).

Because CT is based on X-ray attenuation, the same contrast agents as in radiographic imaging can be used. However, CT is more sensitive to small intensity differences than radiographic projection images and, consequently, contrast agents in small concentrations can also be noticed outside the blood vessels or cavities. This way anatomical differences from an increased or decreased vascularization or diffusion volume and functional diffusion of perfusion differences can be visualized. Figure 3.42 shows an example in which the contrast dye is used to identify tumoral brain tissue and to visualize the cerebral blood vessels. More details about perfusion and diffusion images are given in Chapters 4 and 5.

## Biologic effects and safety

Radiation doses are relatively high in CT. For example, the effective dose of a CT of the head is 1–2 mSv and of the chest, abdomen or pelvis on the order of 5–8 mSv each. A low-dose lung CT is responsible for an effective dose of 1.5–2 mSv and a whole-body screening for 7 mSv or more. This is on the order of 10 to 100 times higher than a radiographic image of the same region.

The possible harm is too high to be neglected, and the patient dose must be kept as low as possible. Taking the required image quality into account, this can be done by a correct use of the equipment and by keeping the equipment in optimal condition. The dose can be limited by a low integrated tube current (mA s) and a limited scan range. Some scanners apply a modulated tube current to reduce the dose. They use a larger tube current in views with higher attenuation. Optimal condition of the equipment requires a daily calibration of the CT scanner by performing a number of blank scans (i.e., scans with only air inside the gantry). Image quality and constancy must be checked by phantom

**59**

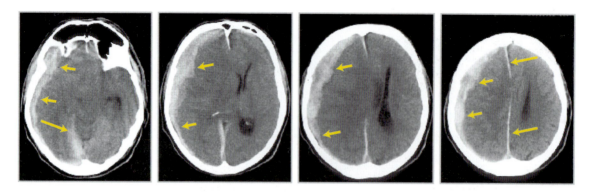

**Figure 3.37** Subsequent CT slices through the brain show a subdural hemorrhage as a hyperdense region along the inner skull wall (short arrows). This blood collection causes an increased pressure on the brain structures with an important displacement of the midsagittal line (long arrows). (Courtesy of Professor G. Wilms, Department of Radiology.)

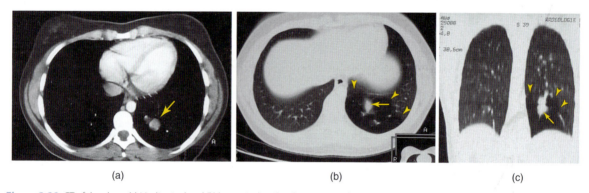

(a)                                          (b)                                          (c)

**Figure 3.38** CT of the chest. **(a)** Mediastinal and **(b)** lung window/level settings, and **(c)** coronal resliced image. The images show a congenital malformation of the lung located in the left lower lobe. Notice the two components of the lesion: a dense multilobular opacity (arrow) surrounded by an area of decreased lung attenuation (arrow heads). (Courtesy of Professor J. Verschakelen, Department of Radiology.)

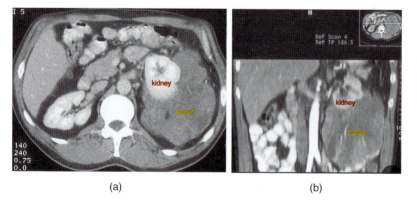

(a)                                          (b)

**Figure 3.39** **(a)** Axial CT slice through the kidney showing a perirenal liposarcoma in the nephrographic phase after intravenous injection of contrast medium. **(b)** Reformatted coronal CT slice at the level of the aorta of the same patient. (Courtesy of Professor R. Oyen, Department of Radiology.)

measurements. Maintenance and safety inspections must occur several times a year.

A useful indicator of the absorbed dose before starting an examination with a specific scanning protocol is the *CT dose index* (CTDI). It is defined as the dose absorbed by a standard cylindric acrylic phantom for one 360° rotation of the X-ray tube

$$\mathrm{CTDI} = \frac{1}{n\,\Delta z} \int_{-\infty}^{\infty} D(z)\,\mathrm{d}z. \qquad (3.45)$$

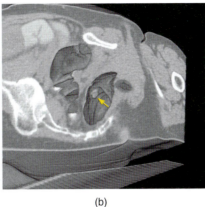

**Figure 3.40** **(a)** A CT slice through the colon shows a polyp (arrow). **(b)** A virtual colonoscopy program creates a depth view of the colon with polyp (arrow) and allows the clinician to navigate automatically along the inner wall. (Courtesy of Dr. M. Thomeer, Department of Radiology, and G. Kiss, Lab. Medical Image Computing.) 3D visualization is discussed further in Chapter 8.

(a)        (b)

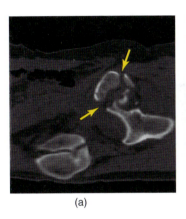 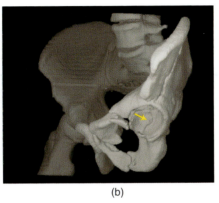

**Figure 3.41** **(a)** On a sagittal reformatted CT image, an anteroposterior course of an acetabular fracture is visible. **(b)** A 3D view on the acetabular surface more clearly localizes the transtectal course of the fracture extending into the posterior column. (Courtesy of Professor M. H. Smet, Department of Radiology, and Professor J. Van Cleynenbreugel, Lab. Medical Image Computing.)

(a)        (b)

$D(z)$ is the radiation dose profile along the $z$-axis, $n$ the number of detector rows and $n\,\Delta z$ the total detector width. Two different standard phantoms exist, i.e., a head phantom with a diameter of 16 cm and a body phantom with a diameter of 32 cm. By using a large integration interval the scattered radiation outside the scanned slab is taken into account as well. Hence, the CTDI value also reflects the absorbed dose obtained by circular scanning a series of adjacent slices.

For practical reasons the measurement along the $z$-axis is typically limited to 100 mm, yielding the standardized $\text{CTDI}_{100}$ value. It is assumed that the scatter is negligible beyond this integration interval. This is a valuable assumption for older systems. For cone-beam CT, however, an integration interval of 100 mm is not sufficient.

The CTDI varies across the image plane and is higher at the periphery than in the center of the FOV. Therefore a weighted CT dose index $\text{CTDI}_w$ was introduced

$$\text{CTDI}_w = \frac{1}{3}\text{CTDI}_c + \frac{2}{3}\text{CTDI}_p, \qquad (3.46)$$

where $\text{CTDI}_c$ and $\text{CTDI}_p$ are the CTDI values in the center and at the periphery respectively. The relative areas of the center and the periphery are approximated by one third and two thirds.

The CTDI value was originally defined for circular scan protocols. For helical scanning, however, the pitch influences the absorbed dose and should be taken into account. The volume CT dose index $\text{CTDI}_{vol}$ was introduced as the weighted CTDI divided by the pitch

$$\text{CTDI}_{vol} = \frac{\text{CTDI}_w}{\text{pitch}}. \qquad (3.47)$$

Note that in practice the $\text{CTDI}_{vol}$ value does not necessarily change with the pitch because the mA s per rotation is often increased proportional to the pitch to

**61**

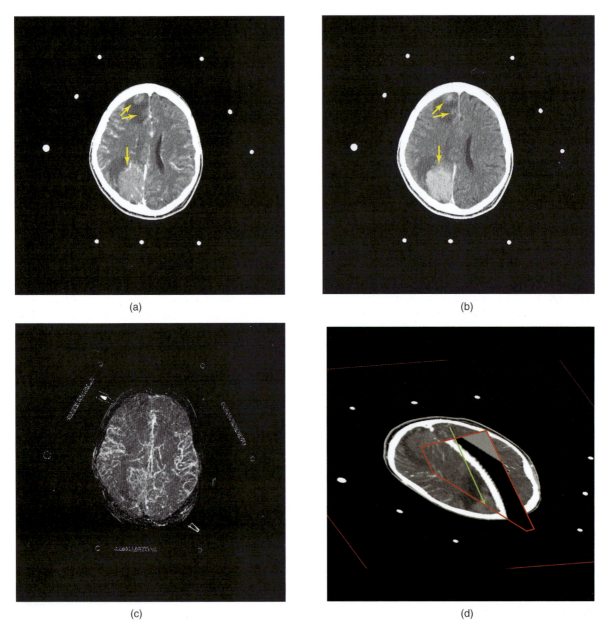

(a)

(b)

(c)

(d)

**Figure 3.42** CT images through the brain used for neurosurgical planning. **(a)** CT slice immediately after contrast injection. The arrows show brain lesions surrounded by oedema. The nine bright spots around the patient are markers used for surgical planning. (More details are presented in Chapter 8.) **(b)** Late postcontrast image. After 10 minutes the tumoral lesions have absorbed the contrast and light up in the image. **(c)** By subtracting the CT images before and immediately after contrast injection, the cerebral blood vessels are visualized. In this image, the whole vessel tree is shown by a maximum intensity projection (MIP), explained in Chapter 4, p. 87. **(d)** All these images are used subsequently to calculate a safe trajectory (long arrow) through the blood vessels and toward one of the lesions in order to take a biopsy of the tumoral tissue. (Courtesy of Professor B. Nuttin, Department of Neurosurgery.)

maintain the CNR. A few examples of $CTDI_{vol}$ values are given in Table 3.1.

The $CTDI_{vol}$ is an indication of the absorbed dose, expressed in Gy, i.e., J/kg. This value is independent of the scan length. Therefore, dose-length product (DLP)

is often used. It multiplies the $CTDI_{vol}$ with the scan length $L$

$$DLP = CTDI_{vol} \cdot L. \tag{3.48}$$

**Table 3.1** Examples of the tube charge (*C*), volume CT dose index (CTDI$_{vol}$), scan length (*L*), dose-length product (DLP), normalized effective dose per DLP (*k*) for adults (from different literature sources), and effective dose (*E*); the exams were chosen arbitrarily during clinical routine on a 64-slice CT scanner

| Exam | *C* (mAs/rotation) | CTDI$_{vol}$ (mGy) | *L* (cm) | DLP (mGy cm) | *k* (mSv/mGy cm) | *E* (mSv) |
|------|------|------|------|------|------|------|
| Head | 380 | 55.75 | 10.8 | 602 | 0.0021–0.0023 | 1.26–1.38 |
| Neck | 185 | 14.20 | 25.8 | 367 | 0.0054–0.0059 | 1.98–2.17 |
|      | 222 | 17.00 | 28.8 | 490 | 0.0054–0.0059 | 2.65–2.89 |
| Chest | 135 | 10.36 | 35.6 | 369 | 0.014–0.019 | 5.17–7.01 |
|       | 140 | 10.69 | 29.2 | 312 | 0.014–0.019 | 4.37–5.93 |
| Abdomen | 150 | 11.57 | 30.3 | 350 | 0.015–0.017 | 5.25–5.95 |
|         | 175 | 13.49 | 25.6 | 345 | 0.015–0.017 | 5.18–5.87 |
| Pelvis | 164 | 19.60 | 26.6 | 522 | 0.015–0.019 | 7.83–9.92 |

Table 3.1 gives some examples of DLP values. Although the DLP is a better indication of the biological sensitivity for a particular examination than the CTDI$_{vol}$, it does not distinguish between different organs. To determine the effective dose, the individual organ doses should be multiplied with their corresponding radiation weighting factors. In the literature average regional conversion factors *k* exist that relate DLP to effective dose. Table 3.1 shows examples of such conversion factors for an adult. An estimated effective dose *E* can then be calculated as

$$E = k \cdot \text{DLP}. \tag{3.49}$$

Note that these values are valid for standard phantoms but they do not distinguish between individual patients.

## Future expectations

CT will remain an important modality for the visualization of the skeleton, calcifications, the lungs and the gastrointestinal tract. To a certain extent, CT will also be the only alternative for patients with implants (e.g., intracranial aneurysm clip, pacemaker, cochlear stimulator) who are not allowed to enter the MR room (p. 103). An increased use can be expected for screening (heart, chest, colon), perfusion imaging and vascular and cardiac imaging.

Until recently all manufacturers were competing to have the largest number of detector rows, also referred to as the slice wars. Today the different vendors have slightly different priorities and pursue different solutions.

From a technical viewpoint the tendency is toward dose reduction, increased volume coverage, higher contrast-to-noise ratio and improved spatial and temporal resolution. Progress in multi-source technologies may lead to dramatic changes in CT architectures. New developments in multi-energy imaging will enhance tissue characterization, automatic segmentation, monochromatic imaging and improved beam hardening correction (e.g., blooming). Ultimately photon counting at higher count rates and with high-energy resolution will be exploited for multi-energy CT with optimal dose efficiency.

# Magnetic resonance imaging

## Introduction

Magnetic resonance imaging (MRI) is a relatively recent medical imaging modality. Although the physical phenomenon of nuclear magnetic resonance (NMR) has been known since the early 1940s [14, 15], its practical application to the field of medical imaging was only realized in 1973 when Paul C. Lauterbur made the first NMR image [16] by introducing gradients in the magnetic field. In 1974 Peter Mansfield presented the mathematical theory for fast scanning and image reconstruction, needed in clinical practice, and showed how extremely rapid imaging could be obtained by very fast gradient variations. Lauterbur and Mansfield shared the Nobel Prize in Medicine or Physiology in 2003.

A difficulty is that NMR cannot totally be explained using "classical" physics (i.e., the physical theories based on the laws of Newton and Maxwell). In 1905, Einstein demonstrated in his special theory of relativity that Newton's laws are only approximately valid. Later in the twentieth century the theory of quantum mechanics was developed to explain physical phenomena on the atomic and subatomic scale. A concise description of the basis of NMR, the property of spin angular momentum, needs the theory of quantum electrodynamics, which combines the special theory of relativity and quantum mechanics. This theory is beyond the scope of this text. A simplified discussion of NMR based on classical and quantum mechanics suffices to explain the principles of MRI.

## Physics of the transmitted signal

In essence, MRI measures a magnetic property of tissue. The following section describes the behavior of a

single particle with angular momentum and magnetic moment in an external magnetic field. This problem is studied from the viewpoints of classical and quantum mechanics. The next section (p. 67) discusses what happens when matter (such as human tissue), which contains a huge quantity of particles, is placed in an external magnetic field.

## Angular momenta and magnetic moments
### A qualitative description

In classical mechanics, angular momentum is employed when discussing the rotation of an object about an axis. For example, as shown in Figure 4.1, in celestial mechanics, the description of the motion of the Earth involves two angular momenta: one corresponding to the rotation of the Earth about the Sun, and a second corresponding to its rotation about its own axis (spinning). When at the end of the nineteenth century it became clear that the atom has an inner structure, physicists used mechanical models to explain the atomic phenomena. Hence, in Rutherford's model of the atom, an *orbital angular momentum* is assigned to the orbital motion of the electron about the nucleus. Furthermore, because the electron is a charged particle, its orbital motion implies the existence of a current loop and thus a magnetic moment.

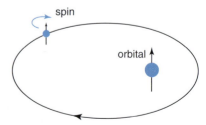

**Figure 4.1** In celestial mechanics, a spin and an orbital angular momentum are associated with the Earth's motion about the Sun. In the classical theory, electron and nucleus replace Earth and Sun, respectively. Because the electron is a charged particle, it also has a magnetic moment. Unfortunately, the classical model is incorrect: spin of elementary particles has no classical analog.

[14] F. Bloch. Nuclear induction. *Physical Review*, 70(7–8): 460–473, 1946.
[15] F. Bloch, W. Hansen, and M. Packard. The nuclear induction experiment. *Physical Review*, 70(7–8): 474–485, 1946.
[16] P. Lauterbur. Image formation by induced local interactions: examples employing nuclear magnetic resonance. *Nature*, 242: 190–191, 1973.

**Table 4.1** Spin values of several nuclei of biomedical interest.
A given nucleus is characterized by a unique spin value (the values are explained on p. 66). Note that the biomedically important nuclei $^{12}_{6}C$ and $^{16}_{8}O$ have no spin and thus no NMR sensitivity [18].

| Nucleus | Spin | $\frac{\gamma}{2\pi}$ (MHz/T) |
|---|---|---|
| $^{1}_{1}H$ | $\frac{1}{2}$ | 42.57 |
| $^{2}_{1}H$ | 1 | 6.54 |
| $^{12}_{6}C$ | 0 | |
| $^{13}_{6}C$ | $\frac{1}{2}$ | 10.71 |
| $^{14}_{7}N$ | 1 | 3.08 |
| $^{15}_{7}N$ | $\frac{1}{2}$ | −4.31 |
| $^{16}_{8}O$ | 0 | |
| $^{17}_{8}O$ | $\frac{5}{2}$ | −5.77 |
| $^{31}_{15}P$ | $\frac{1}{2}$ | 17.23 |
| $^{33}_{16}S$ | $\frac{3}{2}$ | 3.27 |
| $^{43}_{21}Ca$ | $\frac{7}{2}$ | −2.86 |

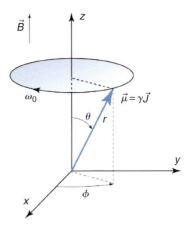

**Figure 4.2** If a particle with angular momentum $\vec{J}$ and magnetic moment $\vec{\mu}$ is suspended without friction in an external magnetic field $\vec{B}$, a precession about $\vec{B}$ occurs. The angular frequency $\omega_0$ of this precession is proportional to $B_0$. For positive $\gamma$, the precession is clockwise.

However, to explain certain experimental facts observed in atomic spectra, Uhlenbeck and Goudsmit postulated in 1925 that the electron must also have a *spin angular momentum* (or *spin* for short) with an associated magnetic moment. However, attempting to give the electron a spatial extension, as in Figure 4.1, and associating this spin with rotation about its own axis, is incorrect. The spin has no classical analog; its origin can only be explained correctly by combining special relativity theory with quantum mechanics [17].

The electron is not the only elementary particle that has spin. The proton and the neutron also possess this property. Consequently, the spin of an atomic nucleus is the vector sum of the spins of its constituent protons and neutrons. The value of the spin thus depends on both the mass number and the atomic number [18]. Because an atomic nucleus is a distribution of charge, a net spin angular momentum is associated with a magnetic moment. Table 4.1 lists the spin values of a number of biomedically important isotopes and shows that the property of spin is more the rule than the exception in nature.

## Classical description

NMR studies the behavior of atomic nuclei with spin angular momentum and associated magnetic moment

[17] P. Dirac. *The Principles of Quantum Mechanics*. Oxford: Clarendon Press, fourth edition, 1958.
[18] P. Morris. *Nuclear Magnetic Resonance Imaging in Medicine and Biology*. Oxford: Oxford University Press, first edition, 1986.

in an external magnetic field. Throughout this text, the direction of the external magnetic field $\vec{B}$ is defined as the z-axis of the coordinate system: $\vec{B} = (0, 0, B_0)$.

Let $\vec{J}$ be a spin angular momentum and $\vec{\mu}$ its associated magnetic moment. The vectors $\vec{J}$ and $\vec{\mu}$ have the same orientation and their relationship can be written as

$$\vec{\mu} = \gamma \vec{J}, \tag{4.1}$$

where $\gamma$ is the *gyromagnetic ratio*, which is a constant for a particular nucleus (see Table 4.1). The interaction between $\vec{B}$ and $\vec{\mu}$ yields a precession motion and a potential energy (Figure 4.2).

*Motion equation*

In classical mechanics, $\vec{J}$ satisfies

$$\frac{d\vec{J}}{dt} = \vec{\tau}, \tag{4.2}$$

where $\vec{\tau}$ is the net external torque acting on the system being studied. In this case,

$$\vec{\tau} = \vec{\mu} \times \vec{B}, \tag{4.3}$$

which, combined with Eqs. (4.2) and (4.1), yields

$$\frac{d\vec{\mu}}{dt} = \vec{\mu} \times \gamma\vec{B}. \tag{4.4}$$

The solution of this equation is

$$\mu_x(t) = \mu_x(0)\cos(\omega_0 t) + \mu_y(0)\sin(\omega_0 t)$$
$$\mu_y(t) = -\mu_x(0)\sin(\omega_0 t) + \mu_y(0)\cos(\omega_0 t) \tag{4.5}$$
$$\mu_z(t) = \mu_z(0),$$

with

$$\omega_0 = \gamma B_0. \tag{4.6}$$

The constants $\mu_x(0)$, $\mu_y(0)$, and $\mu_z(0)$ are the values of the components at $t = 0$. Let $\mu_{xy}(t) = \mu_x(t) + i\mu_y(t)$ and $\mu_{xy}(0) = \mu_x(0) + i\mu_y(0)$. The transverse component can then be written as

$$\mu_{xy}(t) = \mu_{xy}(0)e^{-i\omega_0 t}. \tag{4.7}$$

Equations (4.5) and (4.7) show that the transverse component of $\vec{\mu}$ rotates about the $z$-axis with angular frequency $\omega_0$ and the longitudinal or $z$-component is time independent. Hence, the motion of $\vec{\mu}$ is a *precession* about the $z$-axis with precession frequency $\omega_0$. For positive $\gamma$, the rotation is clockwise.

We can further simplify the description by introducing a reference frame with coordinate axes $x'$, $y'$, $z'$ that rotates clockwise about the $z' = z$-axis with angular frequency $\omega_0$. In this rotating frame, $\vec{\mu}$ stands still. Assuming that the stationary and rotating coordinate frames coincide at $t = 0$, Eq. (4.5) becomes

$$\begin{aligned}
\mu_{x'}(t) &= \mu_x(0) \\
\mu_{y'}(t) &= \mu_y(0) \\
\mu_{z'}(t) &= \mu_z(0).
\end{aligned} \tag{4.8}$$

Therefore, in the rotating frame the effective magnetic field perceived by $\vec{\mu}$ is zero. In the remainder of the text the physical phenomena are described in this rotating reference frame unless explicitly stated otherwise.

*Energy*
The potential energy $E$ is

$$E = -\vec{\mu} \cdot \vec{B} = -\mu B_0 \cos\theta = -\gamma J B_0 \cos\theta. \tag{4.9}$$

$E$ is minimal if $\vec{\mu}$ and $\vec{B}$ are parallel. In the classical theory, $J$ and $\theta$ can have any value, so Eq. (4.9) implies that there are no restrictions on the allowed energy values. Consequently, the atomic axis can have any spatial orientation, and $J_z$ can have any value in the interval $[-J, +J]$.

Unfortunately, the classical description is wrong. In 1921, Stern and Gerlach performed a series of experiments with silver atoms that demonstrated that $J_z$ can only have a limited number of values and the atomic axis can apparently have only a finite number of directions. For silver atoms, only two values are possible. This phenomenon was called *space quantization*.

The correct description of the events on the atomic and subatomic scale requires the use of quantum mechanics.

## Quantum mechanical description
### Motion equation
Quantum mechanics shows that the expectation values of the components of the magnetization vector behave as a classical magnetic moment, that is, they satisfy Eq. (4.6) and Figure 4.2.

### Energy
One of the major differences between classical and quantum mechanics is quantization (i.e., the outcome of a measurement of a physical variable is a multiple of a basic amount (quantum)). When measuring the energy, the quantum theory predicts that the possible energy values are restricted to

$$E = -m\,\gamma\hbar B_0, \quad \text{with } m = -j, -j+1, \ldots, j-1, j. \tag{4.10}$$

By definition $\hbar = h/2\pi$, with $h$ the Planck constant. The energy quantum is $\gamma\hbar B_0$. The constant $j$ is the *spin quantum number*. Depending on the number of protons and neutrons in the nucleus, its value can be $0, 1/2, 1, 3/2, \ldots$ (see Table 4.1). For particles with spin $j = 1/2$, such as the proton (nucleus of $^1_1$H), there are two possible energy values:

$$\begin{aligned}
E_\uparrow &= -\frac{1}{2}\gamma\hbar B_0 \\
E_\downarrow &= +\frac{1}{2}\gamma\hbar B_0.
\end{aligned} \tag{4.11}$$

This phenomenon of quantized energy states in the presence of an external magnetic field is known as the *Zeeman effect* (Figure 4.3). The two states are called "spin up" ($\uparrow$) and "spin down" ($\downarrow$), respectively.

The "spin up" state has the lowest energy and will preferentially be occupied, but quantum mechanics prohibits all spins from being in this state. A proton in the state $E_\uparrow$ can switch to the state $E_\downarrow$ by absorbing a photon with energy equal to

$$E_\downarrow - E_\uparrow = \hbar\gamma B_0. \tag{4.12}$$

For a photon with energy $E = \hbar\omega_{RF}$, the *resonance condition* is described by the *Larmor (angular) frequency*:

$$\omega_{RF} = \gamma B_0. \tag{4.13}$$

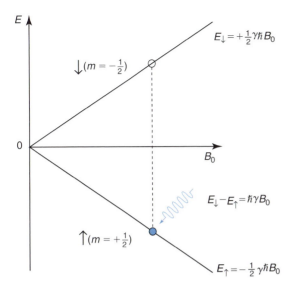

**Figure 4.3** The Zeeman effect for particles with spin $j = 1/2$. In the presence of a time-independent external magnetic field $\vec{B}$ of magnitude $B_0$, the particle can occupy two different energy states, "spin up" ($\uparrow$) and "spin down" ($\downarrow$). The energy difference between the two states is proportional to $B_0$.

Comparing Eq. (4.13) with Eq. (4.6) shows that the Larmor angular frequency is exactly the angular frequency of the precessing magnetic moment, that is,

$$\omega_{RF} = \omega_0. \tag{4.14}$$

If $B_0 = 1$ tesla (T), the Larmor frequency is approximately 42.6 MHz for hydrogen ($^1_1$H). If $B_0 = 1.5$ T, this value becomes approximately 63.85 MHz. The Larmor frequency of this and some other elements can be found in Table 4.1. Electromagnetic waves in this frequency range are called radio-frequency (RF) waves or radio waves for short.

Because hydrogen is abundantly available in the human body, MRI focuses on the visualization of hydrogen-containing tissues (muscles, brain, kidney, CSF, edema, fat, bone marrow, etc.). Other elements are also used for imaging, such as $^{13}$C, $^{19}$F and $^{23}$Na, but not commonly in clinical practice and only for specific applications. Most of these isotopes are present in the body in low concentrations and they are used primarily to label metabolites or pharmaceuticals that are administered to the patient. Hence, the remainder of this chapter deals with the visualization of hydrogen ($^1_1$H), also referred to as protons.

Note that the Larmor frequency slightly depends on the molecular structure the protons $^1_1$H belong to.

Fat molecules are large and surrounded by many electrons, which reduce the effective external field. This way the Larmor frequency of fat is roughly 150 Hz lower at 1 T (220 Hz at 1.5 T) than that of water. This difference normalized to the Larmor frequency of a reference element ($(CH_3)_4Si$), expressed in parts per million (ppm), is called the *chemical shift*. Hence, the chemical shift between fat and water is about 3.5 ppm.

## Dynamic equilibrium: the net magnetization vector of matter

In imaging, each volume element (voxel) is still large enough to contain a huge amount of protons, each proton having its own spin with its associated magnetic moment. In each voxel, a dynamic equilibrium exists in which the spins are distributed over the two possible energy levels. Referring to Figure 4.2, in the spin-up state the magnetic moments point upwards, that is, $\mu_z(t) > 0$, whereas in the spin-down state, the magnetic moments point downward (i.e., $\mu_z(t) < 0$).

The correct description of this dynamic equilibrium must in principle be obtained from statistical quantum mechanics. Fortunately, it can be shown that the expected behavior of a large number of spins is equivalent to the classical behavior of a net magnetization vector representing the sum of all individual magnetic moments [14, 19]. In dynamic equilibrium, each voxel has a net macroscopic magnetization vector $\vec{M}_0$:

$$\vec{M}_0 = \sum_{i=1}^{n_s} \vec{\mu}_i, \tag{4.15}$$

where $n_s$ is the number of spins in the voxel. Because the spin-up state has the lowest energy, more spins occupy this energy level, yielding a net polarization in the direction of the external magnetic field. Hence, the $z$-component of the net magnetization vector and the external field point in the same direction. The larger the external magnetic field, the larger the net magnetization vector (see Eq. (4.102) below) and the signal will be.* A statistical distribution of a large number of

[19] C. Cohen-Tannoudji, B. Diu, and F. Laloë. *Quantum Mechanics.* New York: John Wiley & Sons, first edition, 1977.
* Instead of placing spins in a strong external magnetic field to obtain a sufficient polarization, they can also be premagnetized (hyperpolarized) to produce a high signal, even in a small magnetic field. In MRI this principle is applied to the gases $^{129}$Xe and $^3$He, which can be used for perfusion and ventilation studies respectively.

spins has transverse components in all possible directions of the $xy$-plane. On average, the sum of all these components is zero and, consequently, the net magnetization vector has no $xy$-component in dynamic equilibrium:

$$\vec{M}_0 = (0, 0, M_0). \qquad (4.16)$$

Because all spin vectors possess an angular momentum, it can further be shown that the net macroscopic magnetization *precesses* about the axis of the external magnetic field and $\vec{M}_0$ satisfies Eq. (4.4):

$$\frac{d\vec{M}_0}{dt} = \vec{M}_0 \times \gamma\vec{B}. \qquad (4.17)$$

Figure 4.2 still holds but now for the special case $\theta = 0$. As in the classical description of single spin behavior, $\vec{M}_0$ stands still in a reference frame rotating at the Larmor angular frequency.

## Interaction with tissue

The net magnetization $\vec{M}_0$ in a voxel is proportional to the number of spins in that voxel. Unfortunately, direct measurement of the magnitude $M_0$ is impossible for technical reasons. Only the transverse component of the magnetization can be measured. This can be obtained by disturbing the equilibrium.

## Disturbing the dynamic equilibrium: the RF field

The dynamic equilibrium is disturbed via transmission of photons with the appropriate energy, as prescribed by the Larmor equation (Eq. (4.13)). In the case of a magnetic field of 1 T, this can be realized with an electromagnetic wave at a frequency of 42.57 MHz (see Table 4.1). This is an RF wave. The photons are absorbed by the tissue, and the occupancy of the energy levels changes. The result of this disturbance is that the net magnetization vector has both a longitudinal and a transverse component.

The electromagnetic RF wave is generated by sending alternating currents in two coils positioned along the $x$- and $y$-axes of the coordinate system. This configuration is known in electronics as a quadrature transmitter. The magnetic component of the electromagnetic wave is $\vec{B}_1$; in the stationary reference frame, it can be written as

$$\vec{B}_1(t) = B_1(\cos(\omega_0 t), -\sin(\omega_0 t), 0). \qquad (4.18)$$

The longitudinal component of $\vec{B}_1(t)$ is zero and the transverse component can be written as

$$B_{1_{xy}}(t) = B_1 \cos(\omega_0 t) - iB_1 \sin(\omega_0 t)$$
$$= B_1 e^{-i\omega_0 t}. \qquad (4.19)$$

The net magnetization vector in nonequilibrium conditions is further denoted by $\vec{M}$. With $\vec{M}_0$ replaced by $\vec{M}$ and $\vec{B}$ by $\vec{B} + \vec{B}_1(t)$, Eq. (4.17) becomes

$$\frac{d\vec{M}}{dt} = \vec{M} \times \gamma(\vec{B} + \vec{B}_1(t)). \qquad (4.20)$$

To solve this equation, that is, to find the motion of $\vec{M}$, we resort directly to the rotating reference frame with angular frequency $\omega_0$. The effective field perceived by $\vec{M}$ is the stationary field $\vec{B}_1$. Consequently, $\vec{M}$ precesses about $\vec{B}_1$ with precession frequency

$$\omega_1 = \gamma B_1. \qquad (4.21)$$

At $t = 0$ the effective magnetic field lies along the $x'$-axis, and it rotates $\vec{M}$ away from the $z$-axis to the $y'$-axis (Figure 4.4(a)).

The angle between the $z$-axis and $\vec{M}$ is called the *flip angle* $\alpha$:

$$\alpha = \int_0^t \gamma B_1 \, d\tau = \gamma B_1 t = \omega_1 t. \qquad (4.22)$$

By an appropriate choice of $B_1$ and $t$, any flip angle can be obtained. The trade-off between these two is important. If the up-time of the RF field is halved, $B_1$ has to double in order to obtain the same flip angle. Doubling $B_1$ implies a quadrupling of the delivered power, which is proportional to the square of $B_1$. Via the electric component of the RF wave, a significant amount of the delivered power is transformed to heat, and an important increase in tissue temperature may occur.

In practical imaging, there are two important flip angles.

- *The 90° pulse* This RF pulse brings $\vec{M}$ along the $y'$-axis (Figure 4.4(b)):

$$\vec{M} = (0, M_0, 0). \qquad (4.23)$$

There is no longitudinal magnetization. When RF transmission is stopped after a 90° pulse, $\vec{M}$ rotates clockwise in the transverse plane in the stationary

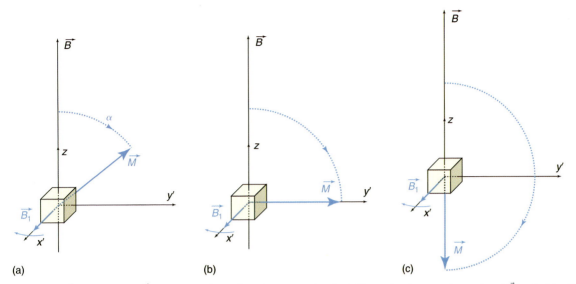

**Figure 4.4 (a)** $\vec{M}$ precesses about $\vec{B}_1$ and is rotated away from the z-axis to the y'-axis. The angle $\alpha$ between the z-axis and $\vec{M}$ is called the *flip angle*. **(b)** $\alpha = 90°$, which is obtained by a 90° RF-pulse. **(c)** $\alpha = 180°$, which is obtained by a 180° RF-pulse, also called an inversion pulse.

reference frame, whereas in the rotating reference frame, it stands still.

- *The 180° or inversion pulse* This RF pulse rotates $\vec{M}$ to the negative z-axis (Figure 4.4(c)):

$$\vec{M} = (0, 0, -M_0). \qquad (4.24)$$

Due to the RF pulse all the individual spins rotate in phase. This phase coherence explains why in nonequilibrium conditions the net magnetization vector can have a transverse component. When the RF field is switched off, the system returns to its dynamic equilibrium. The transverse component returns to zero, and the longitudinal component becomes $M_0$ again. This return to equilibrium is called *relaxation*.

## Return to dynamic equilibrium: relaxation

### Spin–spin relaxation

Spin–spin relaxation is the phenomenon that causes the disappearance of the transverse component of the net magnetization vector. Physically, each spin vector experiences a slightly different magnetic field because of the different chemical environment (protons can belong to $H_2O$, $-OH$, $-CH_3$, ...). As a result of these so-called spin–spin interactions, the spins rotate at slightly differing angular frequencies (Figure 4.5), which results in a loss of the phase coherence (dephasing) and a decrease of the transverse component $M_{tr}(t)$. The dephasing process can be described

by a first-order model. The time constant of the exponential decay is called the *spin–spin relaxation time* $T_2$:

$$M_{tr}(t) = M_0 \sin \alpha \; e^{-t/T_2}. \qquad (4.25)$$

$M_0 \sin \alpha$ is the value of the transverse component immediately after the RF pulse.

$T_2$ depends considerably on the tissue. For example, for fat, $T_2 \approx 100$ ms; for cerebrospinal fluid (CSF), $T_2 \approx 2000$ ms (Figure 4.6(a)). Molecules are continuously in motion and change their motion rapidly. For free protons in fluids, such as CSF, the experienced magnetic field differences are averaged out, yielding little dephasing and long $T_2$ values. For protons bound to large molecules, on the other hand, the magnetic field inhomogeneity is relatively stable, which explains the short $T_2$ relaxation time. Spin–spin relaxation can be considered as an entropy phenomenon and is irreversible. The disorder of the system increases, but there is no change in the energy because the occupancy of the two energy levels does not change.

### Spin–lattice relaxation

Spin–lattice relaxation is the phenomenon that causes the longitudinal component of the net magnetization vector to increase from $M_0 \cos \alpha$ (i.e., the value of the longitudinal component immediately after the RF pulse) to $M_0$. Physically, this is the result of the interactions of the spins with the lattice (i.e., the surrounding

**69**

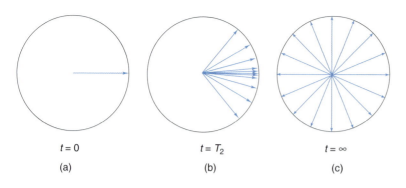

**Figure 4.5** Dephasing of the transverse component of the net magnetization vector with time. **(a)** At $t = 0$, all spins are in phase (phase coherence). **(b)** At $t = T_2$, dephasing results in a decrease of the transverse component to 37% of its initial value. **(c)** Ultimately, the spins are isotropically distributed and no net magnetization is left.

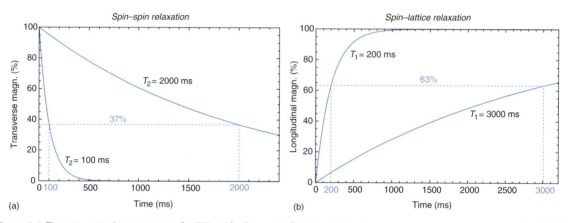

**Figure 4.6** The spin–spin relaxation process for CSF and fat (for $\alpha = 90°$). At $t = T_2$, the transverse magnetization has decreased to 37% of its value at $t = 0$. At $t = 5T_2$, only 0.67% of the initial value remains. **(b)** The spin–lattice relaxation process for water and fat at 1.5 T. At $t = T_1$, the longitudinal magnetization has reached 63% of its equilibrium value. At $t = 5T_1$, it has reached 99.3%.

macromolecules). The spin–lattice relaxation is an energy phenomenon. The energy transferred to the lattice causes an increase of the lattice molecule vibrations, which are transformed into heat (which is much smaller than the heat coming from the RF absorption). The spins then return to their preferred lower energy state, and the longitudinal component of the net magnetization grows toward its equilibrium value. Again, the process can be described by a first-order model with *spin–lattice relaxation time* $T_1$:

$$M_l(t) = M_0 \cos\alpha \; e^{-t/T_1} + M_0 \left(1 - e^{-t/T_1}\right). \quad (4.26)$$

Like $T_2$, $T_1$ is a property that depends considerably on the tissue type. For example, for fat, $T_1 \approx 200$ ms; for CSF, $T_1 \approx 3000$ ms at 1.5 T. (Figure 4.6(b)). Note that $T_1$ depends on the value of the external magnetic field: the higher the field, the higher $T_1$. Furthermore, for each tissue type $T_1$ is always larger than $T_2$.

### Inversion recovery (IR)

Figure 4.7 shows the $T_1$ relaxation for a flip angle $\alpha = 180°$ (inversion pulse). After about 70% of $T_1$,

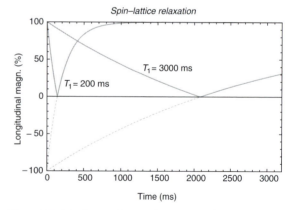

**Figure 4.7** Spin–lattice relaxation for water and fat after an inversion pulse (180°). Negative values are inverted because the magnitude is typically used. After about 70% of $T_1$, called the *inversion time* (TI), the longitudinal magnetization is nulled. Consequently, for fat ($T_1 \approx 200$ ms at 1.5 T) TI $\approx 140$ ms and for CSF ($T_1 \approx 3000$ ms at 1.5 T) TI $\approx 2100$ ms.

called the *inversion time* (TI), the longitudinal magnetization is nulled. Because TI depends on $T_1$ the signal of a particular tissue type can be suppressed by

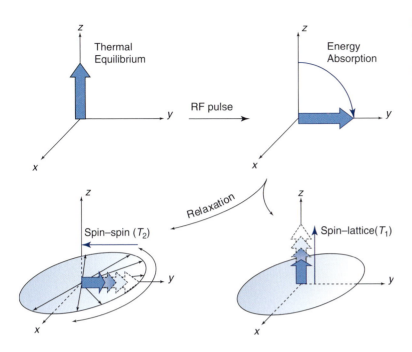

a proper choice of TI. Basic acquisition schemes for imaging (see p. 77) that are preceded by an inversion pulse and inversion time (180°–TI) are called *inversion recovery* (IR) pulse sequences. Suppression of fatty tissue yields so-called STIR images (short TI inversion recovery). Fluid suppression, such as CSF, requires a FLAIR sequence (fluid attenuated inversion recovery), which is characterized by a long TI.

## Signal detection and detector

Figure 4.8 illustrates schematically the relaxation phenomena for an excitation with a 90° pulse. The transverse component of the net magnetization vector in each voxel rotates clockwise at the precession frequency in the stationary reference frame and induces an alternating current in an antenna (coil) placed around the sample in the $xy$-plane. To increase the SNR, a quadrature detector (i.e., two coils in quadrature) is used in practice. As illustrated in Figure 4.9, the coils detect signals $s_x(t)$ and $s_y(t)$, respectively:

$$s_x(t) = M_0 \, e^{-t/T_2} \cos(-\omega_0 t)$$
$$s_y(t) = M_0 \, e^{-t/T_2} \sin(-\omega_0 t). \qquad (4.27)$$

Using the complex notation,

$$s(t) = s_x(t) + i s_y(t)$$
$$= M_0 \, e^{-t/T_2} \, e^{-i\omega_0 t}. \qquad (4.28)$$

This is the signal in the stationary reference frame. The description in the rotating reference frame corresponds technically to demodulation and Eq. (4.28) becomes

$$s(t) = M_0 \, e^{-t/T_2}. \qquad (4.29)$$

If the experiment is repeated after a *repetition time* TR, the longitudinal component of the net magnetization vector has recovered to a value that is expressed by Eq. (4.26), that is,

$$M_l(\text{TR}) = M_0 \left(1 - e^{-\text{TR}/T_1}\right). \qquad (4.30)$$

After a new excitation with a 90° pulse the detected signal becomes

$$s(t) = M_0 \left(1 - e^{-\text{TR}/T_1}\right) e^{-t/T_2}, \qquad (4.31)$$

which depends on the amount of spins or protons and the strength $B_0$ of the external magnetic field (see Eq. (4.102) below), $T_1$, $T_2$, TR and the moment $t$ of the measurement. Note that the amount of spins, $T_1$ and $T_2$ are tissue dependent parameters while $B_0$, TR and $t$ are system or operator dependent. Equation (4.31) holds for a flip angle of 90°. For smaller flip angles it must be modified and becomes dependent on $\alpha$ as well, an additional operator dependent parameter.

The signal $s(t)$ contains no positional information. Equation (4.31) does not allow us to recover the signal

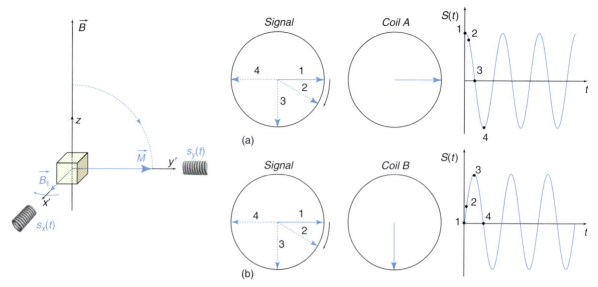

**Figure 4.9** The rotation of the net magnetization vector is detected by means of a quadrature detector. **(a)** The coil along the horizontal axis measures a cosine, and **(b)** the coil along the vertical axis measures a sine.

contribution of each voxel. The next section explains how positional information can be encoded in the signal in order to acquire images of the spin distribution in the human body.

## Imaging

### Introduction

In this section, we show that spatial information can be encoded in the detected signal by making the magnetic field spatially dependent. This is done by superimposing a series of linear magnetic field gradients in the $x$-, $y$-, and $z$-directions onto the $z$-component of the main field. The purposes of the magnetic field gradients are slice selection (or volume selection) and position encoding within the selected slice (or volume).

### Slice or volume selection

In this text, we explain the encoding for a transverse (i.e., perpendicular to the $z$-axis) slice or slab.* Note however that a slice in *any* direction can be selected as well. To select a slice perpendicular to the $z$-axis, a magnetic field that varies linearly with $z$ is superimposed onto the main magnetic field $\vec{B}$. It is

called *a linear magnetic field gradient*:

$$\vec{G} = (G_x, G_y, G_z) = \left(0, 0, \frac{\partial B_z}{\partial z}\right), \qquad (4.32)$$

where $G_z$ is the constant amplitude of the slice-selection gradient. The dimension of a magnetic field gradient is tesla/meter but in practice, millitesla/meter is used, which shows that the value of the superimposed magnetic field is on the order of 1000 times smaller than the value of the main magnetic field. The Larmor frequency now becomes

$$\omega(z) = \gamma(B_0 + G_z z). \qquad (4.33)$$

A slice or slab with thickness $\Delta z$ contains a well-defined range of precession frequencies around $\gamma B_0$

$$\Delta\omega = \gamma G_z \Delta z. \qquad (4.34)$$

Let the middle of the slice be at position $z_0$. An RF pulse with nonzero bandwidth BW $= \Delta\omega$ and centered around the frequency $\gamma(B_0 + G_z z_0)$ is needed to excite the spins (Figure 4.10). A rectangular slice sensitivity profile requires the RF pulse to be a sinc function (cf. example 1 in Appendix A). However, this is impossible because a sinc function has an infinite extent. Therefore, the sinc function is truncated. The resulting slice sensitivity profile will of course no

* A slab is a (very) thick slice. In MRI jargon, slice is usually used for 2D imaging and slab (or volume) for 3D imaging (see p. 79).

longer be a perfect rectangle, implying that spins from neighboring slices will also be excited. Note that by changing the center frequency of the RF pulse, a slice at a different spatial position is selected; table motion is not required.

The thickness of the selected slice or slab is

$$\Delta z = \frac{\Delta \omega}{\gamma G_z} = \frac{\text{BW}}{\gamma G_z}, \qquad (4.35)$$

which shows that the slice thickness is proportional to the bandwidth of the RF pulse and inversely proportional to the gradient in the slice- or volume-selection direction (Figure 4.10). Equation (4.35) shows that any value for $\Delta z$ can be chosen; in practice, however, very thin slices cannot be selected for the following reasons.

- For technical and safety reasons, there is an upper limit to the gradient strength (50–80 mT/m).
- An RF pulse with a (very) small bandwidth is difficult to generate electronically: a small bandwidth implies a large main lobe of the sinc function, which requires a long on-time.

- A very thin slice would imply that few spins were selected. Thus, the signal-to-noise ratio (SNR) would become too small. The SNR could be increased by increasing the field strength. However, there is an upper limit (7 T) to this external magnetic field for technical, safety, and economic reasons.

In practical imaging, the minimum slice thickness (FWHM) used is typically 2 mm on a 1.5 T imaging system and 1 mm on a 3 T imaging system.

## Position encoding: the $\vec{k}$-theorem

To encode the position within the slice, additional magnetic field gradients are used. We will first show what happens if a constant gradient in the $x$-direction is applied, before the general case, called the $\vec{k}$-theorem, is discussed.

We have already shown that the rotating frame is more convenient for our discussion. We therefore continue to use the frame that rotates with angular frequency $\omega_0$. In this frame, the effective magnetic field does not include $B_0$.

After a 90° RF pulse, the transverse component of the net magnetization at every position $(x, y)$ in the slice is (see Eq. (4.31))

$$M_{\text{tr}}(x, y, t) = M_0(x, y)\left(1 - e^{-\text{TR}/T_1}\right) e^{-t/T_2}. \quad (4.36)$$

If a constant gradient $G_x$ in the $x$-direction is applied at $t = \text{TE}$ (Figure 4.11(a)), the transverse component of the net magnetization does not stand still in the rotating frame but rotates at a temporal frequency that differs with $x$:

$$\omega(x) = \gamma G_x x, \quad \text{for } t \geq \text{TE}. \qquad (4.37)$$

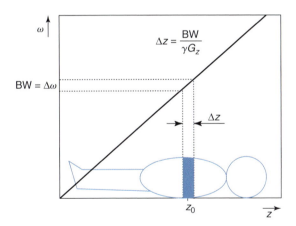

**Figure 4.10** Principle of slice selection. A narrow-banded RF pulse with bandwidth BW = $\Delta\omega$ is applied in the presence of a slice-selection gradient. The same principle applies to slab selection, but the bandwidth of the RF pulse is then much larger. Slabs are used in 3D imaging (see p. 79).

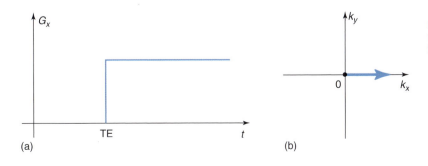

**Figure 4.11** When a positive gradient in the $x$-direction is applied **(a)**, the spatial frequency $k_x$ increases **(b)**.

For $t \geq$ TE this circular motion can be described using complex notation:

$$M_{tr}(x, y, t) = M_0(x, y) \left(1 - e^{-TR/T_1}\right)$$
$$\cdot e^{-t/T_2} e^{-i\gamma G_x x(t-TE)}. \qquad (4.38)$$

The receiver measures a signal from the excited spins in the whole plane, which corresponds to an integration over the entire $xy$-space for ($t \geq$ TE):

$$s(t) = \iint\limits_{-\infty}^{+\infty} \rho(x, y) \left(1 - e^{-TR/T_1}\right) e^{-t/T_2}$$
$$\cdot e^{-i\gamma G_x x(t-TE)} \, dx \, dy, \qquad (4.39)$$

where $\rho(x, y)$ is the net magnetization density in $(x, y)$ at time $t = 0$, which is proportional to the spin or proton density in $(x, y)$. For ease of reading, we will call $\rho$ simply the spin or proton density.

It can be shown that the measured signal $s(t)$ describes a trajectory in the Fourier domain of the image $f(x, y)$ to be reconstructed, that is,

$$s(t) = \mathcal{F}\{f(x, y)\}(k_x, 0), \text{ for } t \geq \text{TE}, \qquad (4.40)$$

if $k_x$ is defined as

$$k_x = \frac{\gamma}{2\pi} G_x (t - \text{TE}) \qquad (4.41)$$

and $f(x, y)$ is the weighted spin density, defined as

$$f(x, y) = \rho(x, y) \left(1 - e^{-TR/T_1}\right) e^{-TE/T_2}. \qquad (4.42)$$

Figure 4.11 shows how the application of a gradient $G_x$ changes the spatial frequency $k_x$ (Eq. (4.41)) over time.

*Proof of Eq. (4.40)*
Using the definition of $k_x$ given by Eq. (4.41), Eq. (4.39) becomes (for $t \geq$ TE)

$$s(t) = \iint\limits_{-\infty}^{+\infty} \rho(x, y) \left(1 - e^{-TR/T_1}\right) e^{-t/T_2} e^{-2\pi i k_x x} \, dx \, dy. \qquad (4.43)$$

Compare this equation with the 2D Fourier transform of a function $f(x, y)$ (Eq. (A.49))

$$F(k_x, k_y) = \iint\limits_{-\infty}^{+\infty} f(x, y) e^{-2\pi i (k_x x + k_y y)} \, dx \, dy. \qquad (4.44)$$

The two equations are equivalent if $k_y = 0$ and if $f(x, y)$ is defined as

$$f(x, y) \equiv \rho(x, y) \left(1 - e^{-TR/T_1}\right) e^{-t/T_2}. \qquad (4.45)$$

However, this equivalence holds only if $e^{-t/T_2}$ is constant because the Fourier transform requires that $f(x, y)$ is time independent. This means that, during the short time of the measurement, $s(t)$ must not be influenced by the $T_2$ relaxation, yielding the definition given by Eq. (4.42). Under this condition $s(t)$ describes the trajectory along the $k_x$-axis of the Fourier transform of $f(x, y)$ as defined in Eq. (4.40).

To reconstruct $f(x, y)$ from the measured signal, values in the Fourier domain for nonzero $k_y$ are also needed. They can be obtained by applying a gradient in the $y$-direction. To understand how and in which order the different gradients have to be applied to sample the whole Fourier space, the $\vec{k}$-theorem is needed. The $\vec{k}$-theorem is a generalization of the special case discussed above. It is not restricted to planar data, but can be applied to signals measured from 3D volumes, i.e., in the case of slab or volume selection (see p. 72), as well.

### $\vec{k}$-theorem

The position vector $\vec{r} = (x, y, z)$ and the magnetization density are 3D functions. The angular frequency can be written as

$$\omega(\vec{r}, t) = \gamma \vec{G}(t) \cdot \vec{r}(t), \qquad (4.46)$$

and the measured signal therefore becomes

$$s(t) = \iiint\limits_{-\infty}^{+\infty} \rho(x, y, z) \left(1 - e^{-TR/T_1}\right) e^{-t/T_2}$$
$$\cdot e^{-i\gamma \int_0^t \vec{G}(\tau) \cdot \vec{r}(\tau) \, d\tau} \, dx \, dy \, dz. \qquad (4.47)$$

The $\vec{k}$-theorem states that the time signal $s(t)$ is equivalent to the Fourier transform of the image $f(x, y, z)$ to be reconstructed, that is,

$$s(t) = \mathcal{F}\{f(x, y, z)\}(k_x, k_y, k_z), \qquad (4.48)$$

if $\vec{k}(t)$ is defined as

$$\vec{k}(t) = \frac{\gamma}{2\pi} \int_0^t \vec{G}(\tau) \, d\tau \qquad (4.49)$$

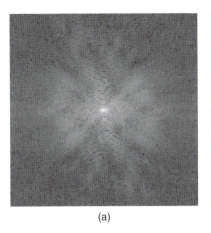

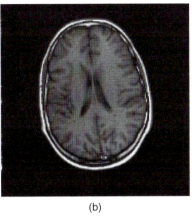

(a)                              (b)

**Figure 4.12** Illustration of the $\vec{k}$-theorem. **(a)** Modulus of the raw data measured by the MR imaging system (for display purposes, the logarithm of the modulus is shown). **(b)** Modulus of the image obtained from a 2D inverse FT of the raw data in (a).

and

$$f(x, y, z) = \rho(x, y, z) \left(1 - e^{-TR/T_1}\right) e^{-TE/T_2}, \quad (4.50)$$

where $\rho(x, y, z)$ is the spin or proton density and $f(x, y, z)$ is the weighted spin density. Note that $f(x, y, z)$ is a real image, i.e., the phase image is theoretically zero.

Equation (4.48) holds only for static spins, i.e., $\vec{r}(t) = \vec{r}$. As will be explained below, motion yields signal loss and other artifacts.

*Proof of Eq. (4.48)*
Using the definition of $\vec{k}(t)$ (Eq. (4.49)), Eq. (4.47) can be rewritten as

$$s(t) = \int\limits_{-\infty}^{+\infty}\!\!\!\int\int \rho(x, y, z) \left(1 - e^{-TR/T_1}\right)$$
$$\cdot\, e^{-t/T_2}\, e^{-2\pi i \vec{k}\cdot\vec{r}}\, dx\, dy\, dz \quad (4.51)$$

if $\vec{r}(t) = \vec{r}$, which implies that the spins to be imaged do not move as a consequence of breathing, blood flow, and so forth.

Compare this equation with the 3D FT of a function $f(x, y, z)$ (Eq. (A.49))

$$F(k_x, k_y, k_z) = \int\limits_{-\infty}^{+\infty}\!\!\!\int\int f(x, y, z)\, e^{-2\pi i \vec{k}\cdot\vec{r}}\, dx\, dy\, dz. \quad (4.52)$$

Equations (4.51) and (4.52) are equivalent if $f(x, y, z)$ is defined as

$$f(x, y, z) \equiv \rho(x, y, z) \left(1 - e^{-TR/T_1}\right) e^{-t/T_2}. \quad (4.53)$$

Because $f(x, y, z)$ must be time independent, $e^{-t/T_2}$ must be constant. Hence, $e^{-t/T_2} = e^{-TE/T_2}$ during the short readout period around $t = $ TE, which implies that the $T_2$ relaxation can be neglected during the period the receiver coil measures the signal.

When all the data have been collected in the Fourier space (or $\vec{k}$-space), the inverse FT yields the reconstructed image $f(x, y, z)$, which represents the *weighted* spin or proton density distribution in the selected slice or volume (Figure 4.12). The spin density $\rho^*$ is weighted by multiplying it with two functions; the former describes the growth of the longitudinal component, and the latter describes the decay of the transverse component. Hence, MR images are not "pure" proton density images but represent a weighted proton density that depends on the tissue dependent parameters $T_1$ and $T_2$, and the operator dependent parameters TR (repetition time) and TE (moment of the measurement). If a short TR is chosen, the image is said to be $T_1$ weighted. If TE is long, it is said to be $T_2$ weighted. A long TR and short TE yield a $\rho$-weighted or proton density weighted image.

Note that we have assumed a 90° RF pulse. For flip angles $\alpha$ smaller than 90° the above equations must be modified and the reconstructed image will depend on $\alpha$ as well, which can also be modified by the operator.

## Dephasing phenomena

The net magnetization vector is the sum of a large number of individual magnetic moments (Eq. (4.15)). If different spin vectors experience a different

---

* Actually $\rho$ is the net magnetization density, which depends not only on the spin density, but also on the strength $B_0$ of the external magnetic field (see Eq. (4.102) below).

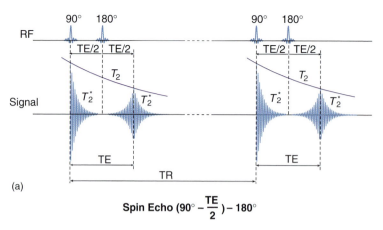

**Spin Echo $\left(90° - \dfrac{\text{TE}}{2}\right) - 180°$**

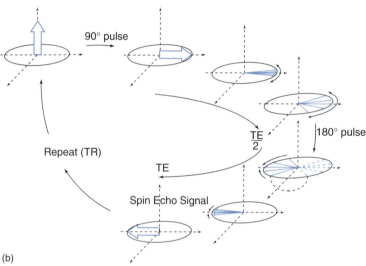

(b)

**Figure 4.13** Immediately after the 90° pulse the signal dephases due to spin–spin interactions and magnetic field inhomogeneities. In **(b)** only the influence of the magnetic field inhomogeneities is shown. This part of the dephasing is restored by the application of a 180° pulse at $t = \text{TE}/2$, which reverses the phases. Because the spins continue to dephase, their dephasing due to magnetic field inhomogeneities is undone at $t = \text{TE}$. The signal is measured around $T = \text{TE}$. At that moment it is only affected by the $T_2$ relaxation, which is irreversible. The time between two 90° RF excitations is the repetition time TR.

magnetic field, they precess with a different Larmor frequency. The resulting dephasing destroys the phase coherence, and the receiver may detect a small and noisy signal! Consequently, it is important to minimize the dephasing phenomena.

Three types of dephasing can be distinguished.

- Dephasing by **spin–spin interactions**. This is an irreversible process described by the time constant $T_2$, as explained on p. 69.

- Dephasing by **magnetic field inhomogeneities**. As will be shown below, this is a reversible process expressed by the time constant $T_2^* < T_2$. The inhomogeneities are due to an inhomogeneous main magnetic field and to differences in the magnetic susceptibility of the tissues.[†]

- Dephasing by **magnetic field gradients**. By definition a gradient causes an inhomogeneous magnetic field, which further reduces $T_2^*$. It is a reversible process.

### Undo dephasing of magnetic field inhomogeneities

To undo this kind of dephasing, a 180° pulse is applied. If this pulse is applied at $t = \text{TE}/2$, an echo-signal, the so-called *spin-echo* (SE), is created at $t = \text{TE}$ (Figure 4.13). Because of the irreversible $T_2$ dephasing, the maximum of the spin-echo is lower than the maximum at $t = 0$. The measurement of a trajectory in $\vec{k}$-space must take place during a short time interval around $t = \text{TE}$. Because of this short time interval, several excitations are typically needed to sample the

[†] The magnetic susceptibility indicates how well a certain substance can be magnetized. The higher this value, the more the substance is able to disturb the homogeneity of the local magnetic field. Iron is a well-known example. It is a so-called ferromagnetic substance and can be magnetized extremely well. Consequently, iron particles in the body are able to disturb the homogeneity of the local field significantly.

complete $\vec{k}$-space. A new excitation starts after a time TR, the repetition time, which can be much longer than the time between excitation and data collection. In the wasted time after the measurement and before TR the same procedure can be repeated to excite other slices and acquire information on their spin distribution. This way trajectories of multiple slices can be measured within one TR. This acquisition method is called *multi-slice imaging*. The number of slices depends on both TR and TE. Note that in practice the slice sensitivity profile is not a perfect rectangle and spins from neighboring slices will also be partially excited. Consequently, these spins are excited twice without giving them the time TR to relax in between, yielding a reduced signal. This phenomenon is called *cross-talk*. It can be avoided by introducing a physical gap between neighboring slices.

### Undo dephasing of magnetic field gradients

This type of dephasing is necessary to sample the $\vec{k}$-space. The phase shift due to a magnetic gradient at the time of the measurement (TE) can be calculated by integrating Eq. (4.46) between excitation and readout:

$$\Phi(\text{TE}) = \int_0^{\text{TE}} \gamma \vec{G}(t) \cdot \vec{r}(t) \, dt. \qquad (4.54)$$

Assuming static spins, i.e., $\vec{r}(t) = \vec{r}$, this equation can be rewritten as

$$\Phi(\text{TE}) = \vec{r} \cdot \int_0^{\text{TE}} \gamma \vec{G}(t) \, dt$$

$$= 2\pi \, \vec{r} \cdot \vec{k}(\text{TE}) \qquad (4.55)$$

The dephasing is undone at $t = \text{TE}$ if $\Phi(\text{TE}) = 0$. Consequently, $\vec{k}(\text{TE}) = 0$ and the measurements are spread around the origin of the $\vec{k}$-space, yielding the best SNR (Figure 4.12). To undo the dephasing effect of a magnetic field gradient, the integral in Eq. (4.55) must be zero, which can be obtained by applying another gradient with the same duration but with opposite polarity. This creates an echo signal at $t = \text{TE}$, called the *gradient-echo* (GE), illustrated in Figure 4.14.

## Basic pulse sequences

Based on the $\vec{k}$-theorem, several practical acquisition schemes have been developed to measure the $\vec{k}$-space. Two basic classes are the spin-echo (SE) pulse sequence and the gradient-echo (GE) pulse sequence.

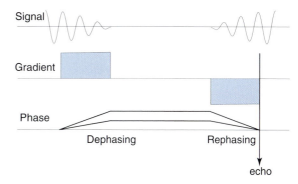

**Figure 4.14** Gradient dephasing can be undone by applying a second gradient with the same amplitude but opposite polarity. The plot labeled "phase" describes the phase behavior at two different spatial positions and shows phase dispersal and recovery that occurs by applying the two gradient pulses.

### The spin-echo pulse sequence

Two-dimensional Fourier transform SE imaging is the mainstay of clinical MRI because SE pulse sequences are very flexible and allow the user to acquire images in which either $T_1$ or $T_2$ (dominantly) influences the signal intensity displayed in the MR images (see also p. 90 below).

The 2D SE pulse sequence is illustrated in Figure 4.15 and consists of the following components.

- A *slice-selection gradient* $G_z$ is applied together with a 90° and a 180° RF pulse. Because the second slice-selection gradient pulse is symmetric around $t = \text{TE}/2$, its initial dephasing effect is automatically compensated after the RF pulse. To undo the dephasing of the first slice-selection gradient, the polarity of this gradient can be reversed during its application. For technical reasons, however, it is easier to apply the second gradient a little longer. Indeed, a positive gradient after the 180° pulse has the same effect as a negative gradient before the 180° pulse.

- The "ladder" in Figure 4.15 represents $G_y$, which is called the *phase-encoding gradient*. Applying $G_y$ before the measurement yields a $y$-dependent temporal phase shift $\phi(y)$ of $s(t)$:

$$\phi(y) = \gamma G_y y T_{\text{ph}}, \qquad (4.56)$$

where $T_{\text{ph}}$ is a constant time interval, representing the on-time of the phase-encoding gradient $G_y$. In practical imaging, $G_y$ has a variable amplitude:

$$G_y = m g_y, \qquad (4.57)$$

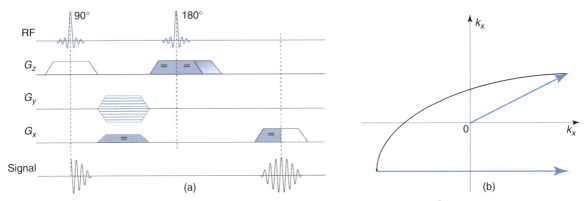

**Figure 4.15** **(a)** Schematic illustration of a 2D spin-echo pulse sequence. **(b)** Associated trajectory of the $\vec{k}$-vector for one positive phase-encoding gradient value $G_y$. By modifying this value, a different line in $\vec{k}$-space is traversed.

where $m$ is a positive or negative integer and $g_y$ is constant. Using Eq. (4.49) yields

$$k_y = \frac{\gamma}{2\pi} m g_y T_{\mathrm{ph}}. \qquad (4.58)$$

Each rung of the ladder thus prepares the measurement of a different trajectory in the $\vec{k}$-space. Note that the dephasing of this gradient must not be compensated because it is mandatory for position encoding.

- During the application of $G_x$, which is called the *frequency-encoding gradient*, the signal $s(t)$ is measured. To undo the dephasing effect of $G_x$ during readout, a compensating gradient is applied before the measurement, typically before the 180° pulse, which reverses the sign of $\vec{k}$ (see Figure 4.15(b)). This way, a horizontal line centered around $k_x = 0$ is measured.

An image is obtained by sampling the complete $\vec{k}$-space and calculating the inverse Fourier transform. This way the acquired raw data form a matrix of, say, 512 by 512 elements (lower and higher values are also possible). By applying 512 different gradients $G_y = m g_y$, $m \in [-255, +256]$, 512 rows of the $\vec{k}$-space can be measured. Per row 512 samples are taken during the application of the gradient $G_x$. Each position in the $\vec{k}$-space corresponds to a unique combination of the gradients $G_x$, $G_y$ and the time they have been applied at the moment of the measurement. Hence, the gradients $G_x$ and $G_y$ are in-plane encoding gradients for the position in the $\vec{k}$-space.

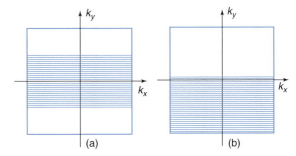

**Figure 4.16** **(a)** Truncated Fourier and **(b)** half Fourier imaging. Only the parallel horizontal lines are measured. In practice, half Fourier imaging acquires a few lines of the upper half-plane as well and requires a phase-correction algorithm during reconstruction. A detailed discussion is beyond the scope of this book.

Physically, the gradients encode by means of the angular frequency and initial phase of the magnetization vector during the measurement. The relationship between a gradient and the angular frequency $\omega$ is given by Eq. (4.46). From this equation the initial phase can be derived (Eq. (4.56)). Application of a gradient $G_x$ during the measurement yields an angular frequency $\omega$ that depends on $x$. A gradient $G_y$ is applied before the measurement starts, which causes an initial phase shift dependent on $y$. This explains why $G_y$ is called the phase-encoding gradient and $G_x$ the frequency-encoding gradient.

To shorten the acquisition time, fewer phase-encoding steps could be applied (e.g., 384 instead of 512 with $m \in [-192, +191]$). This is called *truncated Fourier imaging* (see Figure 4.16(a)). A drawback of acquiring less rows is that the reconstructed images

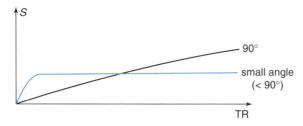

**Figure 4.17** For (very) short repetition times, the steady-state signal formed by low flip angles exceeds that recovered with 90° pulses.

have a lower spatial resolution in the phase-encoding direction.

The image $f(x, y, z)$ (Eq. (4.50)) to be reconstructed is a real function and, according to Eq. (A.66), the Fourier transform of a real function is *Hermitian*. Hence, it is in principle sufficient to measure half of the $\vec{k}$-space, for example, for $m \in [-255, 0]$ (see Figure 4.16(b)). This is called *half Fourier imaging*. Although half Fourier imaging halves the acquisition time, it reduces the SNR of the reconstructed images.

### The gradient-echo pulse sequence

As explained below on p. 90, the major drawback of SE imaging is its need for relatively long imaging times, particularly in $\rho$- and $T_2$-weighted imaging protocols whose TR is long to minimize the influence of the $T_1$ relaxation. One approach to overcome this problem is the use of GE pulse sequences. As compared with SE sequences, they differ in two respects, which have a profound impact on the resulting images.

- *Their flip angle is typically smaller than 90°* Usually, a value between 20° and 60° is used. Nevertheless, it can be shown that for (very) short TR, the steady-state signal is larger than the signal obtained with 90° pulses (Figure 4.17). The flip angle can be used to influence the contrast in the image, as shown on p. 90 below.

- *They have no spin-echo because there is no 180° pulse* Rephasing is done by means of gradient reversal only. This implies that the signal characteristics are influenced by $T_2^*$ (Figure 4.18).

The GE sequences could in principle be used with the same TR and TE values as in SE sequences. However, in that case, there is no difference in acquisition time. Moreover, because of the absence of the 180° pulse and the resulting $T_2^*$ dephasing effect, $T_2^*$-weighted images would be obtained and the signal may be too

low. Therefore, GE sequences are primarily used for fast 2D and 3D acquisition of $T_1$-weighted images.

An example of a 2D GE sequence is the fast low-angle shot (FLASH) pulse sequence shown in Figure 4.19. The feature that distinguishes FLASH from the basic GE sequence is the variable amplitude gradient pulse, called *spoiler*, applied after the data collection. The purpose of the spoiler pulse is to destroy (i.e., dephase) any transverse magnetization that remains after the data collection.[†] Note that the sign of the rephasing gradients in the slice-selection and readout direction is the opposite of that in the SE pulse sequence (see Figure 4.15) because there is no 180° pulse.

## Three-dimensional imaging

On p. 73 we saw that very thin slices cannot be selected. However, several radiological examinations (e.g., wrist, ankle, knee) require thin slices, and 3D imaging offers the solution to this problem. In 3D imaging techniques, a volume or slab instead of a slice is selected. The $z$-position is then encoded in the signal by a second phase-encoding gradient ladder $ng_z$,

$$\phi(y, z) = \gamma (mg_y y T_{\text{ph}} + ng_z z T_{\text{ss}}), \qquad (4.59)$$

where $T_{\text{ss}}$ is the on-time of the phase-encoding gradient in the slab-selection direction. Different values of $n$ correspond to different planes in the $\vec{k}$-space. The most important difference between 2D and 3D pulse sequences is that 3D sequences have two phase-encoding gradient tables, whereas 2D sequences have only one (Figure 4.20). In 3D imaging, reconstruction is done by means of a 3D inverse Fourier transform, yielding a series of 2D slices (16, 32, 100, …). For example, if a slab with thickness 32 mm is divided into 32 partitions, an effective slice thickness of 1 mm is obtained. Such thin slices are impossible in 2D imaging. The SNR of 3D imaging is also better than in 2D imaging because each excitation selects all the spins in the whole volume instead of in a single slice.

The drawback of 3D imaging is an increase in acquisition time, as will be shown on p. 81 below. It will be shown that 3D SE sequences are much slower than 3D GE pulse sequences.

[†] The reasons for the variability of the amplitude are beyond the scope of this book.

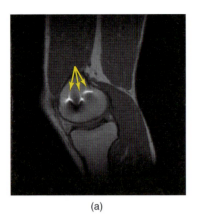 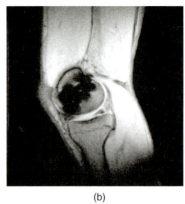

(a)　　　　　　　　　　　　　(b)

**Figure 4.18** The effect of the 180° pulse. **(a)** Sagittal spin-echo image of a knee in which a small ferromagnetic particle causes local magnetic field inhomogeneities. The 180° pulse of the SE compensates for the resulting dephasing. Note, however, that the magnetic field deviation still causes a geometric distortion in the area of the particle (white patterns). **(b)** Gradient-echo image of the same slice. There is no compensation for magnetic field inhomogeneities ($T_2^*$ instead of $T_2$) causing a complete signal loss in the area of the ferromagnetic substance. (Courtesy of Dr. P. Brys, Department of Radiology.)

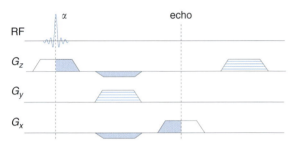

**Figure 4.19** The 2D FLASH pulse sequence is a GE sequence in which a spoiler gradient is applied immediately after the data collection in order to dephase the remaining transverse magnetization.

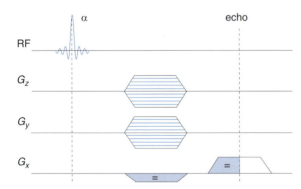

**Figure 4.20** The characteristic feature of any 3D pulse sequence is the presence of two phase-encoding gradient tables. Here a 3D GE sequence is shown, as there is no 180° pulse.

# Chemical shift imaging

Expression (4.47) for the measured signal $s(t)$ can be written as

$$s(t) = \int_{\vec{r}} \rho^*(\vec{r})\, e^{-i\Phi(\vec{r},t)}\, d\vec{r} \qquad (4.60)$$

where

$$\rho^*(\vec{r}) = \rho(\vec{r})\left(1 - e^{-TR/T_1}\right) e^{-TE/T_2} \qquad (4.61)$$

and the phase shift $\Phi(\vec{r}, t)$ is the integral of the angular frequency $\omega(\vec{r}, t)$ (Eq. (4.46)) over time, that is,

$$\Phi(\vec{r}, t) = \int_0^t \omega(\vec{r}, t)dt = \int_0^t \gamma \vec{G}(\tau)\, d\tau \cdot \vec{r} \qquad (4.62)$$

for stationary tissue. Remember that this equation implicitly assumes the use of a rotating coordinate frame at angular frequency $\omega_0$, i.e., the Larmor frequency in the static magnetic field $B_0$.

However, the Larmor frequency slightly depends on the molecular structure the protons belong to. This (normalized) frequency difference is called the chemical shift. Taking the frequency shifts $\omega_s \equiv 2\pi f_s$ into account, Eq. (4.62) has to be rewritten as

$$\Phi(\vec{r}, \omega_s, t) = \int_0^t \gamma \vec{G}(\tau)\, d\tau \cdot \vec{r} + t \cdot \omega_s. \qquad (4.63)$$

Substituting Eq. (4.49) into Eq. (4.63) yields

$$\Phi(\vec{r}, \omega_s, t) = 2\pi(\vec{k}(t) \cdot \vec{r} + t \cdot f_s). \qquad (4.64)$$

The signal $s(t)$ can still be written as a Fourier transform of $\rho^*(\vec{r}, f_s)$

$$s(t) = \mathcal{F}\{\rho^*(\vec{r}, f_s)\}(\vec{k}, t) \qquad (4.65)$$

and the $\vec{k}$-theorem can still be used. As compared to Eq. (4.48), the dimension of the functions has increased by one. The variable $f_s$ has been added to the spatial domain and the variable $t$ to the $\vec{k}$-space.

This way multiple images can be obtained for different frequencies $f_s$, a technique known as *chemical shift imaging* (CSI).

Unfortunately, because the time $t$ continuously increases, samples of the $\vec{k}$-space for all the different values of $\vec{k}$ at a particular $t$-value can be obtained only from repeated excitations with different values of the gradient $\vec{G}$. For example, the reconstruction of a 2D chemical shift image needs two phase-encoding gradient ladders (for $G_x$ and $G_y$) before the measurement, while for regular imaging only one ladder is needed (see Figure 4.15). 3D imaging would require three such ladders (for $G_x$, $G_y$ and $G_z$) instead of two (see Figure 4.20). Consequently, the acquisition time for CSI is an order of magnitude larger than for regular imaging. To reduce this acquisition time, the voxel size in CSI can be increased and the FOV reduced.

## Acquisition and reconstruction time

High-quality images are useless if tens of minutes are required to obtain them. Both acquisition time and reconstruction time must be short. The reconstruction time can be neglected in clinical practice because current computers calculate the inverse Fourier transform in real time.

Obviously, the acquisition time TA equals the number of excitations times the interval between two successive excitations. Hence,

- for 2D pulse sequences

$$TA_{2D} = N_{ph} TR; \qquad (4.66)$$

- for 3D pulse sequences

$$TA_{3D} = N_{ph} N_{ss} TR, \qquad (4.67)$$

where $N_{ph}$ is the number of in-plane phase-encoding steps and $N_{ss}$ is the number of phase-encoding steps in the slab-selection direction.

For example, for a $T_2$-weighted 3D SE sequence with TR $= 2000$ ms, one acquisition and 32 slices, each having 256 phase-encoding steps, TA is more than 4 hours! For a $T_1$-weighted pulse sequence with TR $= 500$ ms, TA is still more than an hour. Obviously, this is practically infeasible because no-one can remain immobile during that time. Three-dimensional imaging is mostly done with GE pulse sequences. For example, if TR is 40 ms, TA reduces to less than six minutes, which is quite acceptable for many examinations.

## Very fast imaging sequences
### Multiple echoes per excitation

Very fast imaging sequences have been developed for multi-slice imaging and have in common that *multiple echoes* are generated and sampled within the same excitation. Equation (4.66) should thus be modified as

$$TA_{2D} = \frac{N_{ph} TR}{ETL}, \qquad (4.68)$$

where ETL is the *echo train length* (i.e., the number of echoes per excitation). Equation (4.68) shows that the acquisition time can be reduced by (1) decreasing TR (cf. GE versus SE sequences), (2) decreasing $N_{ph}$ (cf. truncated and half Fourier imaging), and (3) increasing ETL.

If ETL $> 1$, the rows of the $\vec{k}$-space are sampled at different echo times. The dephasing effect resulting from $T_2$ for SE or from $T_2^*$ for GE sequences cannot be neglected between two different echoes, and the measured signal $S'(k_x, k_y)$ is therefore a filtered version of the signal $S(k_x, k_y)$ that would have been obtained with an acquisition with ETL $= 1$:

$$S'(k_x, k_y) = H(k_x, k_y) S(k_x, k_y), \qquad (4.69)$$

where $H(k_x, k_y)$ is the filter function. Although the conditions of the $\vec{k}$-theorem are violated, in practice the inverse Fourier transform is straightforwardly employed to reconstruct the raw data. A consequence is that the spatial resolution degrades because the reconstructed image is a convolution with the inverse FT of $H(k_x, k_y)$ (see Figure 4.21).

### Examples

Below are two well-known acquisition schemes that are currently used in clinical practice.

- *TurboSE and turboGE* The TurboSE and turboGE sequences are sequences in which 2–128 echoes are generated within the same excitation. Hence, immediately after the first echo, a new phase-encoding gradient is applied to select a different line in the $\vec{k}$-space, a new echo is generated, and so on. The $\vec{k}$-space is divided into 2–128 distinct segments. Within a single excitation, one line of each segment is sampled.

  TurboSE sequences are regularly used for $T_2$-weighted imaging of the brain. For a $256 \times 256$ $T_2$-weighted image (TR $= 2500$ ms) with four

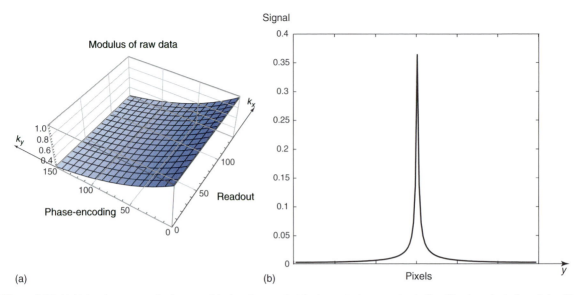

(a)

(b)

**Figure 4.21** Multiple echoes per excitation cause blurring. Assume that the image to be reconstructed is a Dirac impulse in the origin with amplitude equal to 1. **(a)** Modulus of the measured data in the $\vec{k}$-space. Although the raw data are more or less constant in the readout direction, dephasing clearly affects the measurements in the phase-encoding direction. Without $T_2^*$ (or $T_2$, depending on the sequence) the modulus of the raw data would have been constant. **(b)** One column of the modulus of the reconstructed image, which clearly shows that the Dirac impulse has been blurred.

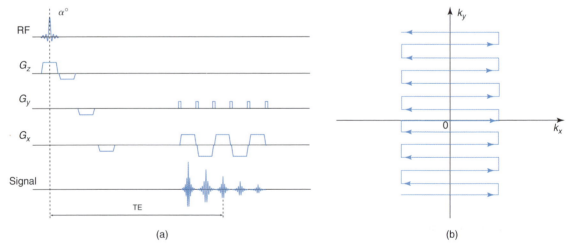

(a)

(b)

**Figure 4.22** **(a)** Schematic representation of the $T_2^*$-weighted blipped GE EPI sequence. A series of gradient-echoes are created and sampled. **(b)** Corresponding trajectory in $\vec{k}$-space. Each "blip" in the phase-encoding direction selects a new row in the raw data matrix.

echoes, for example, the acquisition time TA is

$$\text{TA} = \frac{256 \times 2.5}{4} = 160 \text{ seconds} < 3 \text{ minutes.}$$

(4.70)

- *Echo planar imaging (EPI)* This is the fastest 2D imaging sequence currently available. It is a SE

or GE sequence, and the absence of 180° pulses explains the time gain. All echoes are generated in one excitation (Figures 4.22 and 4.23). Because of the $T_2^*$ dephasing, however, there is a limit to the number of echoes that can be measured above noise level. A typical size of the raw data matrix of EPI images is 128 × 128. The acquisition time TA for one image is 100 ms and even lower! The EPI

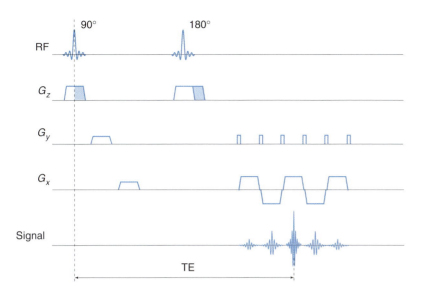

**Figure 4.23** For a $T_2$-weighted SE EPI sequence, a single 180° RF pulse is applied between the 90° RF pulse and the gradient-echo train to sample the $\vec{k}$-space.

sequence is used, for example, in functional MRI (see p. 89) and diffusion and perfusion imaging (see p. 87 and p. 89).

# Imaging of moving spins

## Introduction

In the previous sections we have assumed that the spatial position of the spins does not change. In practice, however, there are many causes of spin motion in the human body such as swallowing, breathing, the beating heart, and blood flow. With adapted MR pulse sequences, motion such as blood flow, diffusion, and perfusion can be visualized (see Table 4.2).

When magnetic field gradients are applied, moving spins experience a change in magnetic field strength, in contrast to the stationary tissues. The total phase shift can be calculated by integrating the angular frequency $\omega(\vec{r}, t)$ (Eq. (4.46)) over time:

$$\Phi(\vec{r}, t) = \int_0^t \gamma \vec{G}(\tau) \cdot \vec{r}(\tau) \, d\tau. \qquad (4.71)$$

Unlike in Eq. (4.55) $\vec{r}(t)$ is not time independent for moving spins. It can be shown that Eq. (4.47) in case of motion can be written as

$$s(t) = \int_{\vec{r}} \rho^*(\vec{r}) \; e^{-i(\vec{v}(\vec{r}) \cdot \vec{m}_1(t) + \vec{a}(\vec{r}) \cdot \vec{m}_2(t) + \cdots)}$$

$$\cdot \; e^{-i\vec{r} \cdot \vec{m}_0(t)} \, d\vec{r} \qquad (4.72)$$

where

$$\rho^*(\vec{r}) = \rho(\vec{r}) \left(1 - e^{-TR/T_1}\right) e^{-TE/T_2} \qquad (4.73)$$

and

$$\vec{m}_l(t) \equiv \int_0^t \gamma \vec{G}(\tau) \frac{\tau^l}{l!} d\tau \quad l = 0, 1, 2, \ldots. \qquad (4.74)$$

$\vec{m}_l$ is the $l$th order gradient moment.

*Proof of Eq. (4.72)*
The exact path $\vec{r}(t)$ followed by the moving spin is unknown. However, any physical motion can be expanded in a Taylor series around $t = 0$. Hence,

$$\vec{r}(t) = \vec{r}(0) + \frac{d\vec{r}}{dt}(0)t + \cdots + \frac{d^l\vec{r}}{dt^l}(0)\frac{t^l}{l!} + \cdots. \qquad (4.75)$$

The position $\vec{r}$, the velocity $\vec{v}(\vec{r})$ and the acceleration $\vec{a}(\vec{r})$ of the spin at time $t = 0$ can be introduced in this equation:

$$\vec{r}(t) = \vec{r} + \vec{v}(\vec{r}) \, t + \vec{a}(\vec{r}) \frac{t^2}{2} + \cdots. \qquad (4.76)$$

Substituting Eq. (4.76) in Eq. (4.71) yields:

$$\Phi(\vec{r}, t) = \vec{r} \cdot \int_0^t \gamma \vec{G}(\tau) \, d\tau + \vec{v}(\vec{r}) \cdot \int_0^t \gamma \vec{G}(\tau)\tau \, d\tau$$

$$+ \; \vec{a}(\vec{r}) \cdot \int_0^t \gamma \vec{G}(\tau) \frac{\tau^2}{2} d\tau + \cdots$$

**Table 4.2** List of motions in the body and their corresponding velocities that can be visualized using appropriate pulse sequences

| Motion type | Velocity range |
| --- | --- |
| Diffusion | 10 μm/s – 0.1 mm/s |
| Perfusion | 0.1 mm/s – 1 mm/s |
| CSF flow | 1 mm/s – 1 cm/s |
| Venous flow | 1 cm/s – 10 cm/s |
| Arterial flow | 10 cm/s – 1 m/s |
| Stenotic flow | 1 m/s – 10 m/s |

*Notes:* MR is capable of measuring six orders of magnitude of flow [20].

or, using the gradient moments as defined in Eq. (4.74),

$$\Phi(\vec{r}, t) = \vec{r} \cdot \vec{m}_0(t) + \vec{v}(\vec{r}) \cdot \vec{m}_1(t)$$
$$+ \vec{a}(\vec{r}) \cdot \vec{m}_2(t) + \cdots . \quad (4.77)$$

Rewriting Eq. (4.47) as

$$s(t) = \int_{\vec{r}} \rho^*(\vec{r}) \; e^{-i\Phi(\vec{r},t)} \, d\vec{r}, \quad (4.78)$$

and substituting Eq. (4.77) into Eq. (4.78), yields Eq. (4.72).

Without motion, only the first-order moment $\vec{m}_0(t)$ in Eq. (4.72) causes a phase shift. This phase shift is needed for position encoding when using the $\vec{k}$-theorem. Motion introduces additional dephasing of the signal $s(t)$. The receiver then detects a smaller and noisier signal. This *motion-induced dephasing* is a fourth cause of dephasing (see also p. 75). If this phase shift is relatively small and almost coherent within a single voxel, it also yields position artifacts such as ghosting (see p. 94 and Figure 4.36).

## Magnetic resonance angiography (MRA)

In the previous section it was shown that motion yields additional dephasing and a corresponding signal loss. However, as we will see, motion-induced dephasing can be reduced by *back-to-back symmetric bipolar pulses of opposite polarity*. They are able to restore

hyperintense vessel signals for blood flowing at a *constant* velocity. In case of constant velocity Eq. (4.72) becomes

$$s(t) = \int_{\vec{r}} \rho^*(\vec{r}) \; e^{-i\vec{v}(\vec{r}) \cdot \vec{m}_1(t)} \; e^{-i\vec{r} \cdot \vec{m}_0(t)} \, d\vec{r} \quad (4.79)$$

and contains only two dephasing factors, one necessary for position encoding and the other introduced by the blood velocity $\vec{v}(\vec{r})$.

Equation (4.55) shows that for *stationary* spins $(\vec{v}(\vec{r}) = 0)$ the net phase shift due to simple bipolar gradient pulses (Figure 4.24(a)) is zero. This is the case at $t = \text{TE}$ in the frequency-encoding and slice-selection directions. For *moving* spins $(\vec{v}(\vec{r}) \neq 0)$, however, a simple bipolar pulse sequence as in Figure 4.24(a) introduces a phase shift because its first gradient moment $\vec{m}_1$ at $t = \text{TE}$ is nonzero:

$$m_1(\text{TE}) = -\gamma \vec{G} (\Delta t)^2 \neq 0. \quad (4.80)$$

Back-to-back symmetric bipolar pulses of opposite polarity on the other hand (Figure 4.24(b)) remove the velocity-induced phase shift at $t = \text{TE}$ while they have no net effect on static spins. Both their zeroth and first-order gradient moments $m_0(\text{TE})$ and $m_1(\text{TE})$ are zero. Higher order motion components are *not* rephased, however, and will still cause dephasing.

The rephasing gradients are applied in the frequency-encoding and slice-selection directions. This technique is known as *gradient moment nulling, gradient moment rephasing* or *flow compensation*. A diagram of a 3D FLASH sequence with first-order flow compensation is shown in Figure 4.25. Technical considerations limit the flow compensation to the first-order or at most the second-order gradient moments. Very complex motion patterns, such as the turbulence in the aortic arch, continue to produce signal dephasing.

### Time-of-flight (TOF) MRA

Time-of-flight (TOF) MRA is a technique that combines motion rephasing with the *inflow effect*. This phenomenon is easy to visualize. First consider a slice or slab with only stationary tissues. With a GE sequence with a very short TR (25–35 ms), the longitudinal component of the magnetization vectors becomes very small after a few excitations because it is not given the time to relax. The signal will be low – an effect called *saturation*. Assume now that the slice is oriented perpendicular to a blood vessel. As blood flows inward, the blood in the slice is not affected by

[20] L. Crooks and M. Haacke. Historical overview of MR angiography. In J. Potchen, E. Haacke, J. Siebert, and A. Gottschalk, editors, *Magnetic Resonance Angiography: Concepts and Applications*, pages 3–8. St. Louis, MN: Mosby – Year Book, Inc., first edition, 1993.

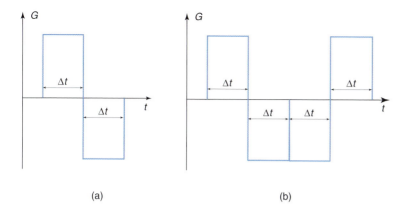

(a)                                        (b)

Figure 4.24 (a) Simple bipolar pulses cannot provide a phase-coherent signal for moving spins. (b) Back-to-back symmetric bipolar pulses of opposite polarity on the other hand restore the phase coherence completely for spins moving at a constant velocity.

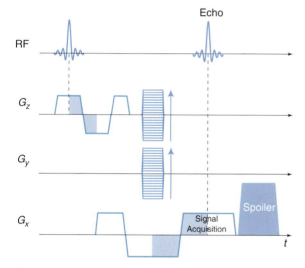

Figure 4.25 Schematic illustration of a 3D FLASH sequence. First-order flow rephasing gradients are applied in the volume-selection and frequency-encoding directions to prevent the dephasing that otherwise would be caused by the corresponding original gradients.

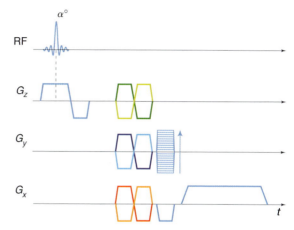

Figure 4.26 Schematic illustration of a PC MRA sequence. Bipolar pulses of opposite polarity are sequentially applied along the three main directions, which requires six different acquisitions.

the saturating effect of the RF pulses. Its longitudinal component remains large and yields a high signal. However, if the blood vessel lies inside the slice or slab, the flowing blood experiences several RF pulses, becomes partly saturated, and yields a lower signal. Hence, the vascular contrast is generated by the difference in saturation between the inflowing spins of the blood and the stationary spins of the tissues in the acquisition volume. The blood vessels appear bright and the stationary tissues dark.

Both 2D and 3D GE-based sequences are used for TOF MRA. They are equipped with rephasing gradients for first- or second-order flow, or both. As long as the refreshment of the spins is significant and the blood flow pattern can be described adequately by

first- and second-order motions, the blood vessels are visible as hyperintense patterns. 3D TOF MRA is for example very suited to visualize the cerebral arteries (as shown in Figure 4.28(b) below).

### Phase-contrast (PC) MRA

In phase-contrast (PC) MRA two subsequent sequences are applied, one with an additional bipolar pulse sequence and another with a reversed bipolar pulse sequence, both before the readout (Figure 4.26).

In case of stationary spins, the reconstructed image $\rho^*(\vec{r})$ (Eq. (4.73)) is a real function and is not influenced by bipolar pulses. Moving spins, however, experience an additional phase shift. If the velocity $\vec{v}(\vec{r})$ is constant, the image that will be reconstructed becomes $\rho^*(\vec{r})e^{-i\vec{v}(\vec{r})\cdot\vec{m}_1(\mathrm{TE})}$ (see Eq. (4.79)), which is a complex function consisting of the magnitude image $\rho^*(\vec{r})$ and the phase image $\Phi(\vec{r},\mathrm{TE}) = \vec{v}(\vec{r})\cdot\vec{m}_1(\mathrm{TE})$. Using a bipolar pulse sequence as in Figure 4.24(a) the

85

phase image can be written as (see Eq. (4.80))

$$\Phi_\uparrow(\vec{r}, \mathrm{TE}) = -\gamma\,(\Delta t)^2\,\vec{v}(\vec{r}) \cdot \vec{G}. \qquad (4.81)$$

For a bipolar pulse with reversed polarity (i.e., $-\vec{G}$ followed by $+\vec{G}$) the phase image is inverted:

$$\Phi_\downarrow(\vec{r}, \mathrm{TE}) = +\gamma\,(\Delta t)^2\vec{v}(\vec{r}) \cdot \vec{G}. \qquad (4.82)$$

Subtracting both phase images yields

$$\Delta\Phi(\vec{r}, \mathrm{TE}) = \Phi_\uparrow(\vec{r}, \mathrm{TE}) - \Phi_\downarrow(\vec{r}, \mathrm{TE})$$
$$= 2\,\gamma\,(\Delta t)^2\vec{v}(\vec{r}) \cdot \vec{G}. \qquad (4.83)$$

Hence, by subtracting the phase images of the two subsequent acquisitions, an image of the phase difference $\Delta\Phi$ is obtained from which the blood velocity can be derived (Figure 4.27). However, Eq. (4.83) shows that only the velocity in the direction of the gradient can be calculated from the measured phase difference. For example, a blood velocity perpendicular to the gradient yields no phase shift at all. To overcome this problem, it is necessary to apply bipolar pulses sequentially along the three gradient axes (Figure 4.26) with the disadvantage of increasing the acquisition time. On the other hand, 3D PC MRA yields better contrast images than 3D TOF MRA in case of slow flow because 3D TOF MRA partly saturates blood flowing at low velocity.

### Contrast-enhanced (CE) MRA

CE MRA relies on the effects of a contrast agent in the blood. It is largely independent of the flow pattern in the vessels. As compared with CT, the physical

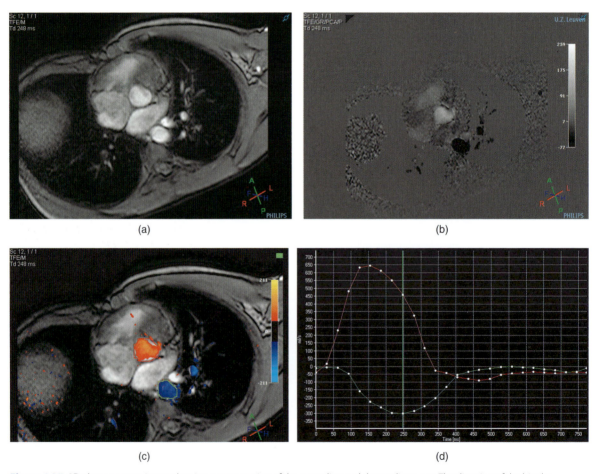

(a)　　　　(b)

(c)　　　　(d)

**Figure 4.27** 2D phase-contrast image showing a cross-section of the ascending and descending aorta. The direction of the bipolar gradients is perpendicular to the image slice in line with the aortic flow. **(a)** Magnitude image. **(b)** Phase difference image. **(c)** The phase difference, which is proportional to the blood velocity in the aorta, is mapped in color onto the magnitude image. The red color is used for ascending flow while blue shows the descending flow. The brightness of the colored pixels represents the local velocity, ranging from 33 up to 106 cm/s. In regions where the velocity is below 33 the magnitude image is shown. **(d)** By acquiring a time series of images, the flux (in ml/s) in the outlined regions is calculated as a function of time. (Courtesy of Professor S. Sunaert, Department of Radiology.)

principle of the contrast agent is different. In MRI, paramagnetic, superparamagnetic, and ferromagnetic substances are used. Chelates of the rare earth metal gadolinium are superparamagnetic and are used most often. Because of their high magnetic susceptibility, they disturb the local magnetic field and decrease $T_2^*$. Furthermore, they have the characteristic of decreasing $T_1$ and $T_2$ of the surrounding hydrogen-containing matter. Depending on the pulse sequence, the contrast generates hypointense (for a $T_2^*$-weighted sequence) or hyperintense (for a $T_1$-weighted sequence) pixels. Contrast-enhanced (CE) MRA employs a 3D GE sequence with short TE and TR, in which the effect of $T_1$ shortening dominates.

Proper timing is important in CE MRA. First, the concentration of the contrast agent in the arteries must be highest at the moment of the measurement. Second, when the contrast agent arrives at the arteries, the central region of the $\vec{k}$-space should be sampled first to obtain the best image contrast. Indeed, a property of the $\vec{k}$-space is that the area around the origin primarily determines the low-frequency contrast, whereas the periphery is responsible for the high-frequency details in the image.

### Visualization of MRA images

In MRA images, the vessels are bright as compared with the surrounding stationary tissues. Although 3D image data can be analyzed by sequential observation of individual 2D slices, considerable experience and training are required to reconstruct mentally the anatomy of the vessels from the large number of slices. Postprocessing can be used to integrate the 3D vessel information into a single image.

Currently, *maximum intensity projections* (MIP) are widely used to produce projection views similar to X-ray angiograms. The principle of this method is illustrated in Figure 4.28. The measured volume is penetrated by a large number of parallel rays or projection lines. In the image perpendicular to these projection lines, each ray corresponds to a single voxel whose gray value is defined as the maximum intensity encountered along the projection ray. Projection images can be calculated for any orientation of the rays. A 3D impression is obtained by calculating MIPs from subsequent directions around the vascular tree and quickly displaying them one after the other.

### Diffusion

Because of thermal agitation, molecules are in constant motion known as Brownian motion. In MRI, this diffusion process can be visualized with an adapted pulse sequence that emphasizes the dephasing caused by random thermal motion of spins in a gradient field. A spin-echo EPI sequence, called *pulsed gradient spin-echo* (PGSE) (see Figure 4.29), is applied to obtain diffusion-weighted images. Because the net magnetization is the vector sum of a large number of individual spin vectors, each with a different motion, the phase incoherence causes signal loss. If $S_0$ represents the signal if no diffusion were present, the signal $S$ in the

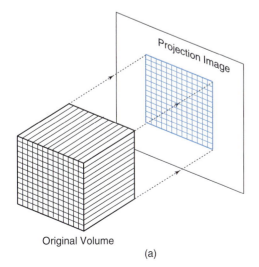

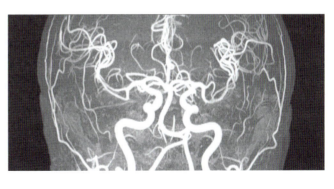

Original Volume

(a)                                    (b)

**Figure 4.28 (a)** Illustration of the MIP algorithm. A projection view of a 3D dataset is obtained by taking the maximum signal intensity along each ray perpendicular to the image. **(b)** MIP of a 3D MRA dataset of the brain.

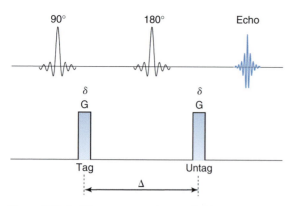

**Figure 4.29** An EPI sequence supplemented with two strong gradient pulses around a 180° RF pulse yields a diffusion-weighted image. The additional pulses have no effect on static spins, but moving spins experience an extra strong dephasing.

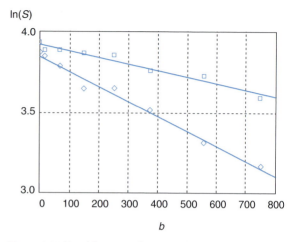

**Figure 4.30** The diffusion coefficient $D$ is found by acquiring a series of images with different $b$ values and calculating the slope of $\ln(S)$ versus $b$. (Reprinted with permission of Mosby – Year Book, Inc.)

presence of diffusion in an isotropic medium is

$$S(b) = S_0\, e^{-bD}$$

$$b = \gamma^2 \delta^2 \left( \Delta - \frac{\delta}{3} \right) G^2. \qquad (4.84)$$

In this equation, $G$ is the gradient amplitude, $\delta$ is the on-time of each of the gradients, and $\Delta$ is the time between the application of the two gradients. $D$ is the *diffusion coefficient*. Figure 4.30 illustrates how it can be calculated from a few values of $b$ and corresponding signal $S(b)$. Note that at least two measurements are needed to calculate $D$, typically one without (i.e., $b = 0$) and one with a pulsed gradient pair. In practice the measured diffusion coefficient is influenced by contributions from other movement sources, such as microcirculation in the capillaries. The term *apparent diffusion coefficient* (ADC) is therefore used. If it is calculated for every pixel, a so-called ADC map is obtained.

In anisotropic media the mean diffusion distances depend on the orientation. In mathematical terminology $D$ is a tensor, which extends the notion of vector. The imaging technique used to acquire this tensor for every pixel is called *diffusion tensor imaging* (DTI). $D$ is a 3 × 3 symmetric matrix, which can be understood as follows. Typically the Brownian random motion can be described by a multivariate normal conditional probability density function expressing the probability that a species displaces from $r_0$ to $r$ after a diffusion

time $\tau$

$$p(\mathbf{r}|\mathbf{r_0}, \tau) = \frac{1}{(4\pi\tau)^{3/2}\sqrt{|D|}} \cdot e^{-(1/4\tau)(\mathbf{r}-\mathbf{r_0})^{\mathrm{T}} D^{-1}(\mathbf{r}-\mathbf{r_0})} \qquad (4.85)$$

with $D$ a covariance matrix describing the displacement in each direction. Isosurfaces of this multivariate Gaussian probability function have an ellipsoidal shape. Assume for a moment that the principal axes of this ellipsoid are oriented along the axes of the 3D coordinate system, then $D$ can be written as

$$D = \Lambda = \begin{pmatrix} \lambda_1 & 0 & 0 \\ 0 & \lambda_2 & 0 \\ 0 & 0 & \lambda_3 \end{pmatrix}. \qquad (4.86)$$

If the ellipsoid has a different orientation, $D$ changes into a symmetric matrix, that is,

$$D = \begin{pmatrix} D_{xx} & D_{xy} & D_{xz} \\ D_{xy} & D_{yy} & D_{yz} \\ D_{xz} & D_{yz} & D_{zz.} \end{pmatrix}. \qquad (4.87)$$

The relationship between Eq. (4.87) and Eq. (4.86) is

$$D = Q \cdot \Lambda \cdot Q^{\mathrm{T}} \qquad (4.88)$$

where $Q = [\mathbf{q_1}\ \mathbf{q_2}\ \mathbf{q_3}]$ is the 3 × 3 unitary matrix of eigenvectors $\mathbf{q}_k$ of $D$, and $\Lambda$ is the diagonal matrix of corresponding eigenvalues $\lambda_k$ (with $\lambda_1 \geq \lambda_2 \geq \lambda_3$).

For anisotropic diffusion, Eq. (4.84) can now be generalized as follows:

$$S(b) = S_0\, e^{-b g^T D g}$$

$$b = \gamma^2 \delta^2 \left( \Delta - \frac{\delta}{3} \right) |G|^2 \qquad (4.89)$$

with $g = G/|G|$ the unit vector in the direction of G. Because matrix $D$ has six degrees of freedom, its calculation requires measurements of $S(b)$ in at least six different noncollinear directions g, together with the blank measurement $S_0$. Increasing the number of measurements improves the accuracy of $D$. The eigenvalues $\lambda_k$ and eigenvectors $q_k$ can be calculated using *principal component analysis* (PCA). More details about PCA are given in Chapter 7, p. 180.

A popular representation of the anisotropic diffusion in each voxel is its principal direction $q_1$ and the so-called *fractional anisotropy* (FA)

$$FA = \frac{1}{\sqrt{2}} \frac{\sqrt{(\lambda_1 - \lambda_2)^2 + (\lambda_2 - \lambda_3)^2 + (\lambda_1 - \lambda_3)^2}}{\sqrt{\lambda_1^2 + \lambda_2^2 + \lambda_3^2}}.$$

$$(4.90)$$

Using color coding both the principal direction $q_1$ and the fractional anisotropy FA can be visualized by the hue and brightness respectively. Figure 4.31 shows a color image of the anisotropic diffusion in the white matter fibers of the brain. These fibers can also be tracked (see Figure 7.16) and visualized as 3D bundles (see Figure 8.9). This technique, called *tractography*, is particularly useful for showing connectivities between different brain regions.[†]

**Perfusion**

Blood perfusion of tissues refers to the activity of the capillary network, where exchanges between blood and tissues are optimized. Oxygen and nutrients are transported to the cells, and the waste products are eliminated. The blood flow is therefore the important parameter for perfusion. As we have seen, blood can be visualized using a contrast agent such as gadolinium chelate, which is injected intravenously as a bolus. It disturbs the local magnetic field and decreases $T_2^*$ in the neighborhood. $T_1$ and $T_2$ of the surrounding hydrogen-containing matter are also decreased. A large signal drop can be obtained when the passage of contrast agent through brain gray matter is imaged using a $T_2$ or $T_2^*$ sensitive EPI sequence (see Figure 4.48 below). Figure 4.49 shows another example of a perfusion study, this time using $T_1$-weighted images. In these images perfused regions appear bright because of their decreased $T_1$.

Quantification of perfusion is still an active area of research. Parameters of interest are the time-to-peak (signal loss), the maximum signal loss, the area under the curve, and so on. However, as in nuclear medicine, there is a strong tendency to describe the behavior of the capillary network via a multicompartment model and to relate its parameters to the obtained perfusion curve. This yields a more objective assessment of the performance of the capillary network. These models are beyond the scope of this book.

## Functional imaging

In 1990, investigators demonstrated the dependence of brain tissue relaxation on the oxygenation level in the blood, which offers a way to visualize the brain function. The brain's vascular system

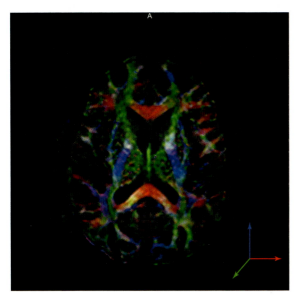

**Figure 4.31** Color coded fractional anisotropy (FA) map. The hue represents the main direction of the diffusion and the brightness the fractional anisotropy. (Courtesy of Professor S. Sunaert, Department of Radiology.)

[†] The tensor model does not hold for fibers crossing, bending, or twisting within a single voxel. High angular resolution diffusion imaging (HARDI) such as diffusion spectrum imaging (DSI) and Q-ball imaging (QBI) have been proposed to resolve multiple intravoxel fiber orientations. These methods require hundreds of measurements, which is more than is used typically in DTI. More details of these pulse schemes are beyond the scope of this textbook.

provides oxygen to satisfy the metabolic needs of brain cells. The oxygen is transported through the blood vessels by means of hemoglobin molecules. In the arteries, each hemoglobin molecule carries a maximum of four oxygen molecules and is called *oxyhemoglobin* (oxygen-rich hemoglobin). At the capillary level, the hemoglobin molecule delivers part of its oxygen molecules to the neurons and becomes *deoxyhemoglobin* (oxygen-poor hemoglobin). Oxyhemoglobin is diamagnetic, whereas deoxyhemoglobin is a paramagnetic substance that produces microscopic magnetic field inhomogeneities that decrease the transverse relaxation time of the blood and the surrounding tissue. This implies that the oxygen concentration in the blood influences the MR signal. This phenomenon is called the BOLD (*blood oxygenation-level dependent*) effect. When brain cells are activated, the blood flow has to increase in order to meet the higher oxygen consumption rate of the neurons. Actually, the blood flow overcompensates the neuronal need for oxygen and, as a consequence, the oxygen concentration *increases* in the capillaries, venules, and veins. Hence, the transverse relaxation time $T_2^*$ of brain tissue is longer when it is active than when it is at rest. Gradient-echo images, such as EPI, are very sensitive to changes in $T_2^*$ and are widely used to detect brain activation.

In a typical functional MRI (fMRI) investigation, the brain function is activated when the patient in the MR scanner performs a certain task. For example, when the subject's hand repeatedly opens and closes, the primary motor cortex is activated. Two image sequences are acquired, one during the task and one during rest (i.e., when the hand does not move). The active brain areas become visible after subtraction of the two images. However, the result is very noisy because of the low sensitivity of the method. The difference in MR signal between task and rest is only 2 to 5% of the local image intensity. To increase the SNR, longer periods of activation (e.g., 30 s) are alternated with equally long periods of rest, and during the whole length of the investigation (e.g., 6 min), images are taken every few seconds (2–10 s). This dataset is processed statistically (see Chapter 7), leaving only those brain areas that show statistically significant activation. Any functional brain area can be visualized by fMRI, such as the sensorimotor cortex (Figure 4.47) and the visual cortex, but also areas responsible for higher order processes such as memory, object recognition, or language.

**Table 4.3** The values of TR and TE determine whether the resulting images are $\rho$, $T_1$, or $T_2$ weighted

| Type | Repetition time TR | Echo time TE |
|---|---|---|
| $\rho$-weighted | long | short |
| $T_1$-weighted | short | short |
| $T_2$-weighted | long | long |

## Image quality

### Contrast

For a SE sequence, Eq. (4.50) shows that the signal is proportional to

$$\rho\left(1 - e^{-\mathrm{TR}/T_1}\right)e^{-\mathrm{TE}/T_2}. \tag{4.91}$$

Although exceptions exist, we have assumed here that $\alpha = 90°$. The parameters in this equation that influence the image contrast can be subdivided into *tissue-dependent* and *technical* parameters. The tissue-dependent parameters are the relaxation times $T_1$ and $T_2$ and the spin or proton density $\rho$.[†] They are physical and cannot be changed. The technical parameters are the repetition time TR and the echo time TE. They are the pulse sequence parameters and can be tuned by the operator in order to adapt the contrast in the image to the specific application. By varying TR and TE, $\rho$-, $T_1$- or $T_2$-weighted images are obtained. Table 4.3 summarizes the parameter settings and their weighting effect.

Commonly used values at 1 T for TR lie between 2000 and 2500 ms for $\rho$- and $T_2$-weighted images and between 400 and 800 ms for $T_1$-weighted images. The echo time TE varies between less than 1 and 20 ms for $T_1$- and $\rho$-weighted images and between 80 and 120 ms for $T_2$-weighted images. Remember that $T_1$ increases with increasing field strength.

For GE sequences with $\alpha < 90°$, the signal also depends on $\alpha$ and on $T_2^*$. For example, the signal intensity for the FLASH sequence in steady state is proportional to

$$\rho\, e^{-\mathrm{TE}/T_2^*}\, \frac{\left(1 - e^{-\mathrm{TR}/T_1}\right)\sin\alpha}{1 - e^{-\mathrm{TR}/T_1}\cos\alpha}. \tag{4.92}$$

Figure 4.32 illustrates this equation. More details can be found in the specialized literature.

---

[†] Actually $\rho$ is the net magnetization density, which depends not only on the spin density, but also on the strength $B_0$ of the external magnetic field (see Eq. (4.102) below).

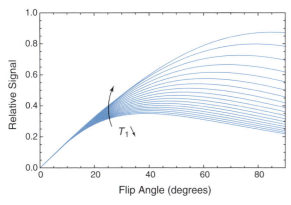

Figure 4.32 Relative signal of the FLASH sequence as a function of the flip angle for $T_1$ values ranging from 200 to 2000 ms. Note that for each $T_1$, there is a maximum signal for $\alpha < 90°$.

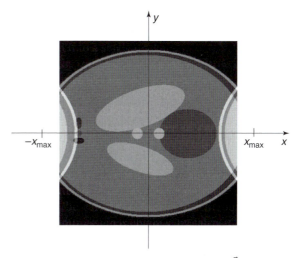

Figure 4.33 In this simulation the distance $k_x$ in the $\vec{k}$-space was chosen too large, yielding aliasing in the readout direction.

## Resolution

### Resolution in the Fourier space

Let $\Delta k_x$ denote the sampling distance in the $k_x$-direction of the Fourier space. To avoid aliasing in the image space, the Nyquist criterion (see Appendix A, p. 228) must be satisfied. It states that

$$\Delta k_x \leq \frac{1}{2x_{max}}, \tag{4.93}$$

where $x_{max}$ is the border of the FOV in the $x$-direction:

$$x_{max} = \frac{FOV_x}{2}. \tag{4.94}$$

Combining both equations yields

$$\Delta k_x \leq \frac{1}{FOV_x}. \tag{4.95}$$

The $\vec{k}$-theorem relates $\Delta k_x$ to $G_x \Delta t$:

$$\Delta k_x = \frac{\gamma}{2\pi} G_x \Delta t. \tag{4.96}$$

Hence, $G_x \Delta t$ is restricted to

$$G_x \Delta t \leq \frac{2\pi}{\gamma FOV_x}. \tag{4.97}$$

In practice, $\Delta t$ is fixed and $G_x$ is scaled to the field of view. An example of aliasing in the readout direction is shown in Figure 4.33.

For $\Delta k_y$ and $T_{ph}$, a similar restriction can be derived:

$$\Delta k_y \leq \frac{1}{FOV_y},$$

$$\Delta k_y = \frac{\gamma}{2\pi} g_y T_{ph}, \tag{4.98}$$

$$g_y T_{ph} \leq \frac{2\pi}{\gamma FOV_y}.$$

Hence, $g_y T_{ph}$ must be sufficiently small. In practice, $T_{ph}$ is fixed and $g_y$ is scaled to the field of view.

### Resolution in the image space

The spatial resolution can be described by the FWHM of the PSF: the smaller the width of the PSF, the larger the spatial resolution. Currently, the FWHM of the PSF is less than 1 mm for conventional sequences. The resolution of fast imaging sequences (EPI, HASTE) is worse because multiple echoes per excitation cause blurring (see Figure 4.21).

The PSF defines the highest frequency $k_{max}$ available in the signal. When sampling the $\vec{k}$-space, the highest measured frequency must preferably be at least as high. Using the $\vec{k}$-theorem in the $x$-direction, this means that

$$k_{max} \leq \frac{\gamma}{2\pi} G_x \frac{T_{ro}}{2} = \frac{\gamma}{2\pi} G_x \frac{N_x \Delta t}{2}. \tag{4.99}$$

As discussed above, $G_x$ is scaled with the field of view and $\Delta t$ is fixed. Hence, the only remaining variable

91

which influences the resolution in the $x$-direction is the number of samples $N_x$.

In the $y$-direction, a similar conclusion can be derived:

$$k_{max} \leq \frac{\gamma}{2\pi} N_{ph}\, g_y\, \frac{T_{ph}}{2}. \qquad (4.100)$$

In practice, $T_{ph}$ is fixed and $g_y$ is scaled to the field of view; $N_{ph}$ is variable but it is proportional to the acquisition time and is thus limited as well.

## Noise

Let $n_\uparrow$ and $n_\downarrow$ denote the number of spins with energy $E_\uparrow$ and $E_\downarrow$, respectively. It can be shown that [18]

$$n_\uparrow - n_\downarrow \approx n_s \frac{\gamma \hbar B_0}{2 k_B T} = 3.3 \times 10^{-6} n_s, \qquad (4.101)$$

where $n_s = n_\uparrow + n_\downarrow$, $k_B$ is Boltzmann's constant, and $T$ is the absolute temperature of the object. Hence, $n_\uparrow > n_\downarrow$, but the fractional excess in the low-energy state is very small. It can be shown that the amplitude of the net magnetization vector is quite small:

$$M \approx \frac{(\hbar \gamma)^2 n_s B_0}{4 k_B T}. \qquad (4.102)$$

To get an idea of the magnitude of $M$, for a bottle of water of 1 L at $T = 310$ K and $B_0 = 1$ T, $n_s \approx 6.7 \times 10^{25}$ and $M \approx 3 \times 10^{-6}$ J/T. Hence, it is not surprising that MR images suffer from noise. The most important noise sources are the thermal noise in the patient and in the receiver part of the MR imaging system. Consequently, the lower the temperature, the less the noise. From Eq. (4.102) it follows that cooling the subject would also yield a higher signal. Unfortunately, this cannot be applied to patients.

Remember that 3D imaging has a better SNR than 2D imaging (p. 79). Furthermore, the SNR of very fast imaging sequences (multiple echoes per excitation, see p. 81) is worse as compared with the conventional sequences.

## Artifacts

Artifacts find their origin in technical imperfections, inaccurate assumptions about the data and numerical approximations.

- The external magnetic field $\vec{B}$ is assumed to be homogeneous to avoid unnecessary dephasing. Dephasing causes signal loss and geometric

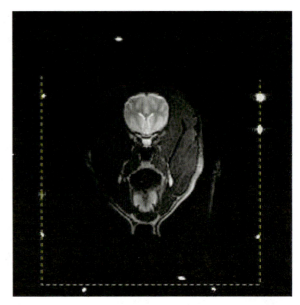

**Figure 4.34** Image obtained with a $T_2$-weighted TurboSE sequence on a 1.5 T system. The circular rods of the reference frame, used for stereotactic neurosurgery (see Chapter 8), should lie on straight lines. Nonlinearities of the magnetic field have caused a pronounced geometric distortion. It can be shown that the distortion is inversely proportional to the gradient strength. For stereotactic surgery, geometric accuracy is of utmost importance, and this image is therefore useless. (Courtesy of Professor B. Nuttin, Department of Neurosurgery and Professor S. Sunaert, Department of Radiology.)

deformations (Figure 4.34) as will be explained below.

The flip angle should be constant throughout the entire image volume to ensure a spatially homogeneous signal. If the RF field is inhomogeneous, the flip angle $\alpha$ slowly varies throughout the image space, causing a low-frequency signal intensity modulation. In Figure 4.35, this *bias field* was separated and removed from the image by postprocessing for proper segmentation of the white brain matter.

In practice the slice sensitivity profile (SSP) is not rectangular, yielding cross-talk between neighboring slices in multi-slice imaging. This can be avoided by introducing a sufficiently large gap (e.g., 10% of the slice width, which is defined as the FWHM of the SSP) between subsequent slices.

Other less common artifacts are due to system failure, inappropriate shielding of the magnet room or interaction with unshielded monitoring equipment. With proper care they can be avoided.

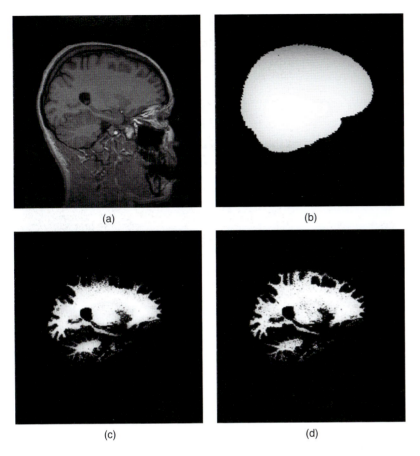

(a)

(b)

(c)

(d)

**Figure 4.35** **(a)** Sagittal image of the brain obtained with a 3D GE pulse sequence. RF field inhomogeneities cause a bias field shown in **(b)**, which is a low-frequency intensity variation throughout the image. This bias field was separated from (a) by image processing. **(c** and **d)** Result of white brain matter segmentation (see Chapter 7) before and after bias field correction, respectively. The result shown in (d) is clearly superior to that in (c). (Images obtained as part of the EC-funded BIOMED-2 program under grant BMH4-CT96-0845 (BIOMORPH).)

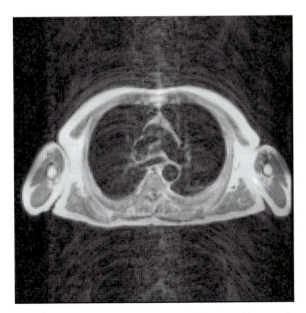

**Figure 4.36** Ghosting is a characteristic artifact caused by periodic motion. In this $T_1$-weighted SE image of the heart, breathing, heart beats, and pulsating blood vessels yield ghosting and blurring.

- The data are assumed to be independent of the $T_2$ relaxation during the measurements. If this is not the case, for example when using multiple echoes per excitation, the spatial resolution decreases (Eq. (4.69)).

  Tissues are assumed to be stationary. Motion yields dephasing artifacts (Figure 4.36).

  Similar to an inhomogeneous external magnetic field, the magnetic susceptibility of tissues or foreign particles and implants yields dephasing (Figure 4.18).

- Digital image reconstruction implies discretization and truncation errors that may produce visual artifacts. Inadequate sampling yields aliasing, known as the *wrap-around* artifact (Figure 4.33). A truncated Fourier transform implies a convolution of the image with a sinc function and yields ripples at high-contrast boundaries. This is the *Gibbs* artifact or *ringing* artifact. A similar truncation artifact is caused in CE MRA when the contrast agent suddenly arrives in the selected slab during the

93

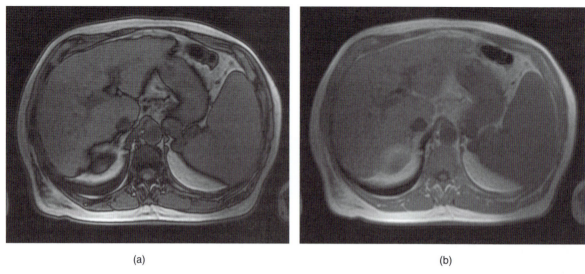

(a)  (b)

**Figure 4.37** Phase cancellation artifact. **(a)** $T_1$-weighted image (GE sequence) in which fat and water are exactly out of phase (i.e., for a specific TE) in voxels that contain both elements. This yields the typical dark edges at water/fat boundaries. **(b)** Phase cancellation is undone by changing the TE to a value where water and fat are in phase. (Courtesy of Professor S. Sunaert, Department of Radiology.)

acquisition of the $\vec{k}$-space. If, for example, the low frequencies in the $\vec{k}$-space are sampled first, when the contrast agent has not yet arrived in the selected volume, and the high-frequency information is acquired next when the blood vessels are filled with contrast, ringing occurs at the blood vessel edges.

The consequences of involuntary phase shifts and dephasing need some more attention. As we have seen, phase shifts are necessary to encode position. Consequently, intervoxel dephasing is unavoidable but yields signal loss. This is particularly the case in the outer regions of the $\vec{k}$-space, where the measured signal is low and noisy. However, during the readout all the spins within a single voxel should precess in phase and with the correct phase, dictated by the spatial position of the voxel.

- If the spins precess in phase, but this phase is not the predicted one, the voxel information is represented at a different spatial position in the reconstructed image.

- In case of intravoxel dephasing, i.e., the spins within the voxel do not precess in phase, the signal detected from this voxel drops down and its assignment is distributed throughout the image domain after reconstruction.

The consequences of phase errors can be summarized as signal loss and position errors, visible as spatial deformation and ghost patterns.

- Signal loss is notable if the effective external magnetic field yields intravoxel dephasing. This is for example the case if magnetic particles are present in the body (Figure 4.18). Another example is the dark edge at water–fat transitions (Figure 4.37). Due to the chemical shift between water and fat, these elements precess at a slightly different Larmor frequency. Consequently, the spins in voxels that contain both elements, can go out of phase, yielding signal loss. Note that this kind of signal loss can be largely undone with a 180° pulse, i.e. by using a SE sequence.

  Velocity induced dephasing is another cause of signal loss, which occurs in blood vessels. Motion compensation can undo this effect for nonturbulent flow.

- Geometric distortions are caused by deviations of the main magnetic field, nonlinear magnetic field gradients (Figure 4.34) and magnetic susceptibility of the tissue. Another cause is the chemical shift between water and fat, yielding a phase difference of 150 Hz per tesla between both and consequently, a mutual spatial misregistration. This is called the *chemical shift artifact* (Figure 4.38).

- *Ghosting* is due to periodic spin motion, such as breathing (Figure 4.36), heart beats, blood vessel pulsation and repeated patient twitches. Because the sampling periods in the phase- and frequency-encoding directions differ substantially (TR versus $\Delta t$), motion artifacts appear particularly in the phase-encoding direction. Ghosting can be explained as follows. Consider a fixed voxel in the image space. The net magnetization in this voxel is not constant but time dependent and periodic as the object moves. In general, any periodic function can be written as a Fourier series of sinusoids. According to the $\vec{k}$-theorem, the time can be replaced by the spatial frequency $k_y$. Consequently, the net magnetization in the fixed voxel can be written as a function of $k_y$, represented by a sum of sinusoids. The inverse Fourier transform of each sinusoid translates the signal some distance $\Delta y$ away from the voxel. The result is a number of ghosts in the $y$-direction (see Figure 4.36).

If the motion is relatively slow, but not periodic, such as continuous patient movements and peristalsis, the images appear blurred. Often, motion cannot simply be represented as purely periodic or continuous, and ghosting and blurring appear simultaneously.

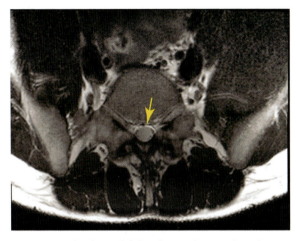

**Figure 4.38** The chemical shift artifact can be seen along the spinal canal. The fat that surrounds the spinal canal, is shifted in the phase-encoding direction with respect to the CSF. (Courtesy of Professor S. Sunaert, Department of Radiology.)

## Equipment

Unlike CT imaging, it is unusual to talk about MR scanner generations. Rather, the image quality has continuously been improved through technical evolutions of the magnets, gradient systems, RF systems, and computer hardware and software.

Throughout the years, improved magnets have resulted in more compact designs with higher main field homogeneities. Superconducting magnets are exclusively used for high field strengths (Figure 4.39(a)).

For lower field strengths, permanent and resistive magnets are employed. They are cheaper than superconducting magnets but have a lower SNR and the field

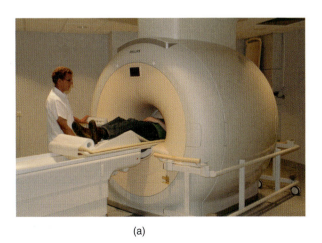

(a)

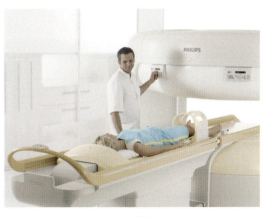

(b)

**Figure 4.39** (a) Whole-body 3 T scanner, designed to visualize every part of the body. This system has a superconducting magnet with a horizontal, solenoid main field. The patient is positioned in the center of the tunnel, which sometimes causes problems for children or for people suffering from claustrophobia. (b) C-shaped 1.5 T open MR system with vertical magnetic field. The open design minimizes the risk of claustrophobia. The increased patient space and detachable table greatly improve handling. The system can also be used for MR-guided procedures. (Courtesy of Philips Healthcare.)

homogeneity is relatively poor. Figure 4.39(b) shows a C-shaped open MR scanner with a vertical magnetic field.

Open MR systems can be used for MR-guided procedures. Interventional MRI (iMRI) (Figure 4.40) provides real time images during surgery or therapy. This way the surgeon is able to follow the surgical instrument during its manipulation. This instrument can be, for example, a biopsy needle, a probe for cyst drainage, a catheter to administer antibiotics, or a laser or a cryogenic catheter for thermotherapy (i.e., to destroy pathological tissue locally by either heating

or freezing it). Note that introduction of an MR unit into an operating room requires some precautions.

- MR-compatible materials must be used for all surgical instruments. Ferromagnetic components are dangerous because they are attracted by the magnetic field and useless because they produce large signal void artifacts in the images.

- Electronic equipment that generates RF radiation must be shielded from the RF field of the MR imaging system and vice versa.

- The combination of electrical leads with the RF field can produce hot spots, which may cause skin burns. Fiberoptic technology is therefore recommended.

The *gradient system* is characterized by its degree of linearity, its maximum amplitude, and its rise time (i.e., the time needed to reach the maximum gradient amplitude). Linearity is mandatory for correct position-encoding. The nonlinearity is typically 1–2% in a FOV with diameter 50 cm. It is worst at the edge of the FOV. The maximum amplitude has increased from 3 mT/m in the early days to 50 mT/m for the current state-of-the-art imaging systems without significant increase in rise time. This is one of the important factors in the breakthrough of ultrafast imaging.

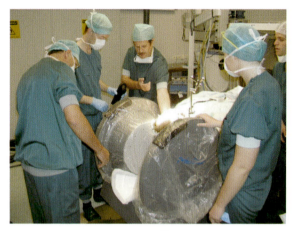

**Figure 4.40** The Medtronic PoleStar® iMRI Navigation Suite, an intra-operative MR image-guidance system, operating at 0.15 T (gradient strength 25 mT/m) suitable for an existing operating room. (Courtesy of Professor B. ter Haar Romeny, AZ Maastricht and TU Eindhoven.)

The *RF system* has improved significantly as well. The sensitivity and in-plane homogeneity of signal detection have increased. Currently, there are special coils for almost every anatomical region (Figure 4.41). They are all designed to detect the weakest MR

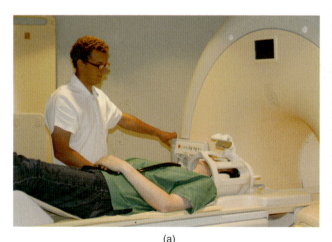

(a)

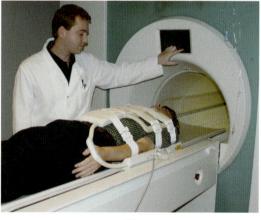

(b)

**Figure 4.41** (a) Head coil and (b) body coil, used to detect optimally the RF signals received from the surrounded body part.

signal possible. The demands on the RF amplifier have also increased. Whereas, for the conventional SE sequences, it was activated twice every TR, ultrafast SE-based sequences such as HASTE (half Fourier single shot turbo spin-echo) require a much higher amplifier performance. Present imaging systems also monitor the deposition of RF power.

As for all digital modalities, MRI has benefited from the hardware and software evolution. Much effort has been spent on decreasing the manipulation time and increasing the patient throughput. Additionally, the diagnosis of dynamic 3D datasets is currently assisted by powerful postprocessing for analysis (e.g., statistical processing of fMRI) and visualization (e.g., MIP of an MRA or reslicing along an arbitrary direction).

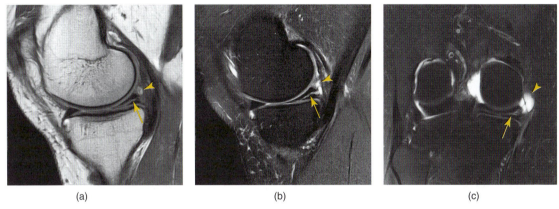

(a)  (b)  (c)

**Figure 4.42** Sagittal proton density image (**a**), and sagittal (**b**) and coronal (**c**) $T_2$ fat-suppressed images of the knee joint, showing a tear in the posterior horn of the medial meniscus (arrow) and a parameniscal cyst (arrowhead). (Courtesy of Dr. S. Pans, Department of Radiology.)

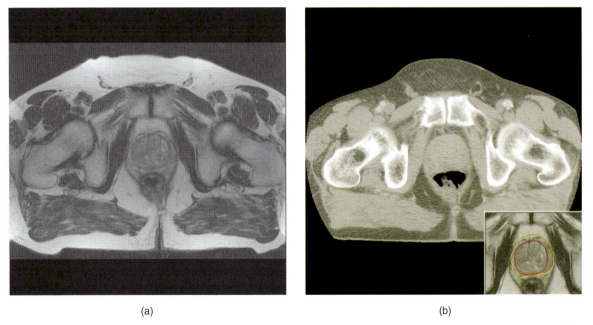

(a)  (b)

**Figure 4.43** (**a**) MR image obtained with a $T_2$-weighted TurboSE sequence (TE = 120 ms, TR = 6 s) through the prostate. (**b**) CT image of the same cross-section. The images of both modalities were geometrically registered with image fusion software (see Chapter 7). The contour of the prostate was manually outlined in both images (see lower right corner; MRI red contour, CT yellow contour). CT systematically overestimates the prostate volume because of the low contrast between prostate tissue and adjacent periprostatic structures, which can only be differentiated in the MR image. (Courtesy of Professor R. Oyen, Department of Radiology.)

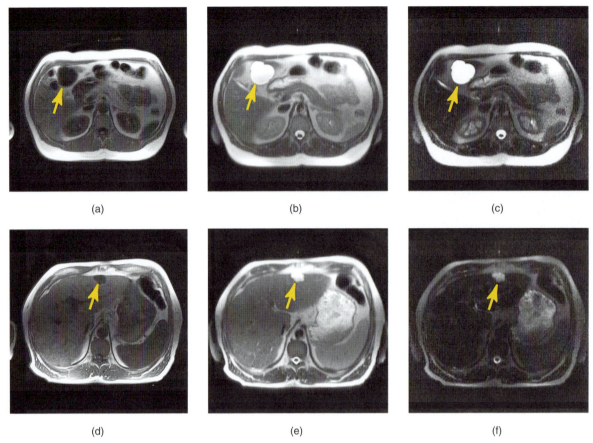

(a)　　　　　　　　　　(b)　　　　　　　　　　(c)

(d)　　　　　　　　　　(e)　　　　　　　　　　(f)

**Figure 4.44** To some extent MRI makes tissue characterization feasible. **(a)** and **(d)** show anatomical images through the liver obtained with a 2D $T_1$-weighted GE sequence. Both detected lesions (arrows) are equally dark. To characterize them, a $T_2$-weighted sequence (HASTE) is used to obtain an image with an early TE train centered around 60 ms (**(b)** and **(e)**) and an image with a late TE train centered around 378 ms (**(c)** and **(f)**). The intensity of the lesion in (b) is only slightly higher than the intensity of the lesion in (e). When measuring around TE = 378 ms, however, the intensity in **(c)** remains almost as high as in (b), but the intensity of the lesion in **(f)** clearly decreases as compared with **(e)**. This intensity decay is characteristic for the type of lesion. (a–c) show a biliary cyst and (d and f) a hemangioma. (Courtesy of Professor D. Vanbeckevoort, Department of Radiology.)

## Clinical use

Magnetic resonance imaging can be applied to obtain anatomical images of all parts of the human body that contain hydrogen, that is, soft tissue, cerebrospinal fluid, edema, and so forth (see Figure 4.42) without using ionizing radiation. The $\rho$-, $T_1$-, and $T_2$-weighted images can be acquired with a variety of acquisition schemes. This flexibility offers the possibility of obtaining a better contrast between different soft tissues than with CT (see Figure 4.43). To a certain extent, the availability of $\rho$-, $T_1$-, and $T_2$-weighted images makes tissue characterization feasible (see Figure 4.44).

As mentioned on p. 89, contrast agents are also used in MRI. There are two biochemically different types of contrast agents. The first type, such as gadolinium compounds, has the same biodistribution as contrast agents for CT and is not captured by the cells. An example is shown in Figure 4.45. The second type, such as iron oxide, is taken up by specific cells, as is the case with contrast agents (radioactive tracers) in nuclear medicine (Chapter 5).

As discussed in the previous sections, special sequences have been developed for blood vessel imaging, functional imaging, perfusion, and diffusion imaging.

Unlike radiography or CT, MRI is able to acquire an image of the blood vessels without contrast injection. However, contrast agents are still used for the visualization of blood with a reduced inflow or

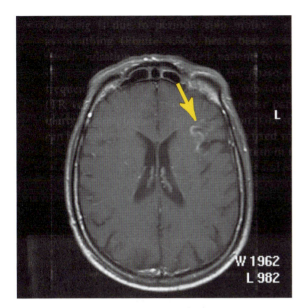

**Figure 4.45** $T_1$-weighted 2D SE image after contrast injection (Gd–DTPA) shows a hyperintense area (arrow) in the left frontal cortical region because of abnormality of the blood–brain barrier after stroke. (Courtesy of Dr. S. Dymarkowski, Department of Radiology.)

with complex motion patterns such as turbulence (Figure 4.46).

The SNR of functional MRI is usually too small simply to visualize the acquired images. Statistical image analysis (see Chapter 7) is then performed on a time series of 3D image stacks obtained with EPI. This way more than a hundred $64 \times 64 \times 32$ image volumes can be acquired in a few minutes. After statistical analysis, significant parameter values are visualized and superimposed on the corresponding $T_1$- or $T_2$-weighted anatomical images (Figure 4.47).

Perfusion images are also time series of 2D or 3D image stacks. Figure 4.48 shows a perfusion study after brain tumor resection to exclude tumor residue or recurrence and Figure 4.49 is an example of a perfusion study after myocardial infarction to assess tissue viability.

Diffusion images reflect microscopically small displacements of hydrogen-containing fluid. A high signal reflects a decreased diffusion (less dephasing). Two examples of impaired diffusion in the brain are shown in Figures 4.50 and 4.51.

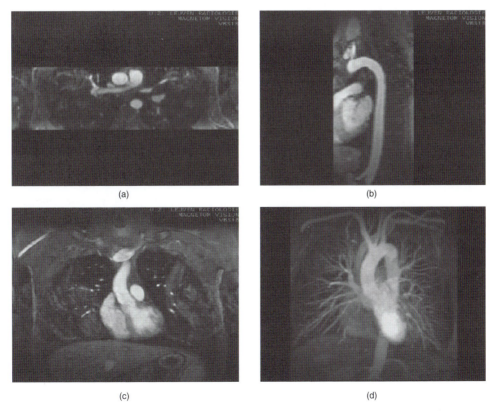

(a)

(b)

(c)

(d)

**Figure 4.46** Contrast-enhanced 3D MR angiography of the thoracic vessels: **(a)** axial, **(b)** sagittal, **(c)** coronal view, and **(d)** maximum intensity projection. (Courtesy of Professor J. Bogaert and Dr. S. Dymarkowski, Department of Radiology.)

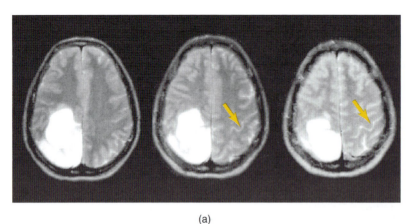

(a)

**Figure 4.47** **(a)** $T_2$-weighted TurboSE axial scan with a hyperintense parietal tumoral lesion. Along the left–central sulcus an "inverted omega" shape (arrow) can be identified, which corresponds to the motor cortex of the hand. This landmark is no longer visible in the right hemisphere because of the mass effect of the parietal lesion. **(b)** Using fMRI of bilateral finger tapping alternated with rest, a parametric color image was obtained and superimposed on the $T_2$-weighted axial sections. The sensorimotor cortex has clearly been displaced in front of the lesion. (Courtesy of Professor S. Sunaert, Department of Radiology.)

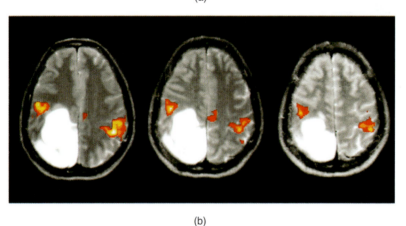

(b)

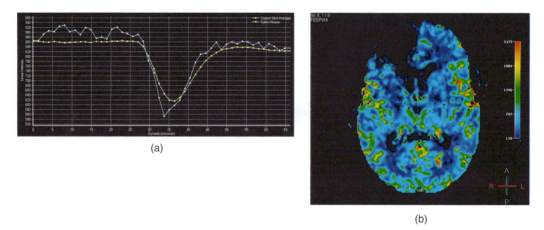

(a)

(b)

**Figure 4.48** **(a)** Typical curve of a perfusion study. A time sequence of $T_2^*$ sensitive echo planar images (EPI) is acquired. The decrease in $T_2^*$ upon the first passage of the contrast agent produces dephasing and a significant signal drop. The smooth yellow line represents the average intensity in the slice as a function of time, while the noisy blue curve shows the intensity in a single pixel. The origin corresponds to the start of the bolus injection in a cubital vein. **(b)** From the curve shown in (a), several color maps can be calculated, such as the cerebral blood volume (CBV), the cerebral blood flow (CBF) and the mean transit time (MTT). In this image the cerebral blood volume (CBV) is shown. (Courtesy of Professor S. Sunaert, Department of Radiology.)

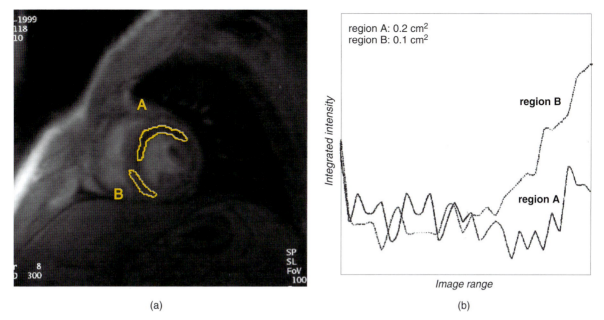

(a)

(b)

**Figure 4.49** Example of anteroseptal myocardial infarction. **(a)** The patency of the coronary arteries can be assessed by means of a first-pass $T_1$-weighted MR image after injection of a contrast agent (Gd–DTPA). Residual obstruction of coronary vessels in this patient yields a large area of hypoperfusion subendocardially in the anteroseptal part of the left ventricular myocardium (region A). **(b)** Integrated intensity of the two regions outlined in (a). The lower curve shows that in region A the signal intensity does not increase any more, in contrast to the signal increase in the normal myocardium (upper curve). Instead of 1D plots, it is clear that parametric images as in Figure 4.48 can also be created. (Courtesy of Professor J. Bogaert and Professor S. Dymarkowski, Department of Radiology, and Professor F. Rademakers, Department of Cardiology.)

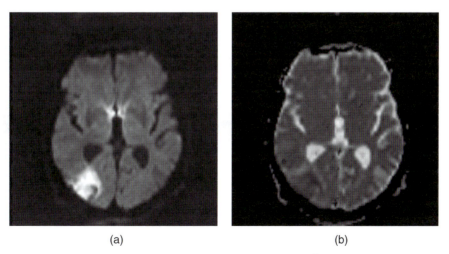

(a)

(b)

**Figure 4.50** Example of acute stroke. **(a)** Native diffusion-weighted image ($b = 1000 \, s/mm^2$) showing a hyperintense area in the posterior watershed area due to restricted diffusion. **(b)** Corresponding ADC map (see p. 88), showing hypointense signal in the same area, confirming the restricted diffusion. The diffusion is restricted due to cytotoxic edema. (Courtesy of Professor S. Sunaert, Department of Radiology.)

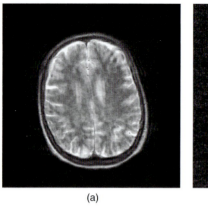

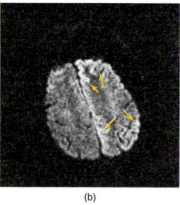

(a)  (b)

**Figure 4.51** **(a)** A $T_2$-weighted transverse TurboSE image does not show any abnormalities in a patient with recent dementia. **(b)** Diffusion-weighted image shows that this patient has Creutzfeldt–Jakob disease. The hyperintense signal (arrows) in the left cortical hemisphere is due to a decreased water diffusion and reflects the spongiform changes in the gray matter with an increased intracellular water content (swollen cells) following inflow from the extracellular space. (Courtesy of Professor P. Demaerel, Department of Radiology.)

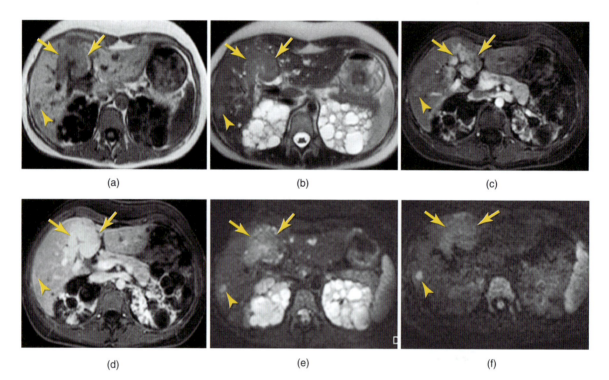

(a)  (b)  (c)

(d)  (e)  (f)

**Figure 4.52** Liver MR examination six months after surgery of bronchial carcinoid. **(a,b)** On the $T_1$- and $T_2$-weighted images a large lesion (arrows) can be seen anterior in the liver and a small nodule is visible at the right lateral side (arrowhead). **(c,d)** The large lesion is visible on both the arterial (c) and venous (d) phase images after contrast application, while the small nodule is nearly invisible. **(e,f)** Diffusion-weighted MR images acquired with respectively $b = 50$ s/mm$^2$ (e) and $b = 1000$ s/mm$^2$ (f). Signal loss is visible in the large lesion when $b$ increases, while the small lesion remains almost unchanged due to a restricted diffusion. For the large lesion an ADC value of 0.00120 mm$^2$/s was found and it was classified as benign. The small lesion, however, presented a low ADC value of 0.00069 mm$^2$/s and was therefore classified as malignant. Histology later confirmed the diagnosis of benign focal nodular hyperplasia in the large lesion, and metastasis of carcinoid tumor in the smaller lesion. (Courtesy of Dr. V. Vandecaveye, Department of Radiology.)

Diffusion imaging is also used to character-ize tumoral tissues. In malignant tumoral deposits, the cells are generally more closely spaced than in normal tissues, leading to an increased restriction of molecular diffusion. An example is shown in Figure 4.52.

## Biologic effects and safety

### Biologic effects

#### RF waves

In normal operating conditions, MRI is a safe medi-cal imaging modality. For example, pregnant women may undergo an MRI examination, but not a CT or PET scan. This is because MRI employs nonionizing RF waves, and the energy of RF photons is much lower than that of ionizing X-ray photons (see Figure 2.1). The absorbed RF energy increases the vibrations of atoms and molecules, which results in small increases of tissue temperature. Furthermore, in conductive elements, such as electrodes, the magnetic component of the RF waves induces a current if not appropriately insulated.

The RF power that can safely be absorbed, is prescribed by the specific absorption rate or SAR value, expressed in watts per kilogram body weight. Based on the body mass entered upon patient registration, the MR system calculates the SAR of each pulse sequence selected by the operator. If the value is too high, the pulse sequence will not start. The user must then change the sequence parameters (e.g., by increasing TR or decreasing the number of slices) until the RF power deposition is within SAR limits. As a rule of thumb the core body temperature rise should be limited to 1°C. Average SAR limits are on the order of 2 to 10 W/kg.

### Magnetic gradients

The magnetic flux $dB/dt$ of a switching magnetic field induces a low-frequency electrical current in conducting material. Fast switching of high-gradient fields may generate a current in tissues such as blood vessels, muscles and particularly nerves, if their stimulation threshold is exceeded. Therefore, modern MRI systems contain a stimulation monitor, and the pulse sequence starts only if the peripheral nerve stimulation threshold is not exceeded. Cardiac stimulation or ventricular fibrillation would require much larger gradient induced electrical fields than currently present and are therefore very unlikely.

Magnetic gradient pulses are obtained by applying pulsed currents in coils. These currents in combination with the static magnetic field yield Lorentz forces. Consequently, the coils make repetitive movements, causing the typical high-frequency drill noise. The loudness should be kept below 100 dB. It can indirectly be reduced by ear plugs or a noise canceling headphone.

### Static magnetic field

Ferromagnetic objects experience a translational force and torque when placed in a magnetic field. Consequently, they can undergo a displacement or cause

malfunction of equipment that contains magnetic components.

Another effect of a static magnetic field is a change in the electrocardiogram (ECG) when the patient is inside the magnet. Because of the external main magnetic field, ions in the blood stream experience Lorentz forces that separate positively and negatively charged ions in opposite directions. This creates a small electric field and a potential difference, which modifies the normal charge distribution. The ECG becomes contaminated (T-wave elevation) by a blood flow related surface potential. This phenomenon is always present but is most obvious when imaging the heart. In these examinations, the pulse sequence is usually triggered, that is, via leads on the patient's chest, the ECG is measured, and the RF excitation is always started at the same time as the heart cycle (this minimizes ghosting from the pulsating heart). When the patient is back out of the magnetic field, the ECG returns to its normal value. As far as is presently known, this small ECG distortion has no negative biological effects for external magnetic fields up to 4 T.

## Safety

*Ferromagnetic objects* must not be brought into the MR examination room because the strong static magnetic field would attract such objects toward the center of the magnetic field. This would destroy the coil and may seriously harm a patient inside the coil. One must be absolutely certain that all materials and equipment (e.g., artificial respirator, scissors, hair pins, paper clips) brought inside the MR examination room are fully MR-compatible. Nonferromagnetic metallic compounds are safe. For example, an aluminum ladder can safely be used when a light bulb inside the MR examination room must be replaced.

Metallic objects *inside the body* are not unusual (e.g., orthopedic fixation screws, hip prostheses, stents, dental fillings, heart valves, pacemakers, and surgical clips). Patients with heart valves, pacemakers, and recent surgical clips (present for less than 3 months) must not be scanned using MRI. Patients with very old prostheses or orthopedic fixation screws must not be scanned if the exact metallic compound is unknown. However, if the implants are recent, it is safe to scan the patient. Caution is particularly needed for patients with a metallic foreign body in the eye or with an intracranial aneurysm clip or coil as even a small movement may lead to hemorrhage.

*Conductive elements*, such as electrodes, may produce burn lesions due to the induced current and must be insulated. Similarly, when positioning the patient, *conducting loops* should be avoided. An example is a patient with his or her hands folded over the abdomen. The RF pulses will cause electrical currents in those conducting loops, which may cause burns. Examples of serious burns caused by improper positioning have already been reported in the specialized MR literature.

Patients with implanted devices with *magnetic or electronic activation* should in principle not be examined using MRI. For example, the RF pulses can reset or modify the pacing of a pacemaker, which may be life threatening for the patient. A cochlear stimulator can be severely damaged.

## Future expectations

Although the contribution of MRI to the total number of radiological examinations is currently limited to only a few percent, it can be expected that this amount will increase continuously in the future because MRI yields high-resolution images of anatomy and function with high specificity and without using harmful ionizing electromagnetic waves.

- With the exception of bone (e.g., skeleton, calcifications) and air (e.g., lungs, gastrointestinal tract) human tissues abundantly contain hydrogen and they can optimally be distinguished by MRI

because of the flexibility of contrast adjustment with proper pulse sequences.

- Other nuclei, such as the isotopes $^{13}$C, $^{19}$F and $^{23}$Na, which are visible in MRI at different resonance frequencies, can be used to label metabolic or pharmaceutical tracers.

- Quantitative analysis of function, perfusion, and diffusion with high resolution and contrast will progress continuously. An example is diffusion-weighted imaging for detection, quantification and therapy response in oncology.

- New contrast agents will become routinely available to study the morphology and function (e.g., hyperpolarized $^{3}$He for dynamic ventilation studies) as well as molecular processes (e.g., ferritin to show gene expressions in vivo (see Figure (5.26)).

From a technical point of view, the development of MRI will focus on a better image quality (higher resolution, better SNR) and shorter acquisition times. This will be obtained with higher external magnetic fields, higher gradients (e.g., gradient head insert coils to avoid cardiac stimulation) in each direction, multiple coils, and reconstruction algorithms that are not based on Fourier theory. As usual in the history of MRI, new pulse sequences will continue to be developed in the future. It can also be expected that the hybrid PET/MR scanner, which exists today and acquires PET and MR images simultaneously, will become an important clinical imaging modality because of its higher specificity than a stand-alone PET or MRI unit.

# 5 Nuclear medicine imaging

## Introduction

The use of radioactive isotopes for medical purposes has been investigated since 1920, and since 1940 attempts have been undertaken to image radionuclide concentration in the human body. In the early 1950s, Ben Cassen introduced the rectilinear scanner, a "zero-dimensional" scanner, which (very) slowly scanned in two dimensions to produce a projection image, like a radiograph, but this time of the radionuclide concentration in the body. In the late 1950s, Hal Anger developed the first "true" gamma camera, introducing an approach that is still being used in the design of all modern cameras: the Anger scintillation camera [21], a 2D planar detector to produce a 2D projection image without scanning.

The Anger camera can also be used for tomography. The projection images can then be used to compute the original spatial distribution of the radionuclide within a slice or a volume, in a process similar to reconstruction in X-ray computed tomography. Already in 1917, Radon published the mathematical method for reconstruction from projections, but only in the 1970s was the method applied in medical applications – first to CT, and then to nuclear medicine imaging. At the same time, iterative reconstruction methods were being investigated, but the application of those methods had to wait until the 1980s for sufficient computer power.

The preceding tomographic system is called a *SPECT* scanner. SPECT stands for single-photon emission computed tomography. Anger also showed that *two* scintillation cameras could be combined to detect *photon pairs* originating after positron emission. This principle is the basis of *PET* (i.e., positron emission tomography), which detects photon pairs. Ter-Pogossian *et al.* built the first dedicated PET system in the 1970s, which was used for phantom studies. Soon afterward, Phelps, Hoffman *et al.* built the first PET scanner (also called PET camera) for human studies [22]. The PET camera has long been considered almost exclusively as a research system. Its breakthrough as a clinical instrument dates only from the last decade.

## Radionuclides

In nuclear medicine, a tracer molecule is administered to the patient, usually by intravenous injection. A tracer is a particular molecule carrying an unstable isotope – a *radionuclide*. In the body this molecule is involved in a metabolic process. Meanwhile the unstable isotopes emit $\gamma$-rays, which allow us to measure the concentration of the tracer molecule in the body as a function of position and time. Consequently, in nuclear medicine the function or metabolism is measured. With CT, MRI, and ultrasound imaging, functional images can also be obtained, but nuclear medicine imaging provides measurements with an SNR that is orders of magnitude higher than that of any other modality.

## Radioactive decay modes

During its radioactive decay a radionuclide loses energy by emitting radiation in the form of particles and electromagnetic rays. These rays are called $\gamma$-rays or X-rays. In nuclear medicine, the photon energy ranges roughly from 60 to 600 keV. Usually, electromagnetic rays that originate from nuclei are called $\gamma$-rays, although they fall into the same frequency range as X-rays and are therefore indistinguishable.

There are many ways in which a radionuclide can decay. In general, the radioactive decay modes can be subdivided into two main categories: decays

[21] S. R. Cherry, J. Sorenson, and M. Phelps. *Physics in Nuclear Medicine*. Philadelphia, PA: W. B. Saunders Company, 3rd edition, 2003.

[22] M. Ter-Pogossian. Instrumentation for cardiac positron emission tomography: background and historical perspective. In S. Bergmann and B. Sobel, editors, *Positron Emission Tomography of the Heart*. New York: Futura Publishing Company, 1992.

with emission or capture of nucleons, i.e., neutrons and protons, and decays with emission or capture of β-particles, i.e, electrons and positrons.

### Nucleon emission or capture

Nucleon emission or capture is not used in imaging because these particles cause heavy damage to tissue due to their high kinetic energy. Instead they can be used in radiotherapy for tumor irradiation.

An example is neutron capture therapy, which exploits the damaging properties of α-particles. An α-particle is a helium nucleus, which consists of two protons and two neutrons. It results from the decay of an unstable atom X into atom Y as follows:

$$_{Z}^{A}X \rightarrow _{Z-2}^{A-4}Y + _{2}^{4}He^{2+}. \tag{5.1}$$

If X has mass number* $A$ and atomic number† $Z$, then Y has mass number $A - 4$ and atomic number $Z - 2$. The α-particle $_{2}^{4}He^{2+}$ is a heavy particle with a typical kinetic energy of 3–7 MeV. This kinetic energy is rapidly released when interacting with tissue. The range of an α-particle is only 0.01 to 0.1 mm in water and soft tissue. In order to irradiate a deeply located tumor, neutron capture therapy can be applied. Neutrons, produced by a particle accelerator, penetrate deeply into the tissue until captured by a chemical component injected into the tumor. At that moment α-particles are released:

$$_{Z}^{A}X + n \rightarrow {}^{A+1}_{Z}X + \gamma \rightarrow _{Z-2}^{A-3}Y + _{2}^{4}He^{2+}. \tag{5.2}$$

The radioactive decay modes discussed below are all used in nuclear medicine imaging. Depending on the decay mode, a β-particle is emitted or captured and one or a pair of γ-rays is emitted in each event.

---

* The mass number is the sum of the number of nucleons, i.e., neutrons and protons.
† The atomic number is the number of protons. Isotopes of a chemical element have the same atomic number (number of protons in the nucleus) but have different mass numbers (from having different numbers of neutrons in the nucleus). Examples are $^{12}C$ and $^{14}C$ (6 protons and 6 respectively 8 neutrons). Different isotopes of the same element cannot have the same mass number, but isotopes of different elements often do have the same mass number. Examples are $^{99}Mo$ and $^{99}Tc$, $^{14}C$ (6 protons and 8 neutrons) and $^{14}N$ (7 protons and 7 neutrons).

### Electron β⁻ emission

In this process, a neutron is transformed essentially into a proton and an electron (called a β⁻-particle):

$$_{Z}^{A}X \rightarrow _{Z+1}^{A}Y + e^{-}$$
$$n \rightarrow p^{+} + e^{-}. \tag{5.3}$$

Because the number of protons is increased, this transmutation process corresponds to a rightward step in Mendelejev's table.

In some cases the resulting daughter product of the preceding transmutation can still be in a *metastable* state $^{Am}Y$. In that case it decays further with a certain delay to a more stable nuclear arrangement, releasing the excess energy as one or more γ-photons. The nucleons are unchanged, thus there is no additional transmutation in decay from excited to ground state.

Because β-particles damage the tissue and have no diagnostic value, preference in imaging is given to metastable radionuclides, which are pure sources of γ-rays. The most important single-photon tracer, $^{99m}Tc$, is an example of this mode. $^{99m}Tc$ is a metastable daughter product of $^{99}Mo$ (half-life = 66 hours). $^{99m}Tc$ decays to $^{99}Tc$ (half-life = 6 hours) by emitting a photon of 140 keV. The half-life is the time taken to decay to half of its initial quantity.

### Electron capture (EC)

Essentially, an orbital electron is captured and combined with a proton to produce a neutron:

$$_{Z}^{A}X + e^{-} \rightarrow _{Z-1}^{A}Y$$
$$p^{+} + e^{-} \rightarrow n. \tag{5.4}$$

Note that EC causes transmutation toward the leftmost neighbor in Mendelejev's table. An example of a single-photon tracer of this kind used in imaging is $^{123}I$ with a half-life of 13 hours.

The daughter emits additional energy as γ-photons. Similar to β⁻ emission it can be metastable, which is characterized by a delayed decay.

### Positron emission (β⁺ decay)

A proton is transformed essentially into a neutron and a positron (or anti-electron):

$$_{Z}^{A}X \rightarrow _{Z-1}^{A}Y + e^{+}$$
$$p^{+} \rightarrow n + e^{+}. \tag{5.5}$$

After a very short time ($\sim 10^{-9}$ s) and within a few millimeters of the site of its origin, the positron hits an electron and *annihilates* (Figure 5.1). The mass of the two particles is converted into energy, which is emitted as two photons. These photons are emitted in opposite directions. Each photon has an energy of 511 keV, which is the rest mass of an electron or positron. This physical principle is the basis of positron emission tomography (PET). An example of a positron emitter used in imaging is $^{18}$F with a half-life of 109 minutes.

As in $\beta^-$ emission and EC, the daughter nucleus may further emit $\gamma$-photons, but they have no diagnostic purpose in PET.

As a rule of thumb, light atoms tend to emit positrons, and heavy ones tend to prefer other modes, but there are exceptions.

## Statistics

In nuclear medicine imaging, the number of detected photons is generally much smaller than in X-ray imaging. Consequently, noise plays a more important role here, and the imaging process is often considered to be stochastic.

The exact moment at which an atom decays cannot be predicted. All that is known is its decay probability per time unit, which is an isotope dependent constant $\alpha$. Consequently, the decay per time unit is

$$\frac{\mathrm{d}N(t)}{\mathrm{d}t} = -\alpha N(t), \tag{5.6}$$

where $N(t)$ is the number of radioactive isotopes at time $t$. Solving this differential equation yields (see Figure 5.2)

$$N(t) = N(t_0)e^{-\alpha(t-t_0)} = N(t_0)e^{-(t-t_0)/\tau}. \tag{5.7}$$

$\tau = 1/\alpha$ is the *time constant* of the exponential decay. Note that $N(t)$ is the expected value. During a measurement a different value may be found because the process is statistical. The larger $N$ is, the better the estimate will be. Using Eq. (5.7) and replacing $t$ by the *half-life* $T_{1/2}$ and $t_0$ by 0 yields

$$N(T_{1/2}) = N(0)e^{-T_{1/2}/\tau} = \frac{1}{2}N(0)$$

$$-T_{1/2}/\tau = \ln\frac{1}{2} = -\ln 2$$

$$T_{1/2} = \tau \ln 2 = 0.69\tau. \tag{5.8}$$

Depending on the isotope the half-life varies between fractions of seconds and billions of years.

Note that the presence of radioactivity in the body depends not only on the radioactive decay but also on biological excretion. Assuming a biological half-life $T_B$, the effective half-life $T_E$ can be calculated as

$$\frac{1}{T_E} = \frac{1}{T_B} + \frac{1}{T_{1/2}}. \tag{5.9}$$

Currently the preferred unit of radioactivity is the becquerel (Bq). The curie (Ci) is the older unit.* One Bq means one expected event per second and 1 mCi = 37 MBq. Typical doses in imaging are on the order of $10^2$ MBq.

It can be shown that the probability of measuring $n$ photons when $r$ photons are expected, equals

$$p_r(n) = \frac{e^{-r}r^n}{n!}. \tag{5.10}$$

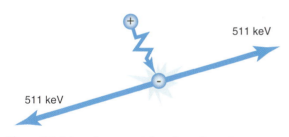

511 keV

511 keV

**Figure 5.1** Schematic representation of a positron–electron annihilation. When a positron comes in the neighborhood of an electron, the two particles are converted into a pair of photons, each of 511 keV, which travel in opposite directions.

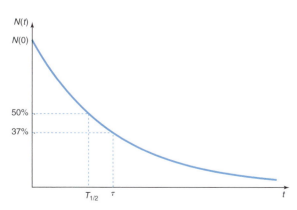

**Figure 5.2** Exponential decay. $\tau$ is the time constant and $T_{1/2}$ the half-life.

* Marie and Pierre Curie and Antoine Becquerel received the Nobel Prize in 1903 for their discovery of radioactivity in 1896.

This is a *Poisson distribution* in which $r$ is the average number of expected photons and $\sqrt{r}$ is the standard deviation. $r$ is also the value with the highest probability. Hence, the signal-to-noise ratio (SNR) becomes

$$\text{SNR} = \frac{r}{\sqrt{r}} = \sqrt{r}. \qquad (5.11)$$

Obviously, the SNR becomes larger with longer measurements.

For large $r$, a Poisson distribution can be well approximated by a Gaussian with the same mean and standard deviation. For small values of $r$, the distribution becomes asymmetrical, because the probability is always zero for negative values.

# Interaction of $\gamma$-photons and particles with matter

## Interaction of particles with matter

Particles, such as $\alpha$- and $\beta$-particles, interact with tissue by losing their kinetic energy along a straight trajectory through the tissue (Figure 5.3). This straight track is called the range $R$. In tissue $R_\alpha$ is on the order of 0.01 to 0.1 mm, while $R_\beta$ is typically a few millimeters.

## Interaction of $\gamma$-photons with matter

As in X-ray imaging, the two most important photon–electron interactions (i.e., Compton scatter and photoelectric absorption) attenuate the emitted $\gamma$-rays.

If initially $N(a)$ photons are emitted in point $s = a$ along the $s$-axis, the number of photons $N(d)$ in the detector at position $s = d$ along the $s$-axis is

$$N(d) = N(a)\, e^{-\int_a^d \mu(s)\,\mathrm{d}s}, \qquad (5.12)$$

where $\mu$ is the linear absorption coefficient. Obviously, the attenuation of a photon depends on the position $s = a$ where it is emitted. Note that it also depends on the attenuating tissue and on the energy of the photons. For example, for photons emitted by $^{99\mathrm{m}}$Tc

(140 keV) the median of the penetration depth in water is about 4.5 cm.

In PET, a pair of photons of 511 keV each has to be detected. Because both photons travel independently through the tissue, the detection probabilities must be multiplied. Assume that one detector is positioned in $s = d_1$, the second one in $s = d_2$, and a point source is located in $s = a$ somewhere between the two detectors. Assume further that during a measurement $N(a)$ photon pairs are emitted along the $s$-axis. The number of detected pairs then is

$$N(d_1, d_2) = N(a)\, e^{-\int_{d_1}^a \mu(s)\,\mathrm{d}s}\, e^{-\int_a^{d_2} \mu(s)\,\mathrm{d}s}$$

$$= N(a)\, e^{-\int_{d_1}^{d_2} \mu(s)\,\mathrm{d}s}. \qquad (5.13)$$

In contrast to SPECT, the attenuation in PET is identical for each point along the projection line.

## Data acquisition

Photon detection hardware in nuclear medicine differs considerably from that used in CT. In CT, a large number of photons must be acquired in a very short measurement. In emission tomography, a very small number of photons is acquired in a longer time interval. Consequently, emission tomography detectors are optimized for sensitivity.

## The detector

### Detecting the photon

Photomultiplier tubes coupled to a scintillation crystal are still very common today. Newer detectors are *photodiodes*, coupled to a scintillator, and *photoconductors* (e.g., CZT), which directly convert X-ray photons into an electrical conductivity (see also p. 35).

A scintillation crystal absorbs the photon via photoelectric absorption. The resulting electron travels through the crystal while distributing its kinetic energy over a few thousand electrons in multiple collisions. These electrons release their energy in the form of a photon of a few electronvolts. These photons are

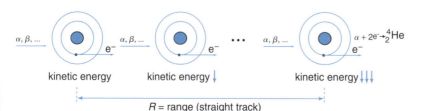

**Figure 5.3** Interaction of particles with matter. The particles are slowed down along a straight track while releasing their kinetic energy.

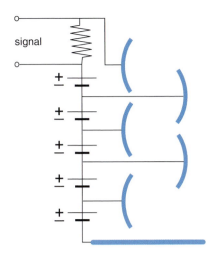

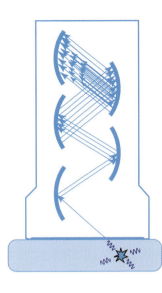

**Figure 5.4** Photomultiplier. Left: the electrical scheme. Right: scintillation photons from the crystal initiate an electric current to the dynode, which is amplified in subsequent stages.

visible to the human eye, which explains the term "scintillation."

Because the linear attenuation coefficient increases with the atomic number $Z$ (see Eq. (2.12)), the scintillation crystal must have a high $Z$. Also, the higher the photon energy, the higher $Z$ should be because the probability of interaction decreases with increasing energy. In single-photon imaging, $^{99m}$Tc is the tracer used most often. It has an energy of 140 keV, and the gamma camera performance is often optimized for this energy. Obviously, PET cameras have to be optimized for 511 keV. Many scintillators exist and extensive research on new scintillators is still going on. The crystals that are most often used today are NaI(Tl) for single photons (140 keV) in gamma camera and SPECT, and BGO (bismuth germanate), GSO (gadolinium silicate) and LSO (lutetium oxyorthosilicate) for annihilation photons (511 keV) in PET.

A *photomultiplier tube* (PMT) consists of a photocathode on top, followed by a cascade of dynodes (Figure 5.4). The PMT is glued to the crystal. Because the light photons should reach the photocathode of the PMT, the crystal must be transparent to the visible photons. The energy of the photons hitting the photocathode releases some electrons from the cathode. These electrons are then accelerated toward the positively charged dynode nearby. They arrive with higher energy (the voltage difference × the charge), activating additional electrons. Because the voltage becomes systematically higher for subsequent dynodes, the number of electrons increases in every stage,

finally producing a measurable signal. Because the multiplication in every stage is constant, the final signal is proportional to the number of scintillation photons, which in turn is proportional to the energy of the original photon. Hence, a $\gamma$-photon is detected, and its energy can also be measured.

### Collimation

In radiography and X-ray tomography, the position of the point source is known and every detected photon provides information about a line that connects the source with the detection point. This is called the projection line. In nuclear medicine, the source has an unknown spatial distribution. Unless some collimation is applied, the detected photons do not contain information about this distribution.

In single-photon detection (SPECT), collimation is done with a mechanical collimator, which is essentially a thick lead plate with small holes (Figure 5.5(a)). The metal plate absorbs all the photons that do not propagate parallel to the axis of the holes. Obviously, most photons are absorbed, and the sensitivity suffers from this approach.

In PET, mechanical collimation is not needed. Both photons are detected with an electronic coincidence circuit (Figure 5.5(b)), and because they propagate in opposite directions, their origin must lie along the line that connects the detection points. This technique is called "coincidence detection" or "electronic collimation." Although in PET two photons instead of one must resist the absorption process, the

109

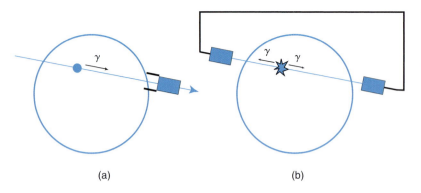

**Figure 5.5** Principle of collimation in **(a)** SPECT and **(b)** PET. In SPECT collimation is done with mechanical collimators, while in PET photon pairs are detected by electronic coincidence circuits connecting pairs of detectors.

(a)　　　　　(b)

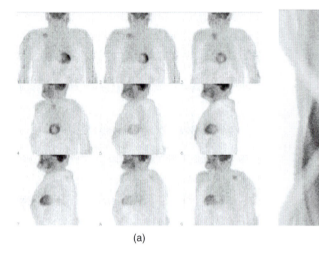

(a)　　　　　(b)

**Figure 5.6** Raw PET data organized as projections **(a)** and as a sinogram **(b)**. Typically, there are a few hundred projections, one for each projection angle, and about a hundred sinograms, one for each slice through the patient's body. (Courtesy of the Department of Nuclear Medicine.)

sensitivity in PET is higher than that of single-photon imaging systems because no photons are absorbed by a lead collimator.

In summary, both in PET and in SPECT, information about lines is acquired. As in CT, these projection lines are used as input to the reconstruction algorithm. Figure 5.6 shows an example of the raw data, which can be organized as projections or as sinograms.

### Photon position

To increase the sensitivity, the detector area around the patient should be as large as possible. A large detector can be constructed by covering one side of a single large crystal (e.g., $50 \times 40 \times 1$ cm) with a dense matrix (30 to 70) of PMTs (a few centimeters width each). Light photons from a single scintillation are picked up by multiple PMTs. The energy is then measured as the sum of all PMT outputs. The position $(x, y)$ where the

photon hits the detector is recovered as

$$ x = \frac{\sum_i x_i S_i}{\sum_i S_i}, \qquad y = \frac{\sum_i y_i S_i}{\sum_i S_i}, \qquad (5.14) $$

where $i$ is the PMT index, $(x_i, y_i)$ the position of the PMT, and $S_i$ the integral of the PMT output over the scintillation duration. In this case, the spatial resolution is limited by statistical fluctuations in the PMT output.

In a single large crystal design, all PMTs contribute to the detection of a single scintillation. Consequently, two photons hitting the crystal simultaneously yield an incorrect position and energy. Hence, the maximum count rate is limited by the decay time of the scintillation event. Multiple, optically separated, crystal modules (e.g., 50 mm × 50 mm), connected to a few (e.g. 2 × 2) PMTs, offer a solution to this problem. The different modules operate in parallel, this way yielding much higher count rates than a single crystal design. PET detectors typically use separate crystal modules while in SPECT, where the count rates are typically lower than in PET, most detectors consist of a single large crystal. More details are given in the section on equipment below (p. 117).

## Number of photons detected

Assume a spatial distribution of tracer activity $\lambda(s)$ along the $s$-axis. In Eqs. (5.12) and (5.13), $N(a)$ must then be replaced by $\lambda(s)\,ds$ and integrated along the projection line $s$. For SPECT, we obtain

$$N(d) = \int_{-\infty}^{+\infty} \lambda(s) e^{-\int_s^d \mu(\xi)\,d\xi}\,ds, \qquad (5.15)$$

and for PET,

$$N(d_1, d_2) = e^{-\int_{d_1}^{d_2} \mu(s)\,ds} \int_{-\infty}^{+\infty} \lambda(s)\,ds. \qquad (5.16)$$

In PET the attenuation is identical for each point along the projection line. Hence, the measured projections are a simple scaling of the unattenuated projections. In SPECT, however, attenuation is position dependent, and no simple relation exists between attenuated and unattenuated projections. Image reconstruction is therefore more difficult in SPECT than in PET, as will be explained on p. 112.

## Energy resolution

As mentioned earlier, an estimate of the energy of the impinging photon is computed by integrating the output of the PMTs. The precision of that estimate is called the "energy resolution." The number of electrons activated in a scintillation event is subject to statistical noise. The time delay after which each electron releases the scintillation light photon is also a random number. Also, the direction in which these light photons are emitted is unpredictable. Consequently, the PMT output is noisy and limits the energy resolution. The energy resolution is usually quantified as the FWHM of the energy distribution and is expressed as a percentage of the photopeak value. It ranges from 10% FWHM in NaI(Tl) to 15% FWHM in LSO and GSO, to over 20% FWHM in BGO. Hence, the energy resolution is 14 keV for a 140 keV photon detected in NaI(Tl) and 130 keV for a 511 keV photon detected in BGO.

## Count rate

In nuclear medicine, radioactive doses are kept low for the patient because of the long exposure times. The detectors have been designed to measure low activity levels and detect individual photons. On the other hand, these devices cannot be used for high activity levels even if this would be desirable. Indeed, the probability that two or more photons arrive at the same time increases with increasing activity. In that case, the localization electronics compute an incorrect single position somewhere between the actual scintillation points. Fortunately, the camera also computes the total energy, which is higher than normal, and these events are discarded. Hence, a photon can only be detected successfully if no other photon arrives while the first one is being detected. The probability that no other photon arrives can be calculated from the Poisson expression (5.10):

$$p(0|\eta N\tau) = e^{-\eta N\tau}, \qquad (5.17)$$

where $\eta$ represents the overall sensitivity of the camera, $N$ the activity in becquerels, and $\tau$ is the detection time in seconds. The detection probability thus decreases exponentially with increasing activity in front of the camera!

Obviously, a high value for $\eta$ is preferred. Therefore, it is important to keep $\tau$ as small as possible. The gamma camera and PET camera must therefore process the incoming photons very quickly. For typical medical applications, the current machines are sufficiently fast.

# Imaging
## Planar imaging

Planar images are simply the raw single-photon projection data. Hence, each pixel corresponds to the projection along a line $s$ (see Eq. (5.15)). Its gray value is proportional to the total amount of attenuated activity along that line. To some extent a planar image can be compared with an X-ray image because all the depth information is lost. Figure 5.7 shows an anterior and posterior whole-body ($^{99m}$Tc-MDP) image acquired with a dual-head gamma camera.

## Fourier reconstruction and filtered backprojection

Assume a spatial distribution of tracer activity $\lambda(s)$ along the $s$-axis. Hence, the number of detected

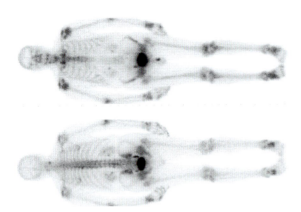

**Figure 5.7** $^{99m}$Tc-MDP study acquired with a dual-head gamma camera. The detector size is about $40 \times 50$ cm, and the whole-body images are acquired with slow translation of the patient bed. MDP accumulates in bone, yielding images of increased bone metabolism. As a result of the attenuation, the spine is more visible in the lower, posterior image. (Courtesy of Department of Nuclear Medicine.)

photons for SPECT is given by Eq. (5.15) and for PET by Eq. (5.16). In both equations, there is an attenuation factor that prevents straightforward application of Fourier reconstruction or filtered backprojection (which are very successful in CT). For example, at 140 keV, every 5 cm of tissue absorbs about 50% of the photons. Hence, in order to apply the projection theorem, this attenuation effect must be corrected.

In Chapter 3 on CT, we have already seen how to measure and calculate the linear attenuation coefficient $\mu$ by means of a transmission scan. In order to measure the attenuation, an external radioactive source that rotates around the patient can be used. The SPECT or PET system thus performs a transmission measurement just like a CT scanner. If the external source in position $d_1$ emits $N_0$ photons along the $s$-axis, the detected fraction of photons at the other side of the patient in position $d_2$ is

$$\frac{N(d_2)}{N_0} = e^{-\int_{d_1}^{d_2} \mu(s)\,ds}. \tag{5.18}$$

This is exactly the attenuation factor for PET in Eq. (5.16). It means that a correction for the attenuation in PET can be performed by multiplying the emission measurement $N(d_1, d_2)$ with the factor $N_0/N(d_2)$. Consequently, Fourier reconstruction or filtered backprojection can be applied.

For SPECT, however, this is not possible. In the literature it has been shown that under certain conditions, the projection theorem can still be used

(i.e., if the attenuation is assumed to be a known constant within a convex body contour (such as the head)). Often, a fair body contour can be obtained by segmenting a reconstructed image obtained without attenuation correction. An alternative solution is to use iterative reconstruction, as discussed below. However, in clinical practice, attenuation is often simply ignored, and filtered backprojection is straightforwardly applied. This results in severe reconstruction artifacts. Nevertheless, it turns out that these images still provide very valuable diagnostic information for an experienced physician.

## Iterative reconstruction

The attenuation problem in SPECT is not the only reason to approach the reconstruction as an iterative procedure. Indeed, the actual acquisition data differ considerably from ideal projections because they suffer from a significant amount of Poisson noise, yielding hampering streak artifacts (cf. Figure 3.21(b) for CT).

Several iterative algorithms exist. In this text, a Bayesian description of the problem is assumed, yielding the popular maximum-likelihood (ML) and maximum-a-posteriori (MAP) algorithms. It is further assumed that both the solution and the measurements are discrete values.

### Bayesian approach

Assume that a reconstructed image $\Lambda$ is computed from the measurement $Q$. Bayes' rule states

$$p(\Lambda|Q) = \frac{p(Q|\Lambda)p(\Lambda)}{p(Q)}. \tag{5.19}$$

The function $p(\Lambda|Q)$ is the posterior probability, $p(\Lambda)$ the prior probability and $p(Q|\Lambda)$ the likelihood. Maximizing $p(\Lambda|Q)$ is called the *maximum-a-posteriori probability* (MAP) approach. It yields the most likely solution given a measurement $Q$.

When maximizing $p(\Lambda|Q)$, the probability $p(Q)$ is constant and can be ignored. Because it is not trivial to find good mathematical expressions for the prior probability $p(\Lambda)$, it is often also assumed to be constant (i.e., it is assumed that a priori all possible solutions have the same probability to be correct). Maximizing $p(\Lambda|Q)$ is then reduced to maximizing the likelihood $p(Q|\Lambda)$. This is called the *maximum-likelihood* (ML) approach.

## Maximum likelihood (ML)

The measurements $Q$ are measurements $q_i$ of the attenuated projections $r_i$ in detector position $i$. The reconstruction image $\Lambda$ is the regional activity $\lambda_j$ in each pixel $j$. The numerical relation between $r_i$ and $\lambda_j$ can be written as

$$r_i = \sum_{j=1,J} c_{ij}\lambda_j, \quad i = 1, I. \tag{5.20}$$

The value $c_{ij}$ represents the sensitivity of detector $i$ for activity in $j$, which includes the attenuation of the $\gamma$-rays from $j$ to $i$. If we have a perfect collimation, $c_{ij}$ is zero everywhere except for the pixels $j$ that are intersected by projection line $i$, yielding a sparse matrix $C$. This notation is very general, and allows us, for example, to take the finite acceptance angle of the mechanical collimator into account, which would increase the fraction of nonzero $c_{ij}$. Similarly, if the attenuation is known, it can be taken into account when computing $c_{ij}$.

Because it can be assumed that the data are samples from a Poisson distribution, the likelihood of measuring $q_i$ if $r_i$ photons on average are expected (see Eq. (5.10)) can be computed as

$$p(q_i|r_i) = \frac{e^{-r_i} r_i^{q_i}}{q_i!}. \tag{5.21}$$

Because the history of one photon (emission, trajectory, possible interaction with electrons, possible detection) is independent of that of the other photons, the overall probability is the product of the individual probabilities:

$$p(Q|\Lambda) = \prod_i \frac{e^{-r_i} r_i^{q_i}}{q_i!}. \tag{5.22}$$

Obviously, this is a very small number: for example, for $r_i = 15$ the maximum value of $p(q_i|r_i)$ is 0.1. For larger $r_i$, the maximum value of $p$ is even smaller. In a measurement for a single slice, we have on the order of 10 000 detector positions $i$, and the maximum likelihood value is on the order of $10^{-10\,000}$.

When calculating the argument $\Lambda$ that maximizes $p(Q|\Lambda)$, the data $q_i!$ are constant and can be ignored. Hence,

$$\arg\max_{\Lambda} p(Q|\Lambda) = \arg\max_{\Lambda} \prod_i e^{-r_i} r_i^{q_i}. \tag{5.23}$$

Because the logarithm is monotonically increasing, maximizing the log-likelihood function also maximizes $p(Q|\Lambda)$, that is,

$$\arg\max_{\Lambda} p(Q|\Lambda) = \arg\max_{\Lambda} \ln p(Q|\Lambda)$$

$$= \arg\max_{\Lambda} \sum_i (q_i \ln(r_i) - r_i)$$

$$= \arg\max_{\Lambda} \sum_i \left( q_i \ln(\sum_j c_{ij}\lambda_j) - \sum_j c_{ij}\lambda_j \right). \tag{5.24}$$

It turns out that the Hessian (the matrix of second derivatives) is negative definite if the matrix $c_{ij}$ has maximum rank. In practice, this means that the likelihood function has a single maximum, provided that a sufficient number of different detector positions $i$ are used.

To solve Eq. (5.24) and calculate $\lambda_j$, the partial derivatives are put to zero:

$$\frac{\partial}{\partial \lambda_j} \sum_i \left( q_i \ln(\sum_j c_{ij}\lambda_j) - \sum_j c_{ij}\lambda_j \right)$$

$$= \sum_i c_{ij} \left( \frac{q_i}{\sum_j c_{ij}\lambda_j} - 1 \right) = 0, \quad \forall j = 1, J. \tag{5.25}$$

This system can be solved iteratively. A popular method with guaranteed convergence is the *expectation-maximization* (EM) algorithm. Although the algorithm is simple, the underlying theory is not and is beyond the scope of this textbook.

Because the amount of radioactivity must be kept low, the number of detected photons is also low, yielding a significant amount of Poisson noise, which strongly deteriorates the projection data. Although the ML–EM algorithm takes Poisson noise into account, it attempts to find the most likely solution, which is an image whose calculated projections are as similar as possible to the measured projections. The consequence is that it converges to a noisy reconstructed image.

To suppress the noise, the measured projections must not be smoothed because this would destroy their Poisson nature used by the reconstruction algorithm. Several alternatives exist as follows.

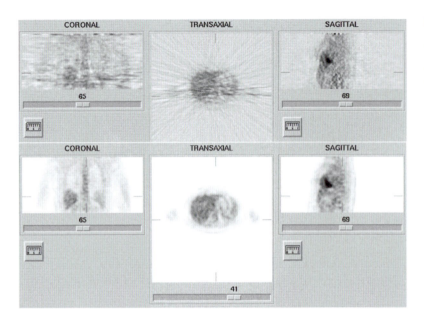

**Figure 5.8** Reconstruction obtained with filtered backprojection (top) and maximum-likelihood expectation-maximization (34 iterations) (bottom). The streak artifacts in the filtered backprojection image are due to the statistical Poisson noise on the measured projection (cf. Figure 3.21(b) for X-ray CT.) (Courtesy of the Department of Nuclear Medicine.)

- The reconstructed image can be smoothed.
- Another approach is to interrupt the iterations before convergence. The ML–EM algorithm has the remarkable characteristic that low frequencies converge faster than high ones. Terminating early has an effect comparable to low-pass filtering. This approach was applied to obtain the image shown in Figure 5.8.
- It is also possible to define some prior probability function that encourages smooth solutions. This yields a *maximum-a-posteriori* (MAP) algorithm, discussed below.

### Maximum-a-posteriori probability (MAP)

The ML approach assumes that the prior probability $p(\Lambda)$ is constant. Consequently, the argument $\Lambda$ that maximizes the posterior probability $p(\Lambda|Q)$ also maximizes the likelihood $p(Q|\Lambda)$. However, if prior knowledge of the tracer activity $\Lambda$ is known, it can be used to improve the quality of the reconstructed image. Starting from Eq. (5.19) the goal then is to find

$$\arg\max_{\Lambda} p(\Lambda\,|Q) = \arg\max_{\Lambda}(\ln p(Q|\Lambda) + \ln p(\Lambda))$$
(5.26)

where $\ln p(Q|\Lambda)$ is defined in Eq. (5.24). $\ln p(\Lambda)$ can be defined as

$$p(\Lambda) = \frac{e^{-E(\Lambda)}}{\sum_{\Lambda} e^{-E(\Lambda)}}.$$
(5.27)

where $E(\Lambda)$ is the so-called Gibbs energy (see also p. 176). Equation (5.26) then becomes

$$\arg\max_{\Lambda} p(\Lambda\,|Q) = \arg\max_{\Lambda}(\ln p(Q|\Lambda) - E(\Lambda)).$$
(5.28)

If, for example, neighboring pixels have similar activity, $E(\Lambda)$ can be defined as

$$E(\Lambda) = \sum_{j}\sum_{k \in N_j} \Phi(\lambda_j, \lambda_k)$$
(5.29)

where $N_j$ is a small neighborhood of $j$ and $\Phi(\lambda_j, \lambda_k)$ is a function that increases with the amount of dissimilarity between $\lambda_j$ and $\lambda_k$. This way Eq. (5.28) yields a smooth solution.

Prior anatomical knowledge can also be taken into account this way. For example, in Figure 5.9 a high-resolution anatomical image was segmented into different tissue classes (gray matter, white matter, cerebrospinal fluid, etc.) using the method of statistical pixel classification explained in Chapter 7, p. 167. During the iterative reconstruction process it can be required that pixels belonging to the same tissue class have a similar tracer activity. This can be obtained by restricting $N_j$ in Eq. (5.29) to the local neighborhood of $j$ with an identical tissue label as that of pixel $j$. This way the tracer activity, measured at low resolution, is iteratively forced back within its expected high-resolution tissue boundaries.

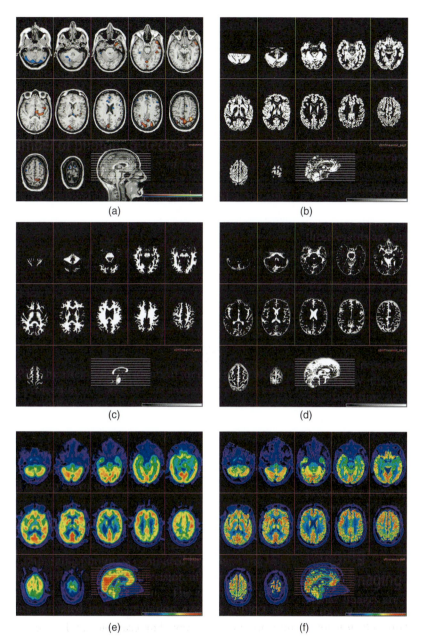

**Figure 5.9** **(a)** $T_1$ MRI image of the brain with overlaid color subtraction SPECT (i.e., ictal minus interictal). The colored patterns are potential indications of epileptic activity. An ictal SPECT shows the brain perfusion during and an interictal SPECT in between epileptic seizures. **(b,c,d)** Segmented images of respectively the gray matter, white matter and CSF. **(e)** PET image obtained by conventional reconstruction. **(f)** PET image obtained by anatomy based MAP reconstruction. (Courtesy of Dr. K. Baete, Department of Nuclear Medicine.)

# 3D reconstruction

In SPECT with parallel hole collimation and in 2D PET the reconstruction problem is two dimensional and the above methods can be applied directly. However, there exist acquisition configurations that do not allow the problem to be reduced to a slice-by-slice reconstruction without approximations.

- There are many different geometries of mechanical collimators in SPECT. One example is the cone-beam collimator. It has a single focal point. Hence, all the projection lines that arrive at the 2D detector intersect in this point, and exact reconstruction from cone-beam data requires true 3D methods.

- In 3D PET all possible projection lines that intersect the detector surface (coincidence lines) are

**115**

used, both parallel and oblique to the transaxial plane. This 3D acquisition has the advantage that more data are obtained from each radioactive pixel, thus reducing the noise.

In these cases, the reconstruction program needs to compute the entire volume using all data simultaneously. This is often called true 3D reconstruction. Three currently used 3D reconstruction approaches are discussed below.

### Filtered backprojection

Filtered backprojection can be extended to true 3D reconstruction for PET. This is only possible if the sequence of projection and backprojection results in a shift-invariant point spread function. That is only true if every point in the reconstruction volume is intersected by the same configuration of measured projection lines, which is not the case in practice. Points near the edge of the field of view are intersected by fewer measured projection lines. In this case, the data may be completed by computing the missing projections as follows. First, a subset of projections that meets the requirement is selected and reconstructed to compute an initial, relatively noisy, reconstruction image. Next, this reconstruction is forward projected along the missing projection lines to compute an estimate of the missing data. Then, the computed and measured data are combined into a single set of data that now meets the requirement of shift-invariance. Finally, this completed dataset is reconstructed with true 3D filtered backprojection.

### ML reconstruction

The ML approach can be applied to the 3D dataset directly. The formulation is very general, and the coefficients $c_{ij}$ in Eq. (5.20) can be used to describe true 3D projection lines. Because the number of calculations in each iteration increases with the number of projection lines, the computational burden becomes quite heavy for a true 3D reconstruction.

### Fourier rebinning

Fourier rebinning converts a set of 3D data into a set of 2D projections. It is based on a property of the Fourier transform of the sinograms. It has also been shown that the Poisson nature of the data is more or less preserved. The resulting 2D set can then be reconstructed with the 2D ML–EM algorithm. In practice, however, the exact rebinning algorithm is not used. Instead, an approximate expression is employed because it is much faster and is sufficiently accurate for most configurations.

## Image quality
### Contrast

The contrast is mainly determined by the characteristics of the tracer and the amount of scatter. The specificity of a tracer for a particular metabolic process is usually not 100%. For example, for most tracers the blood concentration decreases rapidly but is typically not zero during the study. Consequently, the blood concentration produces a "background" tracer uptake, which decreases the contrast. Scattered photons also produce a background radiation that reduces the contrast.

## Spatial resolution

In nuclear medicine the resolution is mostly expressed as the full width at half maximum (FWHM) of the PSF.

In PET, the overall FWHM in the reconstructed image is about 4 to 8 mm. The spatial resolution is mainly limited by the following factors.

- *The positron range* A positron can only annihilate when its kinetic energy is sufficiently low. While reducing its energy by collisions with the electrons of surrounding atoms, the positron travels over a certain distance. The average distance depends on the isotope and is on the order of 0.2 to 2 mm.

- *The deviation from 180°* The annihilation photons are not emitted in exactly opposite directions. There is a deviation of about 0.3°, which corresponds to 2.8 mm for a camera of 1 m diameter.

- *The detector resolution* This is often called the "intrinsic" resolution. The size of the individual detector crystals is currently about 4 mm × 4 mm. This limits the intrinsic resolution to about 2 to 3 mm. If the detection is done with a single large crystal, the resolution is usually about 4 mm.

In SPECT, the overall FWHM in the reconstructed image is about 1 to 1.5 cm. The spatial resolution is affected by the following.

- *The detector resolution* This is comparable to PET.
- *The collimator resolution* The collimator is designed to select photons that propagate along a thin line. However, it has finite dimensions and, as

a result, it accepts all the photons that arrive from within a small solid angle. Therefore, the FWHM of the PSF increases linearly with increasing distance to the collimator. At 10 cm, the FWHM is on the order of 1 cm, and in the image center around 1.5 cm. The collimator resolution dominates the SPECT spatial resolution.

## Noise

We have already seen that Poisson noise contributes significantly to the measurements. The ML–EM reconstruction algorithm takes this into account and inherently limits the influence of this noise by terminating the procedure after a few tens of iterations.

Another noise factor is due to Compton scatter. It produces a secondary photon that is deflected from the original trajectory into a new direction. Some of the scattered photons reach the detector via this broken line. Such a contribution to the measurement is undesired, and a good camera suppresses this as much as possible. The system can reject scattered photons based on their energy. As compared to primary photons, the scattered photons have a lower energy, which is measured by the detector electronics. However, the energy resolution is finite (10% for Na(Tl)), and some of the scatter is unavoidably accepted. The remaining scatter has a negative effect on the image contrast and the accuracy of quantitative measurements.

## Artifacts

There are many possible causes of artifacts in SPECT and PET. Malfunction of the camera is an important cause and quality control procedures are mandatory to prevent this. However, some artifacts are inherent to the imaging and reconstruction process. The most important influencing factors are attenuation, scatter, noise, and patient motion.

- *Attenuation* Accurate correction for attenuation is only possible if a transmission scan is available. Previously, in stand-alone PET, these were obtained by rotating line sources containing the positron-emitting germanium. This procedure was time consuming and was not performed in some centers. The reconstruction process then assumes that there is no attenuation, which yields severe artifacts. A striking artifact in images which are not corrected for attenuation is the apparent high tracer uptake in the lungs and the skin. There will also be a nonhomogeneous distribution in organs

in which the real distribution is homogenous. In modern combined PET/CT scanners, a whole-body CT scan is obtained and used to construct a 511 keV attenuation map which is used for attenuation correction. This correction might introduce artifacts by itself, specifically if there is a misalignment between the emission data and the CT. Figure 5.10 shows a coronal slice of a whole-body study reconstructed without and with attenuation correction. The study was done to find regions of increased FDG uptake ("hot spots"). Although both images clearly show the hot spots, the contours of the tumor and organs are less accurately defined in the study without attenuation correction. A striking artifact in Figure 5.10(a) is the apparent high tracer uptake in the lungs and the skin.

- *Compton scatter* Scattered photons yield a relatively smooth but nonuniform background uptake.
- *Poisson noise* Using filtered backprojection the statistical noise yields streak artifacts, comparable to those in CT (see Figure 3.21(b)). Iterative reconstruction (p. 112) on the other hand tends to keep the spatial extent of such artifacts quite limited.
- *Patient motion* SPECT and PET are more subject to patient motion than the other imaging modalities because of the longer acquisition time. Pure blurring because of motion appears only if all the projections are acquired simultaneously (i.e., in PET without preceding transmission scan). In attenuation-corrected PET, patient motion destroys the required registration between the emission and transmission data, which results in additional artifacts at the edges of the transmission image (Figure 5.10(c)). In SPECT, patient motion yields inconsistent projections and severe artifacts as well. Many researchers have investigated motion correction algorithms, but the problem is difficult, and so far no reliable method has emerged that can be applied in clinical routine.

## Equipment
### Gamma camera and SPECT scanner

Most gamma cameras use one or more large NaI(Tl) crystals (Figure 5.11). A lead collimator is positioned in front of the crystal. It collimates and also protects the fragile and very expensive crystal. Note, however, that the collimator is fragile as well, and the thin lead

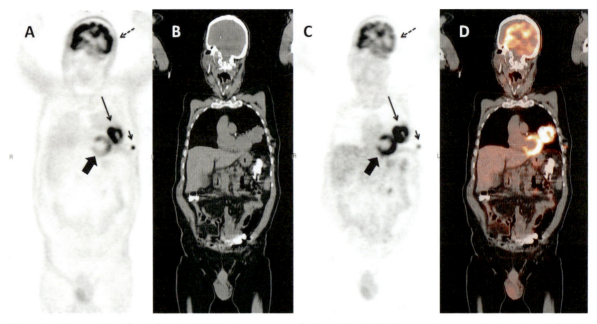

**Figure 5.10** Coronal slice of a whole-body PET/CT study reconstructed without **(a)** and with **(c)** attenuation correction based on whole-body CT **(b)**. The relative intensity of the subcutaneous metastasis (small arrow) compared to the primary tumor (large arrow) is much higher in the noncorrected image than in the corrected one, because the activity in this peripheral lesion is much less attenuated than the activity in the primary tumor. A striking artifact in (a) is the apparent high uptake in the skin and the lungs. Note also that regions of homogenous uptake, such as the heart (thick arrow), are no longer homogenous, but show a gradient. Attenuation correction can lead to artifacts if the correspondence between the emission and transmission data is not perfect. The uptake in the left side of the brain (dotted arrow) is apparently lower than in the contralateral one in (c). The fused data set **(d)** representing the attenuation-corrected PET image registered on the CT image shows that the head did move between the acquisition of the CT and the emission data, resulting in an apparent decrease in activity in the left side of the brain. Courtesy of the Department of Nuclear Medicine

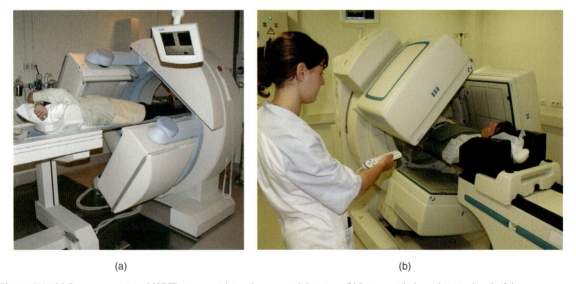

(a)                                                        (b)

**Figure 5.11 (a)** Gamma camera and SPECT scanner with two large crystal detectors. **(b)** System with three detector heads. If the gamma camera rotates around the patient it behaves like a SPECT scanner. Today, the difference between gamma units and SPECT systems has therefore become rather artificial. (Courtesy of the Department of Nuclear Medicine.)

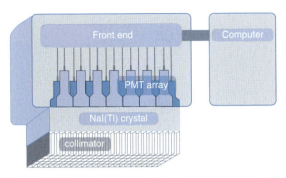

**Figure 5.12** Schematic representation of a gamma camera with a single large scintillation crystal (52 × 37 cm) and parallel hole collimator.

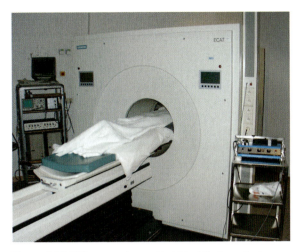

**Figure 5.13** PET scanner. A movable table shifts the patient through the circular hole in the gantry. The external design is similar to that of a CT scanner and to some extent to that of an MRI scanner. (Courtesy of the Department of Nuclear Medicine.)

septa are easily deformed. At the other side of the crystal, an array of PMTs is typically attached to it. Front end electronics interface this PMT array to the computer (Figure 5.12).

For SPECT the detectors are mounted on a flexible gantry (Figure 5.11) since they must rotate over at least 180° around the patient. In addition, the detectors must be as close to the patient as possible because the spatial resolution decreases with the distance from the collimator. Obviously, the sensitivity is proportional to the number of detector heads, and the acquisition time can be decreased with increasing number of detector heads. For some examinations, the body part is too large to be measured in a single scan. Similar to CT, the computer then controls the table and slowly shifts the patient to scan the complete volume.

A camera cannot detect more than one photon at a time, because all PMTs together contribute to that single detection. From the PMT outputs, the front end electronics calculate four values, usually called $x$, $y$, $z$, and $t$.

- $(x, y)$ are the position coordinates. They are computed using Eq. (5.14).
- $z$ is a measure of the photon energy and is computed as $\sum_i S_i$. Because the PMT output is a pulse with a duration of a few hundred nanoseconds, $S_i$ is the integration of this pulse over time: $S_i = \int_{t_0}^{t_1} s_i(t)\, dt$.

  The energy $z$ of detected photons is compared with an energy window $[z_{\min}, z_{\max}]$, which depends on the tracer used. If $z > z_{\max}$, two or more photons hit the crystal simultaneously, messing up the computation of $(x, y)$. If $z < z_{\min}$, the photon is due to Compton scatter and must be discarded.

Some tracers emit photons at two or a few different energy peaks. In this case, multiple energy windows are used.

- $t$ is the detection time and is computed as the moment when the integration of $\sum_i \int_{t_0}^{t} s_i(t)\, dt$ reaches a predefined fraction of $z$.

## PET scanner

Most PET cameras (Figure 5.13) consist of a complete ring (diameter $\approx$ 1 m) of BGO, GSO or LSO crystal modules. In PET, no detector rotation is therefore required. Table motion, however, may still be needed and is comparable to that of a gamma camera.

The detectors are typically small scintillation crystals (e.g., 4 mm × 4 mm) glued together in modular 2D arrays (e.g., 13 × 13) and connected to PMTs (e.g., 2 × 2, a few centimeters width each). These modules are packed on a ring around the field of view. A PET scanner can contain multiple neighboring rings of modules, this way increasing the axial field of view. For example, three rings of 13 × 4 mm each yield an axial FOV of about 16 cm.

The computation of the crystal coordinates $(x, y)$, the energy $z$ and the time $t$ is comparable to that for a large single-crystal detector but is restricted to a single module. This way multiple photons can be detected at the same time by different crystal modules. The detection time $t$ is determined with an accuracy in the range of 1 to 10 ns (in 1 ns light travels about 30 cm), which is

**119**

short as compared to the scintillation decay constant* (300 ns for BGO, 30–60 ns for GSO and 40 ns for LSO; 230 ns for NaI(Tl) in SPECT). The events are discarded only if a single photon is detected or if more than two photons hit the camera within the uncertainty interval. For example, if two photon pairs arrive simultaneously (i.e., within the coincidence timing resolution) at four different modules, they are rejected. Note that, if two photons are detected by the same module within the scintillation decay interval, they are also rejected. This last situation, however, does not happen frequently because of the large amount of crystal modules.

An important problem is the presence of so-called *randoms*. Randoms are photon pairs that do not originate from the same positron but nevertheless hit the camera within the short time interval during which the electronic detection circuit considers this as a coincidence ($\approx$ 1–10 ns). The probability of a random increases with the square of the radioactivity and cannot be ignored. The number of randoms can be estimated with the *delayed* window technique, shown schematically in Figure 5.14. The camera counts the number of detected photon pairs that are obtained with a minimal delay. This short delay time is chosen sufficiently large to guarantee that the two photons do not belong to a single annihilation. This number of guaranteed randoms can be considered independent of the time delay. Consequently, the same amount of randoms can be assumed to appear

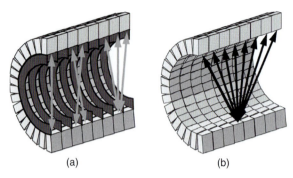

**Figure 5.15** Schematic representation of a PET detector ring cut in half. **(a)** When septa are in the field of view, the camera can be regarded as a series of separate 2D systems. **(b)** Retracting the septa increases the number of projection lines and hence the sensitivity of the system, but true 3D reconstruction is required.

during the measurement of true annihilation pairs and must be subtracted in order to calculate the true coincidences.

Older PET cameras are usually equipped with retractable septa (see Figure 5.15(a)). When the septa are in the field of view, the camera operates in the so-called "2D-mode," and the detector is considered to be a concatenation of independent rings. Only projection lines within parallel planes can be accepted, as the septa absorb photons with oblique trajectories. Recent systems do not contain septa and all the available projection lines are accepted (see Figure 5.15(b)). Reconstruction from these data requires true 3D reconstruction algorithms.

## Hybrid systems

PET and SPECT systems can be combined with a CT or even a MR system. Among these combinations, the PET/CT system (Figure 5.16) is currently the most popular and has become quite common in clinical practice. In this case the CT image is used for attenuation correction. A potential problem is the registration mismatch between the transmission and the emission image due to patient motion during the long duration of the examination (half an hour and more). Nonrigid registration may offer a solution (see Chapter 7, p. 183) but is not straightforward. Another, technical, problem is due to the energy dependence of the linear attenuation coefficient. In PET, for example, the photon energy is 511 keV while an X-ray source in CT transmits an energy spectrum with a maximum energy defined by the tube voltage. For example, a tube with a voltage of 140 kV yields X-ray photons

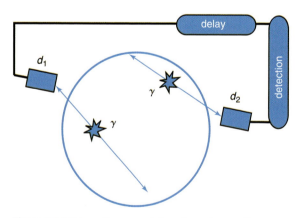

**Figure 5.14** Schematic representation of a random and its detection. One of the two photons is detected with a small time delay.

* Time constant assuming exponential decay, i.e., the moment when the light intensity has returned to $e^{-1}$ of its maximum value.

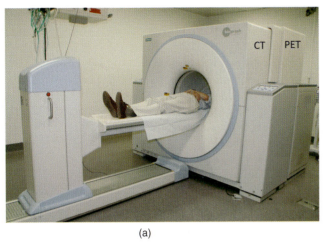 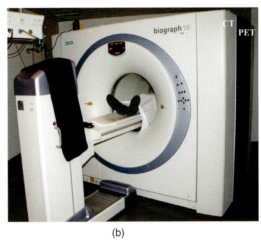

(a)             (b)

**Figure 5.16** A CT and a PET system are linked and integrated into a single gantry and share a common patient bed. Two hybrid PET/CT scanners are shown here. (Courtesy of the Department of Nuclear Medicine.)

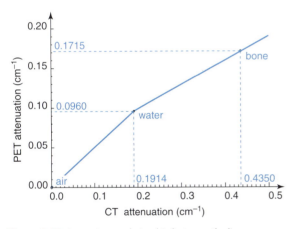

**Figure 5.17** Approximate relationship between the linear attenuation coefficient in CT, operating at 140 kV, and PET. The energy spectrum of the X-ray photons is approximated by a single effective energy of 70 keV. The energy of the PET photons is 511 keV. Tissue is assumed to be a linear mixture of either air and water, or water and bone. The result is a piecewise linear conversion function.

with energy 140 keV and lower. To calculate the attenuation coefficient for the emission image, the X-ray energy spectrum is typically approximated by a single average or *effective* energy. For example, for a voltage of 140 kV the maximum X-ray photon energy is 140 keV and the effective energy is assumed to be 70 keV. Furthermore, the relationship between the attenuation coefficient at 70 keV and at 511 keV is assumed to be piecewise linear (Figure 5.17).

# Time-of-flight (TOF) PET

If the uncertainty in measuring the difference in arrival times of a photon pair is limited to 1 ns or less, it becomes interesting to use this time difference to localize the position of the annihilation along the *line of response* (LOR). The uncertainty $\Delta x$ in the position along the LOR can be calculated from the uncertainty $\Delta t$ in measuring the coincidence, that is,

$$\Delta x = \frac{1}{2} c \, \Delta t. \tag{5.30}$$

More specifically, $\Delta t$ and $\Delta x$ are the FWHM of the uncertainty distributions in time and space respectively (Figure 5.18). A coincidence timing uncertainty $\Delta t$ of 600 ps, for example, yields a positional uncertainty $\Delta x$ of 9 cm along the LOR. Further reducing $\Delta t$ to 100 ps reduces this positional uncertainty $\Delta x$ to 1.5 cm. This information can be fed to the reconstruction algorithm to improve the image quality. Indeed, instead of knowing that the annihilation took place somewhere along the LOR, the expected position along that LOR can now be expressed within a range defined by the spatial uncertainty distribution (FWHM = $\Delta x$).

TOF PET requires proper reconstruction tools. Although ML-based statistical reconstruction can still be used, other algorithms have been developed such as 3D list-mode TOF reconstruction and algorithms that place the events directly into the image space rather

**121**

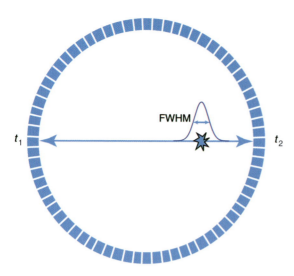

**Figure 5.18** Principle of TOF PET. The position of the annihilation can be calculated from the difference between the arrival times of both photons. The uncertainty in measuring this time difference can be represented by a statistical distribution with FWHM $= \Delta t$. The relationship between $\Delta t$ and $\Delta x$ (FWHM of the spatial uncertainty distribution) is given by Eq. (5.30).

than into the projection space. This theory was pioneered in the 1980s and has recently resurged due to the improvements in detector materials (LSO, LYSO, LaBr$_3$) and electronic stability. A detailed discussion of these advances, however, is beyond the scope of this textbook.

## Clinical use

Nuclear medicine is based on the tracer principle. Small amounts of radioactive-labeled molecules are administered to measure functional parameters of different organs selectively (e.g., perfusion, metabolism, innervation). Many different tracers exist, and the number is still increasing. While gamma cameras need gamma-emitting tracers, PET needs positron emitters. Single-photon emitting atoms tend to be quite heavy. Typical organic molecules do not contain such atoms and must therefore be modified by binding the radioactive atom to the organic molecule. Most molecules are labeled with $^{99m}$Tc (half-life 6 hours) because it is inexpensive and has ideal physical characteristics (short half-life; daughter of $^{99}$Mo, which has a half-life of 66 hours and is continuously available; ideal $\gamma$-ray energy of 140 keV, which is high enough to leave the body but not too high to penetrate the crystal). Other important $\gamma$-emitting radionuclides are $^{123}$I

(half-life 13 hours), $^{131}$I (half-life 8 days), $^{111}$In (half-life 3 days), $^{201}$Tl (half-life 3 days), and $^{67}$Ga (half-life 3 days). Positron emitting tracers are light, have a short half-life, and can be included in organic molecules without modifying their chemical characteristics. The most used in nuclear medicine are $^{11}$C (half-life 20 min), $^{13}$N (half-life 10 min), $^{15}$O (half-life 2 min), and $^{18}$F (half-life 109 min). With the exception of $^{18}$F they have to be produced by a cyclotron in the hospital because of their short half-life.

The most important clinical applications in nuclear medicine are studies of bone metabolism, myocardial perfusion and viability, lung embolism, tumors, and thyroid function.

- *Bone metabolism* For the exploration of bone metabolism a $^{99m}$Tc labeled phosphonate can be used. It accumulates in proportion to bone turnover, which is increased by several pathologies, such as tumors, fractures (Figure 5.19), inflammations, and infections. A SPECT/CT scanner, combining metabolic information of the SPECT and anatomic information of the CT, further improves the diagnostic accuracy of bone disorders.

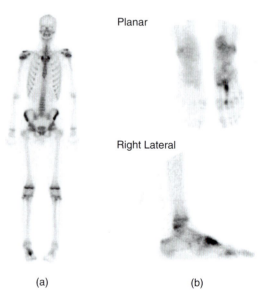

(a)              (b)

**Figure 5.19** Left: whole-body scintigraphy after injection of 25 mCi $^{99m}$Tc-labeled methylene diphosponate. This patient suffers from a stress fracture of the right foot. Right: control scans show an increased uptake in the metatarsal bone II compatible with a local stress fracture. (Courtesy of Professor L. Mortelmans, Department of Nuclear Medicine.)

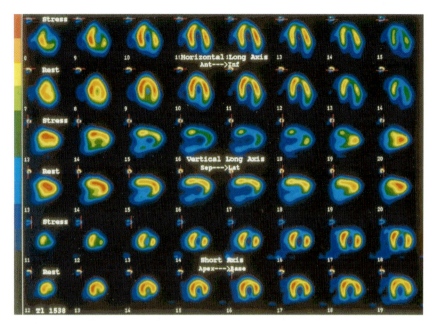

**Figure 5.20** Myocardial perfusion SPECT scan. Rows 1, 3, and 5 show the myocardial perfusion during a typical stress test. Rows 2, 4, and 6 show the rest images acquired 3 hours later. The first two rows are horizontal long-axis slices, the middle two rows are vertical long-axis slices, and the bottom two rows are short-axis slices. This study shows a typical example of transient hypoperfusion of the anterior wall. On the stress images, there is a clear perfusion defect on the anterior wall (horizontal-axis slice 9, vertical long-axis 16 to 18, short-axis slice 13 to 18). The perfusion normalizes on the corresponding rest images. (Courtesy of Professor L. Mortelmans, Department of Nuclear Medicine.)

- *Myocardial perfusion and viability* For myocardial perfusion, tracers are used that are accumulated in the myocardium in proportion to the blood flow. Examples of such tracers are the $\gamma$-emitting tracers $^{201}$Tl and $^{99m}$Tc-Mibi, and the PET tracers $^{13}$NH$_3$ and H$_2^{15}$O. The choice of the imaging modality and tracer depends on factors, such as half-life, image quality, cost, and availability. Often, the imaging process is repeated after several hours to compare the tracer distribution after stress and at rest (Figure 5.20). This procedure answers the question whether there is a transient ischemia during stress. By comparing myocardial perfusion with glucose metabolism, PET is the gold standard to evaluate myocardial viability.

- *Lung embolism* In order to detect lung embolism, $^{99m}$Tc-labeled human serum albumin is injected intravenously. This tracer with a mean diameter of 10–40 $\mu$m sticks in the first capillaries it meets (i.e., in the lungs). Areas of decreased or absent tracer deposit correspond to a pathological perfusion, which is compatible with a lung embolism. The specificity of the perfusion scan can be increased by means of a ventilation scan

(Figure 5.21). Under normal conditions a gas or an aerosol with $^{99m}$Tc-labeled particles is spread homogeneously in the lungs by inhalation. Lung embolism is typically characterized by a mismatch (i.e., a perfusion defect with a normal ventilation). A perfusion CT scan of the lungs has become the first choice technique for diagnosis of lung embolism.

- *Tumors* A very successful tracer for measuring metabolic activity is $^{18}$FDG (fluoro-deoxy-glucose). This molecule traces glucose metabolism. The uptake of this tracer is similar to that of glucose. However, unlike glucose, FDG is only partially metabolized and is trapped in the cell. Consequently, FDG accumulates proportionally to glucose consumption. A tumor is shown as an active area or "hot spot" (Figure 5.22), as in most tumors glucose metabolism is considerably higher than in the surrounding tissue. Whole-body FDG has become a standard technique for the staging of oncologic patients and also for the therapeutic evaluation of chemotherapy and/or radiotherapy.

- *Thyroid function* Captation of $^{99m}$Tc pertechnetate or $^{123}$I iodide shows the tracer distribution

**123**

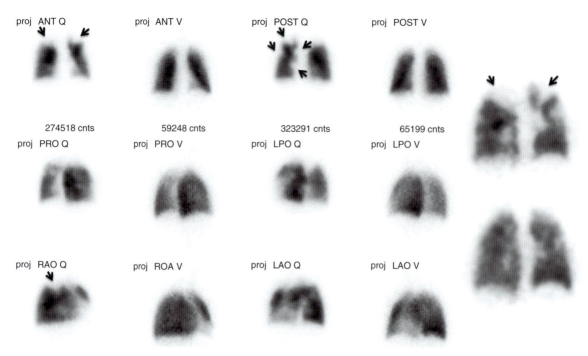

**Figure 5.21** Lung perfusion (Q) and ventilation (V) scan. The second and fourth columns show six planar projections of a ventilation SPECT scan obtained after the inhalation of radioactive pertechnegas distributed homogeneously throughout both lungs. The first and third columns show the corresponding lung perfusion images obtained after injection of $^{99m}$Tc-labeled macroaggregates. Several triangular-shaped defects (arrows) are visible in the perfusion scan with a normal ventilation at the same site. This mismatch between perfusion and ventilation is typical for lung embolism. The fifth column shows a coronal section of the SPECT data set with triangular defects (arrowheads) in the perfusion (upper row) and a normal ventilation (lower row). (Courtesy of Professor L. Mortelmans, Department of Nuclear Medicine.)

within the thyroid, which is a measure of the metabolic function (Figure 5.23). $^{131}$I iodide with a half-life of 8 days is mainly used for treatment of hyperthyroidism (thyroid hyperfunction) or thyroid cancer.

- *Neurological disorders* Brain disorders can be diagnosed using SPECT perfusion scans and PET FDG scans measuring brain metabolism. FDG PET brain scans play an important role in the early and differential diagnosis of dementia (Figure 5.24). New tracers are used for the evaluation of neuroreceptors, transporters, enzymes, etc., allowing more specific diagnosis of several brain disorders. A typical example is the presynaptic dopamine transporter (DAT) scan, measuring the amount of dopamine-producing cells in the substantia nigra and facilitating early and differential diagnosis of Parkinson disease, possibly in combination with postsynaptic dopamine receptor (D2) imaging (Figure 5.25).

## Biologic effects and safety

Unfortunately, tracer molecules are not completely specific for the investigated function and are accumulated in other organs, such as the liver, the kidneys, and the bladder. Furthermore, the radioactive product does not disappear immediately after the imaging procedure but remains in the body for hours or days after the clinical examination is finished. The amount of radioactivity in the body decreases with time because of two effects.

- *Radioactive decay* This decay is exponential. Every half-life, the radioactivity decreases by a factor of two.
- *Biologic excretion* Many tracers are metabolized, and the biologic excretion is often significant as compared with the radioactive decay. It can be intensified with medication. This also means that the bladder receives a high radiation dose, which can

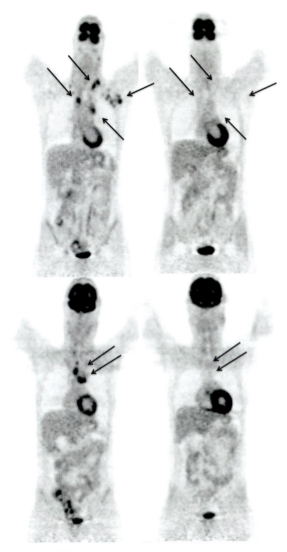

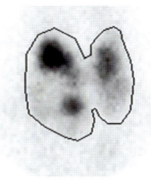

**Figure 5.23** $^{99m}$Tc pertechnetate thyroid scan of a patient with a multinodular goiter. The irregularly enlarged thyroid is delineated. Several zones of normal and increased uptake are visible. Hyperactive zones are seen in the upper and lower pole of the right thyroid lobe. In the right interpolar region there is a zone of relative hypoactivity. (Courtesy of Professor L. Mortelmans, Department of Nuclear Medicine.)

Medicine). Initial tracer concentrations, tracer accumulation, and excretion times must be entered in the simulator, which then computes the radiation load to each organ and derives the effective dose in millisieverts. For the input data, typical values can be used. These values can be defined by repeatedly scanning an injected subject until the radioactivity becomes negligible. Typical doses for a large number of tracers are published by the International Commission on Radiological Protection (ICRP). For example, the effective patient doses of a study of the lung are 0.1–0.5 mSv, the thyroid 0.4–0.7 mSv, bone 1.3 mSv, the myocardium around 5 mSv, and tumors studied with FDG around 6 mSv and gallium 13.0 mSv. Roughly speaking, they have the same order of magnitude as the effective doses for diagnostic radiographic imaging (see p. 31) or CT (see p. 59).

For the patient's entourage, for example the personnel of the nuclear medicine department, it is important to take into account that the radiation dose decreases with the square of the distance to the source and increases with the exposure time. It is therefore recommended that medical personnel stay at a certain distance from radioactive sources, including the patient. Contamination of tracers must be avoided.

## Future expectations

Although continuous technical improvements can be expected (improved TOF and hybrid systems, new detectors, removal of motion artifacts, etc.)

**Figure 5.22** $^{18}$FDG PET scan of a patient suffering from a lymphoma in the mediastinum and the left axilla (left column). The pathological $^{18}$FDG uptake in the lymphomatous lymph nodes (arrows) disappeared after chemotherapy (right column). (Courtesy of Professor L. Mortelmans, Department of Nuclear Medicine.)

amount to more than 50% of the patient's effective dose.

The radiation exposure of a particular organ is a function of the activity in the entire body. Simulation software exists that is based on models for the human body (e.g., the *MIRD model* (medical internal radiation dosimetry) of the Society of Nuclear

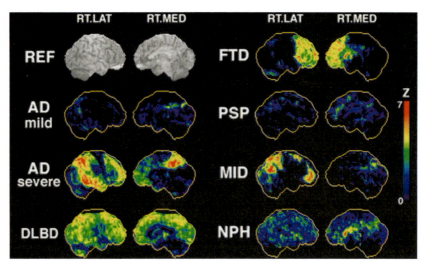

**Figure 5.24** Deviation of FDG uptake with respect to a normal database for different types of "dementias." In the upper left corner, an anatomical MR reference image is shown. AD Alzheimer disease; DLBD Lewy body disease; FTD frontal lobe dementia; PSP progressive supranuclear palsy; MID multi infarct dementia; NPH normal pressure hydrocephalus. (Courtesy of Professor K. Van Laere, Department of Nuclear Medicine.)

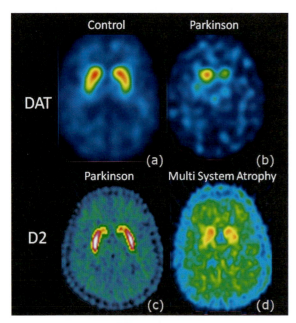

**Figure 5.25** Upper row: $^{123}$I-FP-CIT SPECT scan for presynaptic dopamine transporter (DAT) imaging. Lower row: $^{11}$C-raclopride PET scan for postsynaptic dopamine receptor (D2) imaging. **(a)** Healthy subject. **(b,c)** In an early Parkinson patient a decrease of the dopamine transporter (DAT) is seen in the basal ganglia while the postsynaptic dopamine receptor (D2) is still normal. **(d)** Parkinson patient with multi-system atrophia (MSA). The postsynaptic part of the dopaminergic synapse is also impaired. (Courtesy of Professor K. Van Laere, Department of Nuclear Medicine.)

progression will particularly be stimulated by the development of new generations of tracers.

More clinical indications will be created by labeling new compounds with PET tracers. There is a clear shift from rather aspecific tracers such as FDG to more specific biomarkers that bind to specific receptors. There are also new potentials for therapy with radioactive tracers, especially for the treatment of hematological diseases by means of radioimmunotherapy with labeled antibodies.

Medical imaging is further evolving towards the visualization of biological processes at the cell level. This way cellular function and molecular pathways in vivo can be studied, such as imaging of gene regulation, protein–protein interactions and stem cell tracking. This new discipline, which combines imaging with molecular biology, is called *molecular imaging*. It shifts the focus from imaging the anatomy and function of organs towards imaging the behavior and interaction of molecules. Early disease detection and tracking of gene therapy are among the future applications. Figure 5.26 shows the basic principle of imaging gene expression in vivo. Although this evolution is not limited to nuclear medicine, theoretically emission tomography has the largest potential due to the variety of tracers that can be

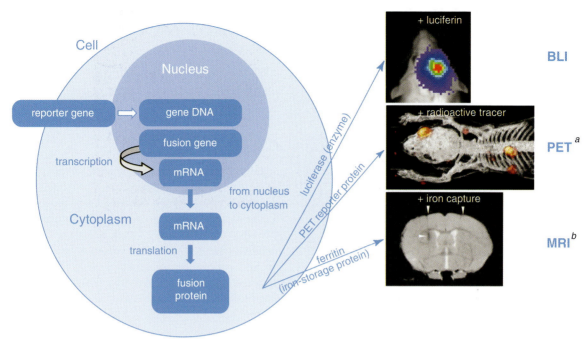

**Figure 5.26** Principle of molecular imaging. A reporter gene is attached to a gene of interest to create a gene fusion, which is copied (transcribed) into a messenger RNA (mRNA) molecule. The mRNA moves from the nucleus to the cytoplasm where its code is used during the synthesis of a protein (translation of mRNA into protein). Depending on the nature of the reporter gene the fusion protein is a reporter protein that is fluorescent (produces light), captures iron (visible in MRI) or interacts with a radioactive tracer (visible in SPECT or PET). (Courtesy of Prof. C. Deroose, Dept. of Nuclear Medicine.)
[a] Reprinted from G. Genove, U. DeMarco, H. Xu, W. F. Goins, and E. T. Ahrens. A new transgene reporter for in vivo magnetic resonance imaging, *Nature Medicine*, **11**(4): 450–454, 2005.
[b] Reprinted from C. M. Deroose, A. De, A. M. Loening, P. L. Chow, P. Ray, A. F. Chatziioannou, and S. S. Gambhir. Multimodality imaging of tumor xenografts and metastases in mice with combined small-animal PET, small-animal CT, and bioluminescence imaging, *Journal of Nuclear Medicine*, **48**(2): 295–303, 2007.

developed. Today most of these techniques are subject to fundamental research. Adapted systems have been developed for imaging small animals, such as mice and rats, in vivo. Because of their small size these scanners are typically labeled with the prefix "micro" (micro-PET/SPECT/CT/MRI/US).

# Chapter

# 6

# Ultrasound imaging

## Introduction

Ultrasound imaging has been used in clinical practice for more than half a century. It is noninvasive, relatively inexpensive, portable, and has an excellent temporal resolution. Imaging by means of acoustic waves is not restricted to medical imaging. It is used in several other applications such as in the field of nondestructive testing of materials to check for microscopic cracks in, for example, airplane wings or bridges, in sound navigation ranging (SONAR) to locate fish, in the study of the seabed or to detect submarines, and in seismology to locate gas fields.

The basic principle of ultrasound imaging is simple. A propagating wave partially reflects at the interface between different tissues. If these reflections are measured as a function of time, information is obtained on the position of the tissue if the velocity of the wave in the medium is known. However, besides reflection, other phenomena such as diffraction, refraction, attenuation, dispersion, and scattering appear when ultrasound propagates through matter. All these effects are discussed below.

Ultrasound imaging is used not only to visualize morphology or anatomy but also to visualize function by means of blood and myocardial velocities. The principle of velocity imaging was originally based on the Doppler effect and is therefore often referred to as Doppler imaging. A well-known example of the Doppler effect is the sudden pitch change of a whistling train when passing a static observer. Based on the observed pitch change, the velocity of the train can be calculated.

Historically, the first practical realization of ultrasound imaging was born during World War I in the quest for detecting submarines. Relatively soon these attempts were followed by echographic techniques adapted to industrial applications for nondestructive testing of metals. Essential to these developments were the publication of *The Theory of Sound* by Lord Rayleigh in 1877 and the discovery of the piezoelectric effect by Pierre Curie in 1880, which enabled easy

generation and detection of ultrasonic waves. The first use of ultrasound as a diagnostic tool dates back to 1942 when two Austrian brothers used transmission of ultrasound through the brain to locate tumors. In 1949, the first pulse-echo system was described, and during the 1950s 2D gray scale images were produced. The first publication on applications of the Doppler technique appeared in 1956. The first 2D gray scale image was produced *in real time* in 1965 by a scanner developed by Siemens. A major step forward was the introduction in 1968 of electronic beam steering using phased-array technology. Since the mid-1970s, electronic scanners have been available from many companies. Image quality steadily improved during the 1980s, with substantial enhancements since the mid-1990s.

## Physics of acoustic waves
### What are ultrasonic waves?

Ultrasonic waves are progressive *longitudinal compression waves*. For longitudinal waves the displacement of the particles in the medium is parallel to the direction of wave motion, as opposed to transverse waves, such as waves on the sea, for which this displacement is perpendicular to the direction of propagation. For compression waves, regions of high and low particle density are generated by the local displacement of the particles. This is illustrated in Figure 6.1. Compression regions and rarefaction regions correspond to high and low pressure areas, respectively.

Wave propagation is possible thanks to both the elasticity and the inertia of the medium: elasticity counteracts a local compression followed by a return to equilibrium. However, because of inertia, this return will be too large, resulting in a local rarefaction, which elasticity counteracts again. After a few iterations, depending on the characteristics of the medium and of the initial compression, equilibrium is reached because each iteration is accompanied by damping. As

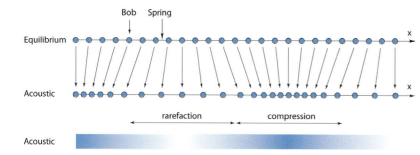

**Figure 6.1** Schematically, a longitudinal wave can be represented by particles connected by massless springs that are displaced from their equilibrium position. (From T.G. Leighton, The Acoustic Bubble, Academic Press, 1994. Reprinted with permission of Academic Press, Inc.)

a consequence of these phenomena, the compression wave propagates.

The word "ultrasonic" relates to the wave frequencies. Sound in general is divided into three ranges: subsonic, sonic and ultrasonic. A sound wave is said to be sonic if its frequency is within the audible spectrum of the human ear, which ranges from 20 to 20 000 Hz (20 kHz). The frequency of subsonic waves is less than 20 Hz and that of ultrasonic waves is higher than 20 kHz. Frequencies used in (medical) ultrasound imaging are about 100–1000 times higher than those detectable by humans.

## Generation of ultrasonic waves

Usually ultrasonic waves are both generated and detected by a *piezoelectric crystal*. These crystals deform under the influence of an electric field and, vice versa, induce an electric field over the crystal upon deformation. As a consequence, when an alternating voltage is applied over the crystal, a compression wave with the same frequency is generated. A device converting one form of energy into another form (in this case electric to mechanical energy) is called a *transducer*.

## Wave propagation in homogeneous media

This paragraph briefly discusses the physical phenomena observed during wave propagation through any homogeneous medium. It is characterized by its *specific acoustic impedance* $Z$. As with any impedance in physics, this is the ratio of the driving force (acoustic pressure $p$) to the particle velocity response ($v$), i.e., $p/v$. For plane, progressing waves it can be shown that

$$Z = \rho c, \qquad (6.1)$$

where $\rho$ is the mass density and $c$ the acoustic wave velocity in the medium. Table 6.1 illustrates that $c$ and consequently also $Z$ typically increase with $\rho$.

**Table 6.1** Values of the acoustic wave velocity $c$ and acoustic impedance $Z$ of some substances

| Substance | $c$ (m/s) | $Z = \rho c$ $(10^6 \text{ kg/m}^2 \text{ s})$ |
|---|---|---|
| Air (25° C) | 346 | 0.000410 |
| Fat | 1450 | 1.38 |
| Water (25° C) | 1493 | 1.48 |
| Soft tissue | 1540 | 1.63 |
| Liver | 1550 | 1.64 |
| Blood (37° C) | 1570 | 1.67 |
| Bone | 4000 | 3.8 to 7.4 |
| Aluminum | 6320 | 17.0 |

### Linear wave equation

Assuming small-amplitude waves (small acoustic pressures $p$) traveling through a nonviscous and acoustically homogeneous medium, the linear wave equation holds

$$\nabla^2 p - \frac{1}{c^2} \frac{\partial^2 p}{\partial t^2} = 0, \qquad (6.2)$$

where $\nabla^2$ is the Laplacian. The velocity $c$ of sound in soft tissue is very close to that in water and is approximately 1540 m/s. In air the sound velocity is approximately 300 m/s and in bone approximately 4000 m/s.

Equation (6.2) is the basic differential equation for the mathematical description of wave propagation. A general solution of the linear wave equation in one dimension is

$$p(x, t) = A_1 f_1(x - ct) + A_2 f_2(x + ct), \qquad (6.3)$$

where $f_1(x)$ and $f_2(x)$ are arbitrary functions of $x$ that are twice differentiable. This can easily be verified by substituting Eq. (6.3) into the wave equation Eq. (6.2). This solution is illustrated in Figure 6.2 for $f_1(x) = f_2(x) = f(x)$ and $A_1 = A_2$. It represents the

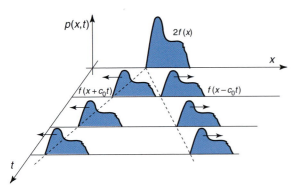

**Figure 6.2** Schematic representation of a solution of the linear wave equation. This solution represents the superposition of a left and right propagating wave.

superposition of a left and right progressive wave with velocity $c$.

The shape of the waveform is irrelevant for the wave equation. In other words, any waveform that can be generated can propagate through matter. A simple example is the following sinusoidal plane wave

$$
\begin{aligned}
p(x, t) &= p_0 \sin\left(\frac{2\pi x}{\lambda} - \frac{2\pi t}{T}\right) \\
&= p_0 \sin\left(\frac{2\pi}{\lambda}(x - ct)\right),
\end{aligned} \quad (6.4)
$$

where $x$ is the direction of the acoustic wave propagation, $\lambda$ the wavelength, and $T$ the period ($c = \lambda/T$). In practice, the shape of the propagating wave is defined by the characteristics of the transducer.

### Acoustic intensity and loudness

The acoustic intensity $I$ (in units W/m$^2$) of a wave is the average energy per time unit through a unit area perpendicular to the propagation direction. Hence,

$$
I = \frac{1}{T} \int_0^T p(t) \cdot v(t)\, dt. \quad (6.5)
$$

For the plane progressive wave of Eq. (6.4), the acoustic intensity is

$$
\begin{aligned}
I &= \frac{1}{Z \cdot T} \int_0^T p^2(t)\, dt \\
&= \frac{p_0^2}{Z \cdot T} \int_0^T \sin^2\left(\frac{2\pi x}{\lambda} - \frac{2\pi t}{T}\right) dt \\
&= \frac{p_0^2}{2Z}.
\end{aligned} \quad (6.6)
$$

A tenfold increase in intensity sounds a little more than twice as loud to the human ear. To express the *sound level* $L$ (in decibels (dB)) a logarithmic scale was therefore introduced

$$
L = 10 \log_{10} \frac{I}{I_0}, \quad \text{with } I_0 = 10^{12}\ \text{W/m}^2. \quad (6.7)
$$

Using Eq. (6.6) $L$ can also be written as

$$
L = 20 \log_{10} \frac{p}{p_0}, \quad \text{with } p_0 = 20\,\mu\text{Pa}. \quad (6.8)
$$

$I_0$ is the threshold at 1000 Hz of human hearing. Hence, absolute silence for humans corresponds to 0 dB. Increasing the intensity by a factor of ten corresponds to an increase in sound level of 10 dB and approximately twice the perceived loudness in humans. Doubling the intensity causes an increase of 3 dB.

The wave frequency also has an effect on the perceived loudness of sound. To compensate for this effect, the *phon* scale, shown in Figure 6.3, is used. The phon is a unit of the perceived loudness level for pure, i.e., single-frequency, tones. By definition, the number of phons equals the number of decibels at a frequency of 1 kHz. In practice, such as in measuring equipment, the isophones are often approximated by simplified weighting curves. For example, the A-weighting, shown in Figure 6.3(b), is an approximation of the isophones in the range 20–40 phons. A-weighted measurements are expressed in dB(A).

### Interference

Interference between waves is a well-known phenomenon. For an infinite (or a very large) number of coherent sources (i.e., sources with the same frequency and a constant phase shift) the resulting complex interference pattern is called *diffraction*. The shape of this 3D pattern is closely related to the geometry of the acoustic source.

Figure 6.4 shows how two coherent point sources interfere in an arbitrary point P. They can interfere constructively or destructively, depending on the difference in traveled distance with respect to the wavelength.

Figure 6.5 shows the simulated spatial distribution of the maximal pressure generated with a pulse of 5 MHz by a circular source with a diameter of 10 mm. When the point of observation is located far away from the source and on its symmetry axis, the

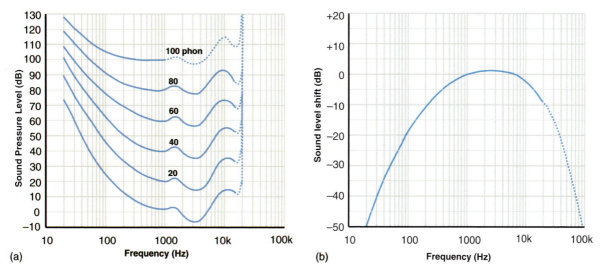

(a)

(b)

**Figure 6.3** **(a)** The phon scale compensates for the effect of frequency on the perceived loudness in humans. By definition, $x$ phon is equal to $x$ dB at a frequency of 1 kHz. 0 phon corresponds to the threshold of audibility for humans, and 120 phon to the pain threshold. An increase of 10 phon corresponds approximately to twice the perceived loudness. **(b)** A-weighting. This curve is an approximation of the isophones in the range 20–40 phons, shown in (a). It expresses the shift of the sound level (in dB) as a function of frequency to obtain an approximation of the perceived loudness level in dB(A).

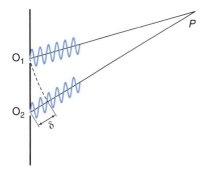

**Figure 6.4** Two coherent point sources, originating from positions $O_1$ and $O_2$ respectively, travel in all directions, but only the direction towards position P is shown. When the waves meet in P, they can amplify each other, i.e., interfere constructively, or depress each other, i.e., interfere destructively. Maximal constructive interference is the case when $\delta = n\lambda$ with $\lambda$ the wavelength, while complete destructive interference happens when $\delta = (n + \frac{1}{2})\lambda$.

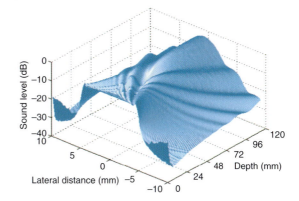

**Figure 6.5** Simulated spatial distribution of the maximal pressure generated by a circular, planar source with a diameter of 10 mm, transmitting a pulse with a center frequency of 5 MHz. (Courtesy of Professor J. D'hooge, Department of Cardiology. Reprinted with permission of Leuven University Press.)

contributions of all wavelets from all point sources will interfere constructively because their phase difference is negligible. Moreover, at such a large distance, moving away from the symmetry axis does not significantly influence the phase differences, and variations in maximal pressure occur slowly. However, when the point of observation comes closer to the source, contributions of different point sources interfere in a complex way because phase differences become significant. This results in fast oscillations of the maximal

pressure close to the source. Points that are at least at a distance where all contributions start to interfere constructively are located in the so-called *far field*, whereas closer points are in the *near field*.

### Attenuation

Attenuation refers to the loss of acoustic energy of the ultrasonic wave during propagation. In tissues, attenuation is mainly due to the conversion of acoustic energy into heat because of viscosity. It results in an

**131**

exponential decay of the amplitude of the propagating wave.

Typically, the attenuation is a function of the wave frequency. Therefore, it is often modeled as a function of the form

$$H(f, z) = e^{-\alpha z} \equiv e^{-\alpha_0 f^n z}, \qquad (6.9)$$

where $f$ is the frequency and $z$ the distance propagated through the medium with attenuation coefficient $\alpha$, which is expressed in nepers (Np) per centimeter. A neper is a dimensionless unit used to express a ratio. The value of a ratio in nepers is given by $\ln(p_z/p_0)$ where $p_z$ and $p_0$ are the amplitudes of the wave at the distances $z$ and 0, respectively.

In the literature, the unit dB/cm is often used. According to Eq. (6.8) the value in decibels is given by $20 \log_{10}(p_z/p_0)$. To use expression (6.9) the conversion from dB/cm to Np/cm needs to be done by dividing $\alpha$ by a factor $20 \log_{10}(e) = 8.6859$.

It has been observed that, within the frequency range used for medical ultrasound imaging, most tissues have an attenuation coefficient that is linearly proportional to the frequency (hence, $n = 1$). The constant $\alpha_0$ can thus be expressed in Np/(cm MHz) or dB/(cm MHz). If $\alpha_0$ is 0.5 dB/(cm MHz) a 2 MHz wave will approximately halve its amplitude after 6 cm of propagation. Some typical values of $\alpha_0$ for different substances are given in Table 6.2.

**Nonlinearity**

The derivation of the wave equation Eq. (6.2), assumes that the acoustic pressure $p$ is only an infinitesimal disturbance of the static pressure. In that case, the *linear* wave equation can be derived, which shows that any waveform propagates through a medium without changing its shape (cf. Figure 6.2). However, if the acoustic pressure increases, this approximation is no longer valid, and wave propagation is associated with distortion of the waveform. This effect is visible in the frequency domain by the generation of higher harmonics (i.e., integer multiples of the original frequency).

To illustrate this phenomenon, a propagating wave was measured as a function of time. Figure 6.6 represents these recorded time signals and their spectra. The origin of the time axis (time = 0) is the moment at which the pulse was generated. The distortion of the waveform and the introduction of harmonic frequencies increase with increasing pressure amplitude, which can be noticed by comparing the top row with

**Table 6.2** Some typical values of $\alpha_0$ for different substances

| Substance | $\alpha_0$ (dB/(cm MHz)) |
| --- | --- |
| Lung | 41 |
| Bone | 20 |
| Kidney | 1.0 |
| Liver | 0.94 |
| Brain | 0.85 |
| Fat | 0.63 |
| Blood | 0.18 |
| Water | 0.0022 |

the central row in the diagram. Furthermore, because nonlinear wave distortion is induced during propagation, the effect increases with propagation distance. This is visible when comparing the bottom and central rows in the diagram, which show the measurement of an identical pulse at a different distance from the source.

The rate of harmonics generation at constant pressure amplitude is different for different media. The nonlinearity of a medium is described by its nonlinearity parameter $B/A$. Table 6.3 gives an overview of some $B/A$ values for different biologic tissues. The larger the value of $B/A$, the more pronounced the nonlinearity of the medium.

*Physical meaning of A and B*

The acoustic pressure $p$ can be expressed as a function of the density $\rho$ using a Taylor expansion around the static density $\rho_0$

$$p = \left(\frac{\partial p}{\partial \rho}\right) \Delta\rho + \frac{1}{2}\left(\frac{\partial^2 p}{\partial \rho^2}\right) \Delta\rho^2 + \cdots \qquad (6.10)$$

where $\Delta\rho = \rho - \rho_0$ is the acoustic density. For small amplitudes of $\Delta\rho$ (and, consequently, of $p$), a first-order approximation of the previous equation can be used:

$$p = \left(\frac{\partial p}{\partial \rho}\right) \Delta\rho. \qquad (6.11)$$

In this case, which is used to derive the linear wave equation, a linear relationship exists between the

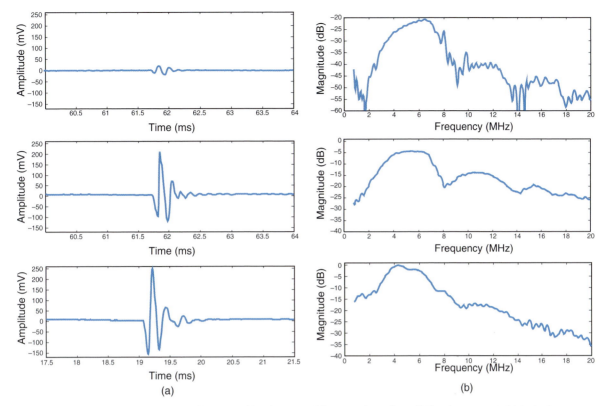

**Figure 6.6** (a) The nonlinear propagation of a wave yields a distortion of the original waveform. (b) This distortion is visible in the frequency domain as higher harmonics. The amount of distortion depends on both the amplitude (central versus top row) and the propagation distance (bottom versus central row). (Courtesy of Professor J. D'hooge, Department of Cardiology. Reprinted with permission of Leuven University Press.)

**Table 6.3** Nonlinearity parameter $B/A$ of some biologic tissues

| Medium | B/A | Medium | B/A |
|--------|-----|--------|-----|
| Pig blood | 6.2 | Liver | 7.5 |
| Spleen | 7.8 | Kidney | 7.2 |
| Muscle | 6.5 | Fat | 11.0 |
| $H_2O$ | 5.0 | | |

acoustic pressure and the acoustic density. However, if the amplitude of $\Delta\rho$ is not small, the second- and higher order terms cannot be neglected. Defining

$$A \equiv \rho_0 \left( \frac{\partial p}{\partial \rho} \right) \tag{6.12}$$

and

$$B \equiv \rho_0^2 \left( \frac{\partial^2 p}{\partial \rho^2} \right). \tag{6.13}$$

Eq. (6.10) can be rewritten as

$$p = \left( \frac{\partial p}{\partial \rho} \right) \Delta\rho + \frac{1}{2} \left( \frac{\partial^2 p}{\partial \rho^2} \right) \Delta\rho^2 + \cdots$$

$$= A \left( \frac{\Delta\rho}{\rho_0} \right) + \frac{B}{2} \left( \frac{\Delta\rho}{\rho_0} \right)^2 + \cdots. \tag{6.14}$$

The larger $B/A$ is, the stronger the nonlinearity effect.

# Wave propagation in inhomogeneous media

Tissues are inhomogeneous media. When inhomogeneities are present, additional phenomena occur, which can be explained using Huygens' principle, as shown in Figure 6.7. This states that any point on a wavefront can be considered as the source of secondary waves, and the surface tangent to these secondary waves determines the future position of the wavefront.

**133**

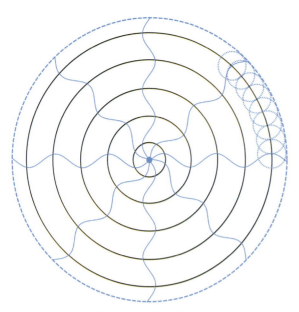

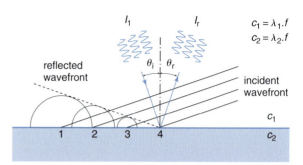

**Figure 6.8** Schematic representation of reflection of an incident wave at a planar interface of two different media. The relationships between the angles $\theta_i$ is given in Eq. (6.15).

**Figure 6.7** Schematic representation of Huygens' principle. The concentric lines in this figure represent the wavefronts, i.e., surfaces where the waves have the same phase. Any point on a wavefront can be considered as the source of secondary waves and the surface tangent to these secondary waves determines the future position of the wavefront.

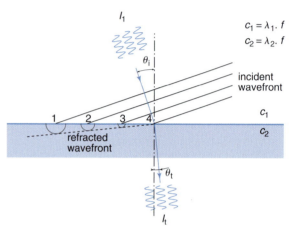

**Figure 6.9** Schematic representation of refraction of an incident wave at a planar interface of two different media. The relationships between the angles $\theta_i$ is given in Eq. (6.15).

A *wavefront* is a surface where the waves have the same phase.

## Reflection and refraction

When a wave propagating in a medium with density $\rho_1$ and sound velocity $c_1$ meets another medium with density $\rho_2$ and sound velocity $c_2$, as illustrated in Figures 6.8 and 6.9, part of the energy of the wave is reflected and part is transmitted. The frequency of both the reflected and refracted waves is the same as the incident frequency. Using Huygens' principle, it can easily be shown that the angles of the traveling (planar) waves with respect to the planar interface have the following relationship, which is *Snell's law*:

$$\frac{\sin \theta_i}{c_1} = \frac{\sin \theta_r}{c_1} = \frac{\sin \theta_t}{c_2}, \tag{6.15}$$

with $\theta_i$, $\theta_r$ and $\theta_t$ the angles of incidence, reflection, and transmission, respectively. The transmitted wave does not necessarily propagate in the same direction as the incident wave. Therefore, the transmitted wave is also called the *refracted wave*. From Eq. (6.15) it

follows that

$$\cos \theta_t = \sqrt{1 - \left(\frac{c_2}{c_1} \sin \theta_i\right)^2}. \tag{6.16}$$

If $c_2 > c_1$ and $\theta_i > \sin^{-1}(c_1/c_2)$, $\cos \theta_t$ becomes a complex number. In this case, it can be shown that the incident and reflected waves are out of phase.

Not only does the direction of propagation at the interface between two media change, but also the amplitude of the waves. In the case of a smooth planar interface, it can be shown that these amplitudes relate as

$$T \equiv \frac{A_t}{A_i} = \frac{2Z_2 \cos \theta_i}{Z_2 \cos \theta_i + Z_1 \cos \theta_t} \tag{6.17}$$

and

$$R \equiv \frac{A_r}{A_i} = \frac{Z_2 \cos\theta_i - Z_1 \cos\theta_t}{Z_2 \cos\theta_i + Z_1 \cos\theta_t}, \qquad (6.18)$$

where $A_i$, $A_r$, and $A_t$ are the incident, reflected, and transmitted amplitudes and $Z_1$ and $Z_2$ the specific acoustic impedances of the two media. The parameters $T$ and $R$ are called the *transmission coefficient* and the *reflection coefficient* and relate as

$$R = T - 1. \qquad (6.19)$$

The reflection is large if $Z_1$ and $Z_2$ differ strongly, such as for tissue/bone and air/tissue transitions (see Table 6.1). This is the reason why in diagnostic imaging a gel is used that couples the transducer and the patient's skin. Note that when a wave propagates from medium 1 into medium 2, $T$ and $R$ are different than when the same wave travels from medium 2 into medium 1. Both coefficients can therefore be assigned indices to indicate in which direction the wave propagates (e.g., $T_{12}$ or $R_{21}$).

The type of reflections discussed in this paragraph are pure *specular reflections*. They occur at perfectly smooth surfaces, which is rarely the case in practice. Reflections are significant in a cone centered around the theoretical direction $\theta_r$. This is the reason why a single transducer can be used for the transmission and measurement of the ultrasonic waves.

## Scattering

From the previous discussion, it must not be concluded that reflections only occur at tissue boundaries (e.g., blood–muscle). In practice, individual tissues are inhomogeneous owing to local deviations of density and compressibility. *Scatter reflections* therefore contribute to the signal, as is illustrated in Figure 6.10.

The smallest possible inhomogeneity is a point and is called a *point scatterer*. A point scatterer retransmits the incident wave equally in *all* directions as if it were a source of ultrasonic waves (Huygens' principle). Waves scattered in the opposite direction to the incident pulse are called *backscatter*. The characteristics of a finite scatterer can be understood by considering it as a collection of point scatterers. Since each point scatterer retransmits the received pulse in all directions, the scattered pulse from a finite scatterer is the interference between the wavelets from the constituting point scatterers. Obviously, this interference pattern depends on the shape and size of the scatterer. Because this pattern is the result of the interference of a very large number of coherent (secondary) sources, it is also known as the *diffraction pattern* of the scatterer.

If the scatterer is much smaller than the wavelength, all contributions interfere constructively, independently of the shape of the scatterer or of the point of observation P (as long as it is far enough from the scatterer). This is illustrated schematically in Figure 6.11(a). On the other hand, if the size of the object is comparable to the wavelength, there is a phase

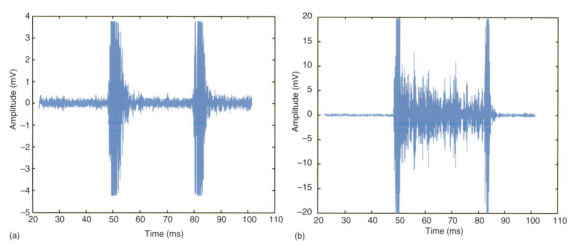

(a)

(b)

**Figure 6.10** **(a)** Reflected signal as a function of time for a homogeneous object in water. Obviously, a large reflection occurs at the interfaces between the two matters. The other apparent reflections within the water and object are caused by acquisition noise (note their small amplitude). **(b)** Reflected signal as a function of time for an inhomogeneous object in water. The reflections show an exponential decay. Deeper regions in the scattering object have a smaller amplitude. This is due to attenuation. Note the different scales in both diagrams. (Courtesy of Professor J. D'hooge, Department of Cardiology. Reprinted with permission of Leuven University Press.)

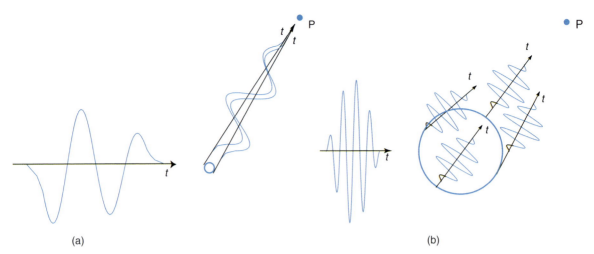

**Figure 6.11** A scatterer can be represented by a collection of point scatterers. Each point scatterer retransmits the incident pressure field in all directions. **(a)** These wavelets interfere constructively at the point P of observation if the scatterer is much smaller than the wavelength. **(b)** They interfere in a complex manner when the size of the scatterer is comparable to or larger than the wavelength.

shift between the retransmitted wavelets, and the interference pattern depends on the shape of the scatterer and the point of observation (see Figure 6.11(b)).

# Wave propagation and motion: the Doppler effect

If an acoustic source moves relative to an observer, the frequencies of the observed and transmitted waves are different. This is the Doppler effect. A well-known example is that of a whistling train passing an observer. The observed pitch of the whistle is higher when the train approaches than when it moves in the other direction.

Consider the schematic representation of a transducer, a transmitted pulse, and a point scatterer in Figure 6.12. Assume that the scatterer moves away from the static transducer with an axial velocity component $v_a = |\vec{v}| \cdot \cos\theta$. If $f_T$ is the frequency of the pulse transmitted by the transducer, the moving scatterer reflects this pulse at a different frequency $f_R$. The frequency shift $f_D = f_R - f_T$ is the Doppler frequency and can be written as

$$f_D = f_R - f_T = -\frac{2v_a}{c + v_a}f_T. \tag{6.20}$$

*Proof of Eq. (6.20)*

The position $P_s(t)$ of the start point of the transmitted pulse at time $t$ can be written as

$$P_s(t) = ct, \tag{6.21}$$

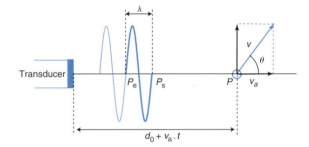

**Figure 6.12** Geometry used to derive an expression for the frequency shift due to the motion of the scatterer (i.e., the Doppler frequency).

where $c$ is the sound velocity within the medium and $t$ the time since the pulse was transmitted.

The position $P(t)$ of the scatterer can be written as

$$P(t) = d_0 + v_a t, \tag{6.22}$$

where $d_0$ is the distance from the transducer to the scatterer at time $t = 0$.

The start point of the ultrasonic pulse meets the scatterer when $P_s(t) = P(t)$, say at time $t_{is}$. Hence, $P_s(t_{is}) = P(t_{is})$. From Eqs. (6.21) and (6.22) it follows that

$$ct_{is} = d_0 + v_a t_{is}$$

$$t_{is} = \frac{d_0}{c - v_a}. \tag{6.23}$$

Without loss of generality, assume that the pulse length equals one wavelength $\lambda$. If $T$ is the period of the transmitted pulse, the position $P_e(t)$ of the end point can be written as

$$P_e(t) = ct - \lambda$$
$$= c(t - T). \tag{6.24}$$

Point $P_e$ meets the scatterer if $P_e(t) = P(t)$, say at time $t_{ie}$. Hence, $P_e(t_{ie}) = P(t_{ie})$. From Eqs. (6.24) and (6.22) it then follows that

$$c(t_{ie} - T) = d_0 + v_a t_{ie}$$
$$t_{ie} = \frac{d_0 + cT}{c - v_a}$$
$$= t_{is} + \frac{c}{c - v_a} T. \tag{6.25}$$

The scatterer reflects the pulse back to the receiver. The position where the points $P_s$ and $P_e$ meet the scatterer are respectively $P_s(t_{is})$ and $P_e(t_{ie})$. These are also the distances these points have to travel back to the transducer. The corresponding travel times $t_{rs}$ and $t_{re}$ are

$$t_{rs} = \frac{P_s(t_{is})}{c} = t_{is}$$
$$t_{re} = \frac{P_e(t_{ie})}{c} = t_{ie} - T, \tag{6.26}$$

which have to be added to $t_{is}$ and $t_{ie}$ respectively to calculate the travel time back and forth of $P_s$ and $P_e$, that is, $t_s = t_{is} + t_{rs}$ and $t_e = t_{ie} + t_{re}$ respectively. Hence,

$$t_s = 2t_{is}$$
$$t_e = 2t_{ie} - T. \tag{6.27}$$

Consequently, the duration $T_R = t_e - t_s$ of the received pulse can easily be obtained from Eq. (6.25):

$$T_R = 2\frac{c}{c - v_a}T - T$$
$$= \left(\frac{c + v_a}{c - v_a}\right)T. \tag{6.28}$$

Substituting $T_R$ by $1/f_R$ and $T$ by $1/f_T$ in this equation, yields the Doppler frequency $f_D$

$$f_D = f_R - f_T = -\frac{2v_a}{c + v_a}f_T. \tag{6.29}$$

In practice, the velocity of the scatterer is much smaller than the velocity of sound and the Doppler frequency can be approximated as

$$f_D \approx -\frac{2|\vec{v}|\cos\theta}{c}f_T. \tag{6.30}$$

For example, if a scatterer moves away from the transducer with a velocity of 0.5 m/s and the pulse frequency is 2.5 MHz, the Doppler shift is approximately $-1.6$ kHz. Note that for $\theta = 90°$ the Doppler frequency is zero.

## Generation and detection of ultrasound

Ultrasonic waves are both generated and detected by a piezoelectric crystal, which deforms under the influence of an electric field and, vice versa, induces an electric field over the crystal after deformation. This crystal is embedded in a so-called *transducer* that serves both as a transmitter and as a detector. Two piezoelectric materials that are often used are PZT (lead zirconate titanate) and PVDF (polyvinylidene fluoride), which are both polymers.

If a piezoelectric crystal is driven with a sinusoidal electrical signal, its surfaces move, and a compression wave at the same frequency is generated and propagates through the surrounding media. However, Eqs. (6.17) and (6.18) show that the transmission and reflection coefficients at the interface between two media depend on the acoustic impedances of the media. Therefore, part of the energy produced by the transducer is reflected inside the crystal and propagates toward the opposite surface. Because this reflected (compression) wave in turn induces electrical fields that interfere with the driving electrical force, it can be shown that the amplitude of the vibration is maximal when the thickness of the crystal is exactly half the wavelength of the induced wave. This phenomenon is called *resonance*, and the corresponding frequency is called the *fundamental resonance frequency*.

Obviously, as much of the acoustic energy as possible should emerge from the crystal through the surface on the image side. Therefore, appropriate materials with totally different acoustic impedance than that of the crystal are used as a backing at the other surface (Figure 6.13). As such, almost all energy is reflected into the crystal. At the front side of the crystal, as much energy as possible should be transmitted into the

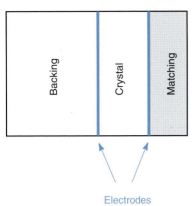

**Figure 6.13**
Schematic illustration of the cross-section of an ultrasonic transducer, which consists of four important elements (i.e., a backing layer, electrodes, a piezoelectric crystal, and a matching layer).

the frequencies involved are in the MHz range and correspond to the frequencies of radio waves in the electromagnetic spectrum.

### M-mode

The A-mode measurement can be repeated. For a static transducer and object, all the acquired lines are identical, but if the object moves, the signal changes. This kind of imaging is called *M-mode* (motion) imaging and yields a 2D image with depth and line number as the dimensions (see Figures 6.14 and 6.15).

### B-mode

A 2D image (e.g., Figure 6.16) can be obtained by translating the transducer between two A-mode

medium. However, because the acoustic impedance of solids is very different from that of fluids (which is a good model for biologic tissue), part of the energy is reflected into the crystal again. This problem is solved by using a so-called matching layer (Figure 6.13), which has an acoustic impedance equal to $\sqrt{Z_c Z_t}$, with $Z_c$ and $Z_t$ being the acoustic impedance of the crystal and the tissue, respectively. It can be shown that if this layer has a thickness equal to an odd number of quarter wavelengths, complete transmission of energy from the crystal to the tissue can be obtained.

An ultrasonic transducer can only generate and receive a limited band of frequencies. This band is called the *bandwidth* of the transducer.

## Gray scale imaging

## Data acquisition

Instead of applying a continuous electrical signal to the crystal, pulses are used to obtain spatial information. Data acquisition is done in three different ways.

### A-mode

Immediately after the transmission of the pulse, the transducer is used as a receiver. The reflected (both specular and scattered) waves are recorded as a function of time. An example has already been shown in Figure 6.10. Note that time and depth are equivalent in echography because the sound velocity is approximately constant throughout the tissue. In other words, *c* multiplied by the travel time of the pulse equals twice the distance from the transducer to the reflection point. This simplest form of ultrasound imaging, based on the *pulse–echo* principle, is called *A-mode* (amplitude) imaging. The detected signal is often called the radiofrequency (RF) signal because

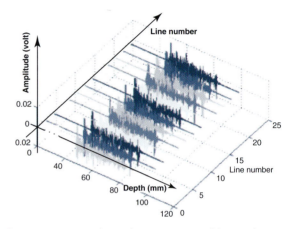

**Figure 6.14** Repeated A-mode measurement yields M-mode imaging. (Courtesy of Professor J. D'hooge, Department of Cardiology. Reprinted with permission of Leuven University Press.)

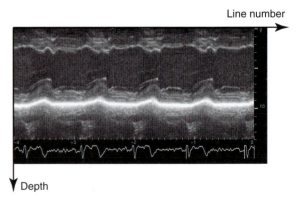

**Figure 6.15** M-mode image of the heart wall for assessment of cardiac wall motion during contraction. The black region is blood, the bright reflection is the pericardium (i.e., a membrane around the heart), and the gray region in between is the heart muscle itself. (Courtesy of Professor J. D'hooge, Department of Cardiology. Reprinted with permission of Leuven University Press.)

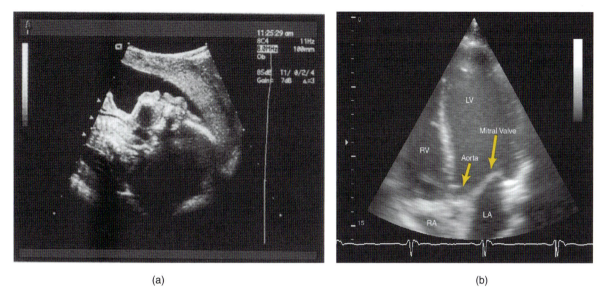

(a)　　　　　　　　　　　　　　　　　　(b)

**Figure 6.16 (a)** B-mode image of a fetus. The dark region is the uterus, which is filled with fluid. (Courtesy of Professor M. H. Smet, Department of Radiology) **(b)** B-mode image of a normal heart in a four-chamber view showing the two ventricles (LV left ventricle; RV right ventricle), the two atria (LA left atrium; RA right atrium) and the origin of the aorta (outflow tract). Besides the anatomy of the whole heart, the morphology of the valves (e.g., mitral valve) can be visualized. (Courtesy of the Department of Cardiology.)

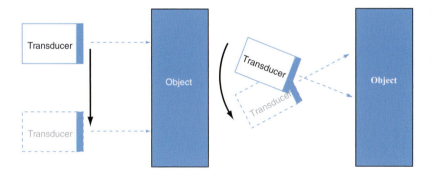

**Figure 6.17** B-mode image acquisition can be done by either translating **(a)** or tilting **(b)** the transducer. (Courtesy of Professor J. D'hooge, Department of Cardiology. Reprinted with permission of Leuven University Press.)

acquisitions. This is illustrated in Figure 6.17(a). This kind of imaging is called *B-mode* imaging, where B stands for brightness (see also p. 140). If this measurement is repeated over time, an image sequence is obtained.

Because bone has a high attenuation coefficient, transmission of sound through bone is minimal. For example, the waves can approach the heart only through the small space between the ribs. This space is often called the *acoustic window*. Because the acoustic window for the heart is relatively small, the translation technique described above cannot be applied to cardiac applications. A possible solution is to scan a sector by tilting the transducer rather than translating it (see Figure 6.17(b)).

The same imaging modes are also used for *second harmonic imaging*. The difference with traditional imaging is that the complete bandwidth of the transducer is not used during transmission but only a low-frequency part. Higher harmonics are generated during wave propagation and are detected with the remaining high-frequency part of the sensitive bandwidth of the transducer. The bandwidth used during transmission can be changed by modifying the properties of the electrical pulses that excite the crystals.

## Image reconstruction

Reconstructing ultrasound images based on the acquired RF data as shown in Figure 6.14, involves

**139**

the following steps: filtering, envelope detection, attenuation correction, log-compression, and scan conversion. All of these steps are now briefly discussed.

## Filtering

First, the received RF signals are filtered in order to remove high-frequency noise. In second harmonic imaging, the transmitted low-frequency band is also removed, leaving only the received high frequencies in the upper part of the bandwidth of the transducer. The origin of these frequencies, which were not transmitted, is nonlinear wave propagation (see p. 132). Figure 6.18 shows fundamental and second harmonic images of the heart.

## Envelope detection

Because the very fast fluctuations of the RF signal (as illustrated in Figure 6.19(a)) are not relevant for *gray scale imaging*, the high-frequency information is removed by envelope detection. Usually this is done by means of a quadrature filter or a Hilbert transformation. A detailed discussion, however, is beyond the scope of this text.

Figure 6.19(a) shows an example of an RF signal and its envelope. If each amplitude along the envelope is represented as a gray value or brightness, and different lines are scanned by translating the transducer, a B-mode (B stands for brightness) image is obtained. Figure 6.19(b) shows an example. Bright pixels correspond to strong reflections, and the white lines in the image represent the two boundaries of the scanned object.

To construct an M-mode image, the same procedure with a static transducer is applied. The result is a gray value image with depth and time as the dimensions, as illustrated in Figure 6.15.

## Attenuation correction

Identical structures should have the same gray value and, consequently, the same reflection amplitudes. However, the amplitude of the incident and reflected wave decreases with depth because of attenuation of the acoustic energy of the ultrasonic wave during propagation (see Eq. (6.9)). To compensate for this effect, the attenuation is estimated. Because time

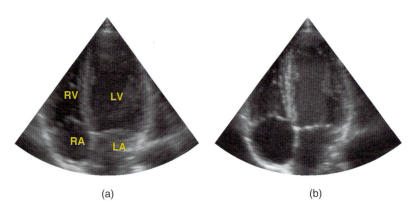

**Figure 6.18** B-mode image of the heart in fundamental (**a**) and second harmonic (**b**) imaging modes. The two ventricular and the two atrial cavities are shown as dark regions. The heart muscle itself is situated between the cavities and the bright specular reflection. Second harmonic imaging yields a better image quality in corpulent patients. (Courtesy of the Department of Cardiology.)

(a)                                          (b)

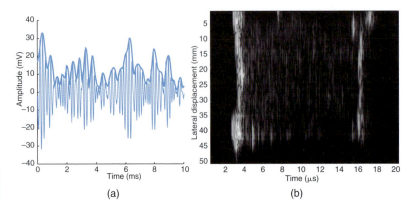

**Figure 6.19** Plotting the amplitudes of the envelope (**a**) as gray values yields an ultrasound image (**b**). (Courtesy of the Department of Cardiology.)

(a)                                          (b)

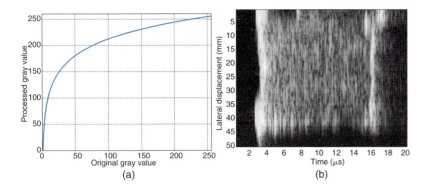

**Figure 6.20** Processing the original gray values as indicated in **(a)** results in a better visualization of the scatter reflections **(b)**. This is an example of a gray level transformation, as discussed in Chapter 1, p. 4. (Courtesy of the Department of Cardiology.)

and depth are linearly related in echography, attenuation correction is often called *time gain compensation.* Typically, a simple model is used – for example, an exponential decay – but in practice several tissues with different attenuation properties are involved. Most ultrasound scanners therefore enable the user to modify the gain manually at different depths.

### Log-compression

Figure 6.19(b) mainly shows the specular reflections. However, the scatter reflections are almost invisible. The reason is the large difference in amplitude between the specular and the scatter reflections, yielding a large dynamic range. In order to overcome this problem, a suitable gray level transformation can be applied (see Chapter 1, p. 4). Typically, a logarithmic function is used (Figure 6.20(a)). The log-compressed version of the image in Figure 6.19(b) is shown in Figure 6.20(b). The scatter or *speckle* can now easily be perceived. Note that different tissues generate different speckle patterns.

### Scan conversion

If the image is acquired by tilting the transducer instead of translating it, samples on a polar grid are obtained. Converting the polar into a rectangular grid needs interpolation. This process is called scan conversion or sector reconstruction.

## Acquisition and reconstruction time

To have an idea of the acquisition time of a typical ultrasound image, a simple calculation can be made. Typically, each line in the image corresponds to a depth of 20 cm. Because the velocity of sound is approximately 1540 m/s and the travel distance to and from the transducer is 40 cm, the acquisition of each line takes 267 μs. A typical image with 120 image lines

then requires an acquisition time of about 32 ms. The reconstruction of the images can be done in real time. Consequently, a temporal resolution of 30 Hz (i.e., 30 images per second) can be obtained. This temporal resolution can be increased at the cost of spatial resolution by decreasing the number of scan lines. However, current clinical scanners are able to acquire multiple scan lines simultaneously with little influence on the spatial resolution (see p. 150 below). This way, frame rates of 70–80 Hz can be obtained.

## Doppler imaging

Doppler imaging is a general term used to visualize velocities of moving tissues. Data acquisition and reconstruction are different from gray scale imaging. Furthermore, the Doppler principle is not always used.

## Data acquisition

In Doppler imaging data acquisition is done in three different ways.

- *Continuous wave (CW) Doppler* A continuous sinusoidal wave is transmitted by a piezoelectric crystal, and the reflected signal is received by a second crystal. Usually, both crystals are embedded in the same transducer. CW Doppler is the only exception to the pulse–echo principle for ultrasound data acquisition. It does not yield spatial (i.e., depth) information.

- *Pulsed wave (PW) Doppler* Pulsed waves are transmitted along a particular line through the tissue at a constant pulse repetition frequency (PRF). However, rather than acquiring the complete RF signal as a function of time, as in the M-mode acquisition (see p. 138), only one sample of each reflected pulse is taken at a fixed time, the so-called *range gate*, after the transmission of the pulse. Consequently, information is obtained from one specific spatial position.

- *Color flow (CF) imaging* This is the Doppler equivalent of the B-mode acquisition (see p. 138). However, for each image line, several pulses (typically 3–7) instead of one are transmitted. The result is a 2D image in which the velocity information is visualized by means of color superimposed onto the anatomical gray scale image.

## Reconstruction

From the acquired data the velocity must be calculated and visualized. This is different for each of the acquisition modes.

### Continuous wave Doppler

To calculate the velocity of a scattering object in front of the transducer, the frequency of the received wave $f_R$ is compared with that of the transmitted wave $f_T$. Equation (6.30) gives the relation between the Doppler frequency $f_D = f_R - f_T$ and the velocity $v_a$ of the tissue. Note that only the axial component of the object's motion can be measured this way.

Cardiac and blood velocities cause a Doppler shift in the sonic range. Therefore, the Doppler frequency is often made audible to the user. A high pitch corresponds to a high velocity, whereas a low pitch corresponds to a low velocity.

If the received signal is subdivided into segments, the frequency spectrum at subsequent time intervals can be obtained from their Fourier transform. The spectral amplitude can then be encoded as a gray value in an image. This picture is called the *spectrogram* or *sonogram*. Typically, scatterers with different velocities are present in one segment, yielding a range of Doppler shifts and a broad instead of a sparse peaked spectrum. Moreover, segmentation of the received signal corresponds to a multiplication with a rectangular function and a convolution of the true spectrum with a sinc function. Consequently, the spectrum appears smoother than it actually should be. This kind of broadening is called intrinsic broadening because it has no physical origin but is due purely to signal processing. An example of a continuous wave spectrogram is given in Figure 6.21. It is clear that a compromise has to be made between the amount of intrinsic spectral broadening and the time between two spectra in the spectrogram. In other words, a compromise has to be made between the

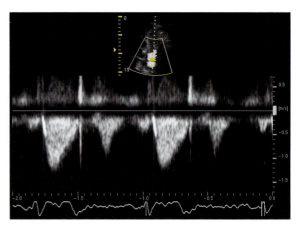

**Figure 6.21** CW Doppler spectrogram showing the velocity profile of the blood flow through a heart valve. (Courtesy of the Department of Cardiology.)

velocity resolution and temporal resolution of the spectrogram.

### Pulsed wave doppler

Pulsed wave (PW) Doppler does not make use of the Doppler principle. Instead, the received signal is assumed to be a scaled, delayed replica with the same frequency (i.e., $f_R = f_T$) as the transmitted pulse. Effects such as diffraction and nonlinearity are also neglected. Assume a transmitted sinusoidal wave

$$p(t) = y_{max} \sin(2\pi f_T t). \qquad (6.31)$$

The received signal then is

$$s(t) = A \sin(2\pi f_T (t - \Delta t)). \qquad (6.32)$$

The interval $\Delta t$ is the time between the transmission and the reception of the pulse and depends on the distance $d$ from the transducer to the scatterer, i.e., $\Delta t = 2d/c$. The PW Doppler system takes only one sample of each of the received pulses at a fixed range gate $t_R$ (Figure 6.22), that is,

$$s(t_R) = A \sin(2\pi f_T (t_R - \Delta t))$$
$$= A \sin(2\pi f_T (t_R - 2d/c)). \qquad (6.33)$$

If the scattering object moves away from the transducer with a constant axial velocity $v_a$, the distance $d$ increases between subsequent pulses with $v_a T_{PRF}$, where $T_{PRF}$ is the pulse repetition period, $T_{PRF} =$

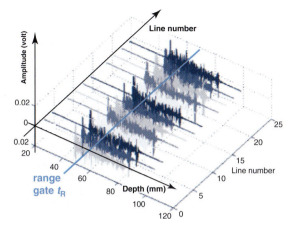

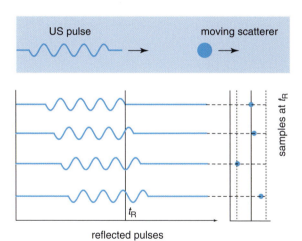

**Figure 6.22** Pulsed wave Doppler uses the M-mode acquisition scheme (see Figure (6.14)) and samples the subsequent reflected pulses at a fixed range gate $t_R$ to calculate the Doppler frequency $f_D$.

**Figure 6.23** Schematic representation of the PW Doppler principle. Pulses are transmitted at a fixed pulse repetition frequency (PRF). They are reflected at a scatterer in motion. Because of this motion, the reflected pulses are dephased. Measuring each reflected pulse at the range gate $t_R$ yields a sampled sinusoidal signal with frequency $f_D$.

1/PRF (see Figure 6.23). Consequently, Eq. (6.33) can be written as

$$s_j(t_R) = A \sin\left(-2\pi f_T\left(\frac{2(d_0 + j \cdot v_a \cdot T_{PRF})}{c}\right) + t_R\right)$$
$$= A \sin\left(-2\pi f_T\left(j \cdot \frac{2 \cdot v_a \cdot T_{PRF}}{c}\right) + \phi\right) \quad (6.34)$$

where $s_j(t_R)$ is the sample of the $j$th pulse. Hence, the values $s_j(t_R)$ in Eq. (6.34) are samples of a slowly

time-varying sinusoidal function with frequency

$$f_D = -\frac{2v_a}{c}f_T, \quad (6.35)$$

which is exactly the Doppler frequency defined in Eq. (6.30). Hence, the velocity of the scattering object at a specific depth, defined by the range gate, can be calculated from the sampled signal $s_j(t_R)$. As in CW Doppler, this signal can be made audible or can be represented as a spectrogram. Often, the spectrogram is displayed together with a B-mode gray scale image in which the position of the range gate is indicated. Such a combined scan is called a *duplex*.

Note that a PW Doppler system as described above is not able to detect the direction of motion of the scattering object. To obtain directional information, not one but two samples, a quarter of a wavelength or less apart, have to be taken each time because this completely determines the motion direction of the waveform as illustrated schematically in Figure 6.24.

Similarly to CW Doppler, the received (sampled) signal is subdivided into segments and their frequency spectrum is obtained by calculating the Fourier transform. The result is also visualized as a spectrogram. An example is shown in Figure 6.25.

### Color flow imaging

Similar to pulsed wave (PW), Doppler color flow (CF) imaging uses ultrasonic pulses and makes the same assumption that the received signal $s(t)$ is a scaled, delayed replica with the same frequency (i.e., $f_R = f_T$) as the transmitted (sinusoidal) pulse. However, instead of calculating $v_a$ from samples of a signal with frequency $f_D$ (see Eq. (6.34)) color flow imaging calculates the phase shift between two subsequent received pulses. Equation (6.34) shows that this phase shift can then be used to calculate the velocity $v_a$:

$$\Delta\phi = 2\pi f_T \frac{2v_a T_{PRF}}{c}. \quad (6.36)$$

The phase shift $\Delta\phi$ can be derived by sampling two subsequent pulses at two specific time instances $t_{R1}$ and $t_{R2}$. It can easily be shown that two samples of a sinusoid completely determine its phase given that they are no more than a quarter of a wavelength apart (see Figure 6.24). Consequently, two such unique couples of samples are sufficient to determine completely the phase shift $\Delta\phi$ between two subsequent pulses.

Another way to calculate $\Delta\phi$ is by cross-correlation of the signals received from both pulses. This method

**143**

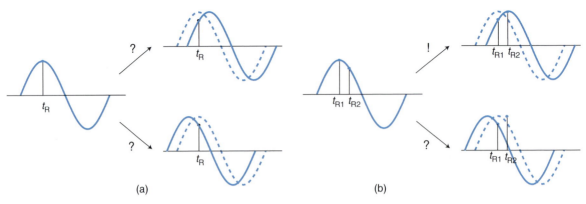

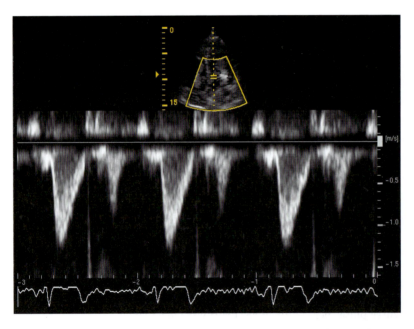

**Figure 6.24** If a single sample is acquired at the range gate, no directional information is obtained (**a**). However, if a second sample is acquired slightly after the first one, the direction of motion is uniquely determined since a unique couple of samples within the cycle is obtained (**b**).

**Figure 6.25** Normal PW Doppler spectrogram of blood flow through the aortic valve. (Courtesy of the Department of Cardiology.)

has the advantage that it does not suffer from aliasing (see Appendix A, p. 230). Moreover, cross-correlation is not limited to one-dimensional signals. It can also be applied to the subsequent ultrasound images of a time sequence. This has the advantage that the real velocity $|\vec{v}|$ instead of the axial velocity $v_a = |\vec{v}| \cos \theta$ is calculated. However, cross-correlation is not commonly available yet in clinical practice.

In practice, the measurements are noisy. To increase the accuracy, more than two pulses (typically three to seven) are used and the results are averaged. By dividing the whole acquired RF line into range gates in which a few samples are taken, this method

permits calculations of the local velocity along the complete line (i.e., for all depths). This process can be repeated for different lines in order to obtain a 2D image. Usually, the velocity information is color coded and displayed on top of the conventional gray scale image (see Figure 6.26, for example), which can be reconstructed simultaneously from the acquired RF signals. Typically, red represents velocities toward the transducer, and blue the opposite.

The color flow technique can also be applied to data acquired along a single image line. In that case, the M-mode gray scale image can be displayed together with the estimated local velocities. This is color flow M-mode.

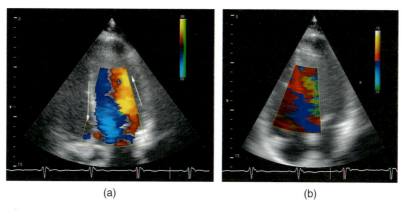

(a)          (b)

**Figure 6.26 (a)** Using color Doppler techniques, blood flow within the ventricles can be visualized. This image shows the flow in a normal left ventricle at the beginning of diastole. Red colors represent flow toward the transducer, coming from the left atrium through the mitral valve and into the left ventricle. Blue colors show the blood within the left ventricle flowing away from the transducer toward the aorta. **(b)** Doppler techniques can be used to acquire the slower, regional velocities of the heart muscle itself. Local velocities in the direction of the transducer are represented in red, and velocities away from the transducer are in blue. (Courtesy of the Department of Cardiology.)

## Acquisition and reconstruction time

Continuous wave and pulsed wave Doppler require a long transmission of either CW or PW ultrasound in tissue. Reconstruction then consists of a simple Fourier transform, which can be done in real time. In practice, changes in velocities over time are investigated, and the received signal is subdivided into small (overlapping) segments whose spectral amplitudes constitute the columns of a spectrogram. Figure 6.21 shows an example of a spectrogram of the heart. One such complete spectrogram is typically acquired in 3 to 4 seconds, which corresponds to 3 to 4 heart cycles.

In color flow imaging, a few pulses are sent along each image line. This means that the time needed to acquire an image is the time required to obtain a B-mode gray scale image times the number of pulses sent along each line. If, for example, three pulses per line are used, an image is obtained in approximately 100 ms. Velocity calculation can be done in real time, resulting in a frame rate of 10 Hz. To increase this frame rate, the field of view (FOV) is usually decreased. The size of the FOV can be selected independent of the FOV of the gray scale image. This way, the velocity calculations are limited to the regions that contain relevant velocity information.

## Image quality
### Spatial resolution

The spatial resolution in ultrasound imaging distinguishes the *axial*, *lateral*, and *elevation* resolution, i.e., the resolution in the direction of wave propagation, the

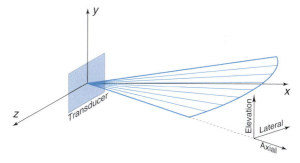

**Figure 6.27** Schematic representation of the axial, lateral and elevation directions.

resolution perpendicular to the axial direction within the image plane, and the resolution perpendicular to the image plane (see Figure 6.27).

### Axial resolution

Resolution can be expressed by the PSF, which determines the minimum distance between neighboring details that can still be distinguished as separate objects. In the axial direction, the width $\Delta x$ of the PSF depends on the duration $\Delta T$ of the transmitted pulse. Because the pulse has to travel back and forth, an object point does not contaminate the received signal of a neighboring point if the distance $\Delta x$ between them is larger than $c\Delta T/2$ (Figure 6.28), which is a measure of the resolution. A typical 2.5 MHz transducer has an axial resolution $\Delta x$ of approximately 0.5 mm.

While in MRI a small bandwidth and, consequently, a long RF pulse for slice selection is needed

**145**

to obtain the best resolution (see Chapter 4, p. 73), in ultrasound a short pulse with large bandwidth is needed. For technical reasons beyond the scope of this text, this bandwidth is limited by the transducer and is proportional to the central frequency. Hence, the resolution can be improved by increasing the transmitted frequency (see for example Figure 6.41(a) below). However, because the attenuation increases with higher frequencies (see Eq. (6.9)), the penetration depth decreases. Hence, a compromise has to be made between spatial resolution and penetration.

In Doppler imaging, the continuous wave (CW) mode does not yield spatial information. The axial resolution of pulsed wave (PW) and color flow (CF) imaging theoretically can be the same as for gray scale imaging. However, it can be shown that the velocity resolution is improved by increasing the

pulse length. Consequently, PW and CF Doppler systems have to make a compromise, and in practice the axial resolution is somewhat sacrificed to the velocity resolution. We note here that no such compromise has to be made when cross-correlation is used for reconstruction (see p. 143). However, cross-correlation is not available in clinical practice today.

### Lateral and elevation resolution

The width of the PSF is determined by the width of the ultrasonic beam, which in the first place depends on the size and the shape of the transducer. Unlike a planar crystal, a concave crystal focuses the ultrasonic beam at a certain distance. At this position, the beam is smallest and the lateral resolution is best.

Figure 6.29 shows an example of the sound field produced by a planar and a curved transducer. Figure 6.30(b) illustrates the finer speckle pattern obtained with a concave crystal as compared with Figure 6.30(a) produced with a planar crystal. Note that focusing can also be obtained electronically by means of a phased-array transducer, as explained on p. 150 below.

It can further be shown that the beam width can be reduced and, consequently, the lateral resolution improved by increasing the bandwidth and the central frequency of the transmitted pulse. Because gray scale images are acquired with shorter pulses than PW and CF Doppler images (see previous paragraph) their lateral resolution is better. On the other hand, the lateral

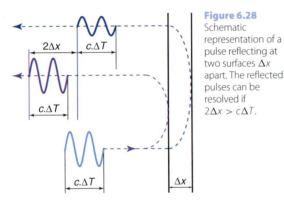

**Figure 6.28**
Schematic representation of a pulse reflecting at two surfaces $\Delta x$ apart. The reflected pulses can be resolved if $2\Delta x > c.\Delta T$.

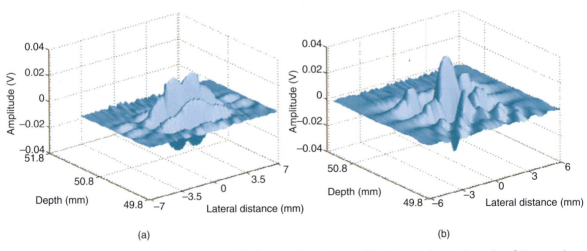

(a)                                                                 (b)

**Figure 6.29** Experimentally measured lateral pressure field of a planar **(a)** and concave **(b)** circular transducer with a radius of 13 mm and a central frequency of 5 MHz. Note the smaller shape in (b), which is due to focusing.

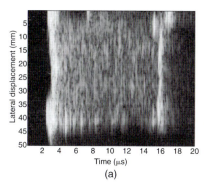

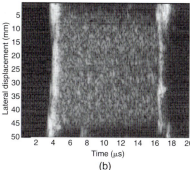

**Figure 6.30** Image obtained with **(a)** a planar and **(b)** a concave transducer. Because of beam focusing, the lateral resolution in (b) is clearly superior to that in (a). (Courtesy of Professor J. D'hooge, Department of Cardiology. Reprinted with permission of Leuven University Press.)

resolution of pulsed Doppler systems is better than that of a continuous wave (CW) system, which has a smaller bandwidth.

Typically, the lateral and elevation resolution in the focal region is on the order of a few millimeters (i.e., an order of magnitude worse than the resolution in the axial direction). Outside this region the beam width increases and the resolution becomes even worse.

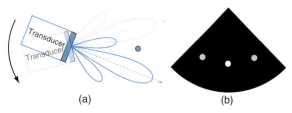

**Figure 6.31** **(a)** A focusing transducer produces side lobes. **(b)** The point scatterer in front of the transducer appears several times in the reconstructed image, once for each lobe.

## Noise

The noisy pattern as observed in Figure 6.30 is almost completely due to scatter reflections. Acquisition noise can be neglected compared with this so-called speckle noise. It can be shown that if sufficient scatterers are present per unit volume and if their position is completely random, the SNR equals 1.92. This is poor compared with other imaging modalities. However, the speckle pattern, here defined as noise, enables the user to distinguish different tissues from each other and thus contains useful information. Therefore, defining the speckle pattern as noise is not very relevant.

## Image contrast

Strongly reflecting structures, such as calcifications or tissue interfaces, yield bright reflections and are called *echogenic* as opposed to *hypogenic* structures with weak reflections, such as blood. The received signal is not only due to specular reflections but also to scatter. The large-amplitude difference between the specular and the scatter reflections yields a large dynamic range. Typically, a logarithmic function is used to overcome this problem (Figure 6.20).

It is important to note that in ultrasound imaging the degree of perceptibility of tissues is not only defined by the contrast (i.e., the difference in brightness in adjacent regions of the image), but also by the difference in speckle pattern or texture.

## Gray scale image artifacts
### Side lobes

A closer look at the pressure field produced by a focused transducer (see Figure 6.29(b)) reveals that the lateral pressure profile shows a *main lobe* and *side lobes*. The amplitudes of these side lobes are much smaller but can nevertheless introduce image artifacts. The reflections from the side lobes can contribute significantly to the reflected signal and introduce information from another direction in the received signal. An extreme situation of a single point scatterer is illustrated in Figure 6.31. Because of the side lobes, two scatterers wrongly appear in the image.

### Reverberations

If a reflected wave arrives at the transducer, part of the energy is converted to electrical energy and part is reflected again by the transducer surface. This latter part starts propagating through the tissue in the same way as the original pulse. That means that it is reflected by the tissue and detected again. These higher order

147

reflections are called *reverberations* and give rise to phantom patterns if the amplitude of the wave is large enough (see Figure 6.41 below). Because the length of the completed trajectory for a reverberation is a multiple $n$ of the distance $d$ between transducer and tissue, they appear at a distance $n \cdot d$.

## Doppler image artifacts

### Aliasing

A common artifact of pulsed Doppler methods (PW and CF) is *aliasing* (see Figure 6.32). Aliasing is due to undersampling (see Appendix A, p. 230). The principle is shown schematically in Figure 6.33.

The following constraint between the range $d_0$ and the velocity $v_a$ can be deduced:

$$|v_a| < \frac{c^2}{8d_0 f_T}. \tag{6.37}$$

For example, given a range gate at a depth of 6 cm and an ultrasonic frequency of 5 MHz, the velocity that can be measured without aliasing is restricted to approximately 1 m/s.

*Proof of Eq. (6.37)*

According to the Nyquist criterion, the sampling frequency PRF must be larger than twice the maximum

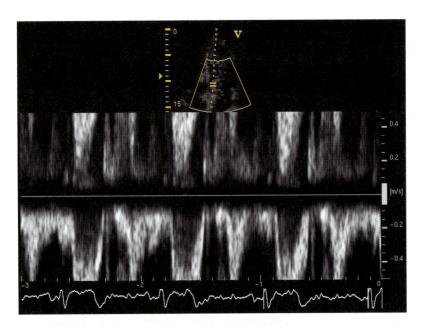

**Figure 6.32** Aliased PW Doppler spectrogram of blood flow through the aortic valve. (Courtesy of the Department of Cardiology.)

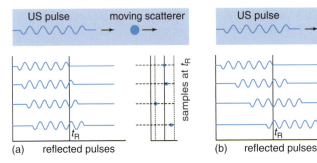

**Figure 6.33** Schematic representation of aliasing encountered in Doppler imaging. **(a)** Same as Figure 6.23. The reflected pulse is sampled fast enough to avoid aliasing. **(b)** The scatterer moves faster than in (a) causing a larger phase difference of the subsequent reflected pulses. Measuring this signal at the range gate $t_R$ results in exactly the same sampled sinusoidal function and Doppler frequency $f_D$ as in (a). Sampling is clearly too slow and the calculated scatterer velocity is too low.

spatial frequency present in the signal, that is,

$$\text{PRF} > 2|f_D| = \frac{4|v_a|}{c} f_T. \tag{6.38}$$

Because the reflected ultrasonic pulse must be received before the next one can be transmitted, a pulse must be able to travel to and from the range gate within the period $T_{PRF}$. Hence, the following relation between $T_{PRF}$ and the depth $d_0$ of the range gate holds:

$$\frac{2d_0}{c} < T_{PRF}. \tag{6.39}$$

Because $T_{PRF} = 1/\text{PRF}$ by definition, it follows that

$$\frac{c}{2d_0} > \text{PRF}. \tag{6.40}$$

From Eqs. (6.38) and (6.40), it follows that

$$\frac{4|v_a|}{c} f_T < \text{PRF} < \frac{c}{2d_0} \tag{6.41}$$

or

$$|v_a| < \frac{c^2}{8d_0 f_T}. \tag{6.42}$$

## Equipment

An ultrasound scanner is small and mobile. This is an important advantage as compared with the other imaging modalities. It consists of a transducer connected to a signal processing box, which displays the reconstructed images on a monitor in real time (Figure 6.34). Laptop and pocket-size ultrasound scanners are also being developed. The wide applicability of these portable devices will certainly play an important role in the further development of ultrasound imaging.

A variety of transducers for 2D and 3D imaging exist for different applications. The most important characteristics are discussed below.

## One-dimensional array transducers

A disadvantage of the acquisition method shown in Figure 6.17 is that it involves a mechanical displacement or rotation of the transducer. This yields several practical difficulties. For example, the displacement between two steps must be kept constant, and the contact with the medium must not be lost. To reduce this

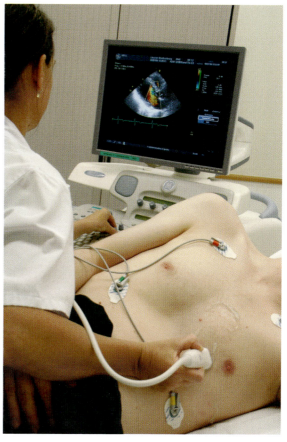

**Figure 6.34** Example of a commercial echocardiographic scanner. (Courtesy of the Department of Cardiology.)

mechanical motion, electronic scanning with an array transducer can be used. An array transducer is a collection of many small identical crystals that can be excited independently. Most common in medical imaging are the *linear-array* and the *phased-array* transducers that consist of a 1D array of crystals (Figure 6.35).

The linear-array transducer moves the ultrasonic beam linearly by firing its elements sequentially. This is the electronic representation of the mechanical translation shown in Figure 6.17(a). Typically, linear arrays are used where the acoustic window is large, which is, for example, often the case in vascular imaging and obstetrics.

For applications in which the acoustic window is small, such as in cardiology where the waves can approach the heart only through the small space in between the ribs, phased-array transducers can be used. The crystals are then used to steer the direction of propagation of the wave by tuning the phases of the

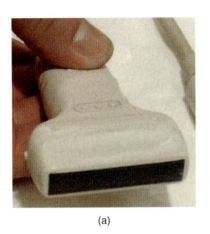 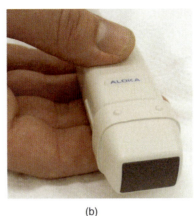

(a)　　　　　　　　　　　(b)

**Figure 6.35 (a)** Linear-array transducer. **(b)** Phased-array transducer. (Courtesy of Professor R. Oyen, Department of Radiology.)

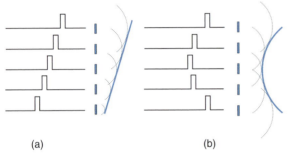

(a)　　　　　　　　　　　(b)

**Figure 6.36** By using an array of crystals, a sound beam can be directed **(a)** or focused **(b)** without mechanical movement of the transducer. A time delay is imposed on the electrical signals that excite the crystals, causing a phase shift of the emitted pulse. This yields the specific tilted or focusing wavefront as shown in this diagram.

waves sent by the different crystals (Figure 6.36(a)). This is the electronic equivalent of tilting the transducer mechanically, as shown in Figure 6.17(b). At the same time, the 1D array of crystals enables the beam to be focused at an arbitrary point along each direction (Figure 6.36(b)). This way the ultrasonic beam can be steered and focused and a sector image is obtained. Electronic focusing is also useful for linear arrays. This can be obtained by firing multiple neighboring elements simultaneously (with phase shift) for each ultrasonic scan line. Because the distance between crystals is relatively large, electronic focusing improves the resolution.

The wavefronts as shown in Figure 6.36 are drawn for the ideal case of an homogeneous medium. For inhomogeneous tissue and in the case of multiple tissues the velocity of the ultrasonic waves is not constant and the wavefront becomes distorted. This

effect is called *phase aberration*. Commercial phased-array devices typically use a constant sound velocity of 1540 m/s. The consequence is a loss of contrast and spatial resolution. Several methods have been proposed for phase aberration correction, but they are not yet used in clinical practice.

Theoretically the focus is a single point at a certain depth. Consequently, an optimal resolution requires many pulses along the same scan line, each focusing at a different depth. In practice, the axial scan line is subdivided into a few segments around a limited number of focal points. The smaller the segments, the better the spatial resolution, however, at the cost of the temporal resolution. Small segments are unacceptable in cardiac applications, but for static organs, such as the liver, this method is very useful.

In principle, it is not necessary to transmit multiple pulses over time in order to change the focal point. Indeed, the individual signals received by the array of crystals can be virtually shifted over time after their reception and before they are added together. Consequently, their phase is artificially modified, and the focal point during reception changes. If they are changed dynamically as a function of time, the focal point is artificially positioned at the depth from which reflections are expected to arrive (because the sound velocity in tissue is known). This technique is called *dynamic focusing*. It improves the lateral resolution significantly without influencing the temporal resolution.

The same principle of virtually shifting and adding the signals of the individual crystals can be used to change the direction of the beam artificially. Different scan lines can then be obtained simultaneously. This way the temporal resolution can be increased from

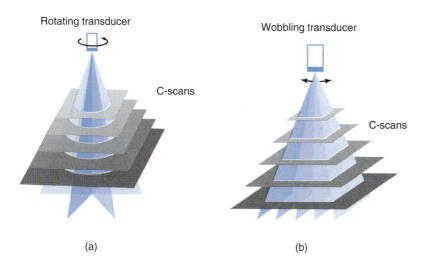

Rotating transducer

Wobbling transducer

C-scans

C-scans

(a)

(b)

**Figure 6.37** One way of acquiring 3D datasets is by rotation **(a)** or wobbling **(b)** of the transducer, resulting in a sampled cone. By reslicing the 3D dataset, C-mode images are obtained.

30 to 70–80 Hz, which is the standard frame rate of current clinical scanners. Higher scan rates require the acquisition of additional scan lines lying further away from the symmetry axis of the emitted beam, where the beam intensity falls off and, consequently, the detected SNR is limited.

## Transducers for 3D imaging

The easiest way to construct a 3D image is to rotate or wobble a phased-array transducer and acquire images sequentially from different scan planes as illustrated in Figure 6.37. Three-dimensional imaging offers the opportunity to obtain slices of any orientation through the scanned volume. Images of planes parallel to the surface of the transducer, as illustrated in Figure 6.37, are known as *C-scans*. Obviously, the patient should not move during the scanning process. An exception is the cyclic rhythm of the cardiac contraction, which can trigger the imaging process.

Again, the mechanical motion can be replaced by its electronic representation using a 2D phased-array transducer. The focal point can be positioned at any point within a *cone* instead of a plane and a 3D image can be obtained. However, the number of 2D slices that can be acquired per second is limited by the frame rate, which in turn is limited by the sound velocity. This way a 3D acquisition cannot be accomplished in real time. Hence, a compromise needs to be made between the spatial resolution and the temporal resolutions. Moreover, because a 2D array of crystals contains about $64 \times 64 = 4096$ crystals, A/D conversion and cabling are technically difficult.

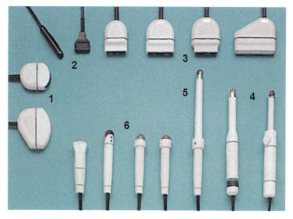

**Figure 6.38** The shape of the transducer is adapted to the application: (1) abdominal transducers – general purpose; (2) intraoperative transducers; (3) small parts transducers (muscles, tendons, skin, thyroid, breast, scrotum); (4) intrarectal transducer (rectal wall, prostate); (5) intravaginal transducer (uterus, ovaries, pregnancy); (6) infants (abdominal, brain). (Courtesy of Professor R. Oyen, Department of Radiology.)

Nevertheless, commercial 3D scanners are already available.

## Special purpose transducers

Several transducers exist for a variety of applications, such as intrarectal, intravaginal, transesophageal and intravascular transducers (see Figure 6.38). Transesophageal probes (Figure 6.39) are used to visualize the heart through the esophagus. Intravascular probes are inserted into an artery or vein to make intravascular ultrasound (IVUS) images. The crystal is mounted on top of a catheter (diameter 1 mm). Complete phased arrays can be built on this small tip.

## Clinical use

Echography is a safe, transportable, and relatively cheap imaging technique that does not require any special infrastructure. In addition, sequences of images are obtained in real time. For these reasons, ultrasound imaging is usually the method of choice if it is clinically relevant. It is useful if the ultrasonic waves are able to reach the tissues under examination and if the specular or scatter reflections, or both, are high enough to be perceived in the image. Consequently,

this method is limited to soft tissues, fluids, and small calcifications that are preferably close to the patient's body surface and not hidden by bony structures.

## Gray scale imaging

The most common investigations include the following.

- *Head* Although ultrasound does not completely penetrate through bone, the brain of a newborn can be visualized (Figure 6.40) because a neonatal skull is immature and not fully ossified at the fontanelles. To obtain images of the retina, high-resolution 20 MHz transducers are used (Figure 6.41). The general drawback of such high-frequency waves is their limited depth penetration because of their high attenuation coefficient. However, for tissues at the surface of the body, such as the retina, this loss of acoustic energy is negligible.

- *Neck* The soft tissues close to the surface, such as the thyroid (Figure 6.42), salivary glands, and lymph nodes, can easily be approached by the ultrasonic waves.

- *Thorax* Air (lungs) and bone (ribs) limit echography of the thorax to soft tissues that surround the lungs, such as the pleura (Figure 6.43) and the diaphragm.

- *Breast* Mammography (Figure 6.44) is mostly combined with an ultrasound examination for differential diagnosis.

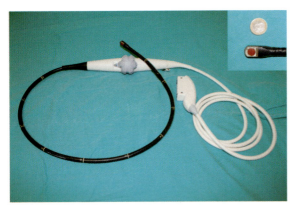

**Figure 6.39** Transesophageal transducer for cardiac imaging. This transducer is swallowed by the patient and makes ultrasound images of the heart from within the esophagus. (Courtesy of the Department of Cardiology.)

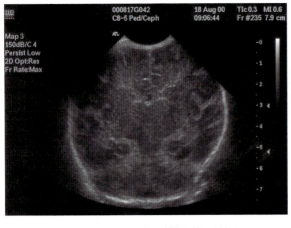

(a)

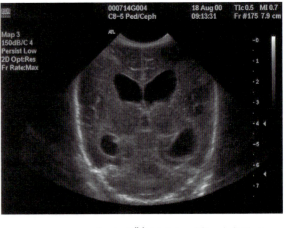

(b)

**Figure 6.40** **(a)** Normal cranial ultrasound. **(b)** Fluid-filled cerebral cavities on both sides as a result of an intraventricular hemorrhage. (Courtesy of Professor M. H. Smet, Department of Radiology.)

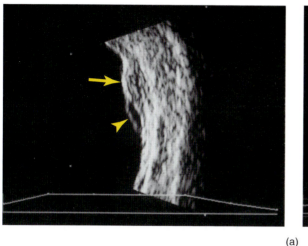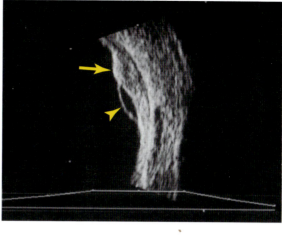

(a)

<br />

Left     AVERAGE  TL = 22.79 mm    T+12.3dB

COR = 0.00 mm  AC = 3.22 mm  L = 4.69 mm  V = 15.05 mm  TL = 22.95 mm

1620 m/s    1532 m/s   1641 m/s   1532 m/s

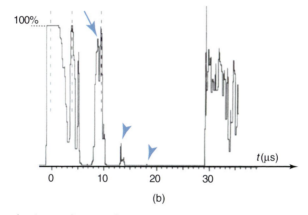

(b)

**Figure 6.41** **(a)** B-scans of the eye showing a malignant melanoma (arrow) with a localized retinal detachment (arrow head) in a 10 MHz (left) and 20 MHz (right) scan. **(b)** A-scan of a patient with cataract (arrow). The dotted lines are automatically recognized as the borders of the anterior chamber (AC), the lens (L), and the vitreous (V). The system calculates the length of each of these regions, taking the estimated sound velocity in the different tissues into account. The total eye length is defined as TL = AC + L + V. The small peaks (arrow heads) in the vitreous are due to reverberations. (Courtesy of Dr. J. Blanckaert, Department of Ophthalmology.)

- *Abdomen* In the abdominal region, all organs such as the spleen, pancreas, and liver (Figure 6.45) are well suited to be visualized by ultrasound imaging.

- *Urogenital tract* (The kidney, bladder, prostate, testicles, uterus, vagina, and ovaries.) Quite often a transrectal transducer is used to visualize the prostate (Figure 6.46(a)). The diagnosis of suspicious lesions can be proved by ultrasound-guided biopsy (Figure 6.46(b)). The visualization of the uterus and ovaries can be optimized by transvaginal scanning.

- *Fetus* Ultrasound imaging of pregnant women has become daily routine and includes an investigation of the fetus (Figure 6.47), the uterus, and the placenta.

- *Vascular system* Dilations (aneurysm, Figure 6.48) and obstructions (stenosis, thrombosis) can be recognized in gray scale images. Often Doppler imaging yields complementary information (the clinical use of Doppler imaging will be discussed in the next section).

- *Musculoskeletal system* Echography can be used to diagnose tears (Figure 6.49), calcifications, and

153

acute inflammations with edema in the muscles, tendinous, and capsular structures.

- *Heart* Cardiac ultrasound includes images of the ventricles and atria (Figure 6.50), the aorta, the valves, and the myocardium.

Note that ultrasound imaging is not only used for diagnostic purposes but also as a guidance during interventions, such as a biopsy of the kidney, the prostate or the liver, and abscess drainage.

## Doppler imaging

Besides static tissues, motion can be visualized and velocities calculated by means of Doppler imaging.

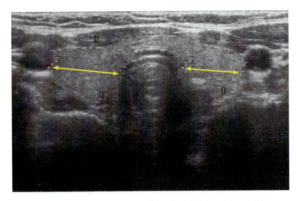

**Figure 6.42** Ultrasound image of the thyroid showing a mild bilateral enlargement (arrows) suggesting an inflammatory disease or hormonal inbalance. (Courtesy of Dr. D. Bielen, Department of Radiology.)

- *Flow imaging* Obviously, Doppler imaging is quite useful for measuring flow in the blood vessels and the heart. Vascular diseases such as atherosclerosis and clots (thrombi) in the big vessels induce local flow disturbances (turbulence, velocity changes) of the blood because of the local stricture of the vessel. In the heart, leaking valves (Figure 6.51) or interventricular shunts can be demonstrated.

- *Strain imaging* This is a more recent application of Doppler imaging. When neighboring pixels move with a different velocity, the spatial velocity gradient can be calculated. This gradient corresponds to the strain rate (i.e., strain per time unit; the tissue lengthening or shortening per time unit). The strain rate can be estimated in real time. The strain (i.e., the local deformation) of the tissue can then be calculated as the integral of the strain rate over time (Figure 6.52).

## Contrast echography

Because the acoustic impedance of air is quite different from that of tissue, ultrasonic waves are almost completely reflected at a tissue–air interface. Consequently, blood injected with microscopic air bubbles significantly scatters and appears brighter than normal – even brighter than tissue (as can be noticed in Figure 6.53). Ultrasound imaging using a solution with microscopic air bubbles (typical diameter 4 μm) injected into the blood circulation is called

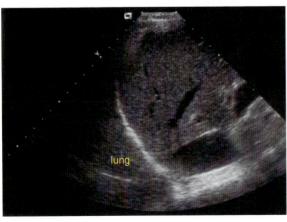

(a)

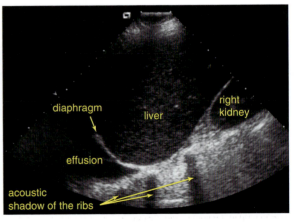

(b)

**Figure 6.43** Ultrasound image of thoracic base: **(a)** normal lung, **(b)** pleural effusion. (Courtesy of Dr. D. Bielen, Department of Radiology.)

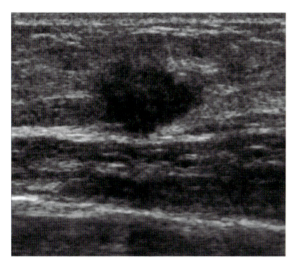

**Figure 6.44** Ultrasound image (10 MHz) of a female breast, showing a hyporeflective lesion with irregular borders, which corresponds to a vast mass with the characteristics of a malignant lesion. (Courtesy of Dr. Van Ongeval, Department of Radiology.)

*contrast echography.* It can be used, for example, to visualize fluid cavities and for the assessment of organ perfusion.

## Biologic effects and safety

Some experimental animal studies in the late 1960s reported that the genetic properties of irradiated tissue change. However, these results have never been confirmed, and in clinical practice the benefits of ultrasound imaging outweigh any potential side effects. Although ultrasound is said to be safe, there are two physical phenomena that can cause tissue damage (i.e., tissue heating and cavitation).

- Ultrasonic energy is absorbed by the tissue and converted to heat. To prevent tissue damage, the thermal index based on the transmitted power has been introduced. This parameter is indicated on

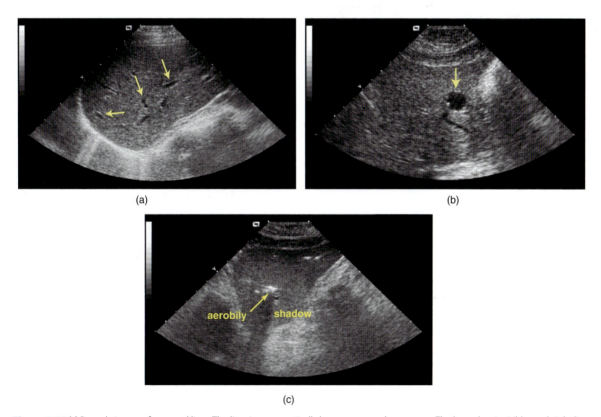

(a)

(b)

(c)

**Figure 6.45** **(a)** B-mode image of a normal liver. The liver is an acoustically homogeneous, large organ. The boundary is visible as a bright line. The little black holes (arrows) inside the liver are cross-sections of blood vessels. **(b)** Liver with cyst visible as a large black hole (arrow). Note the so-called acoustic retroamplification, a hyperechoic region behind the cyst. The origin of this increased reflectivity is the reduced acoustic attenuation in the fluid within the cyst. **(c)** The opposite effect of acoustic retroamplification is observed when air is present in the bile ducts, as in a disease called aerobily. Because air is a perfect reflector for ultrasound, it is visible as a very bright reflection. Because of this extremely high attenuation, deeper regions cannot be imaged and are said to be in the "acoustic shadow" of the air. (Courtesy of Dr. D. Bielen, Department of Radiology.)

**155**

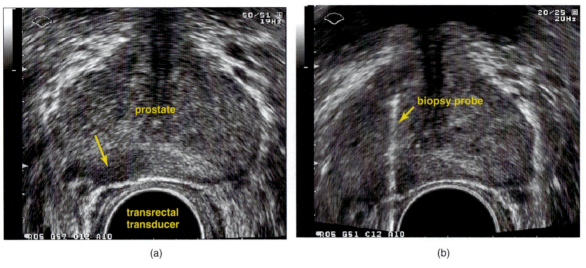

(a)  (b)

**Figure 6.46** Transrectal ultrasound study of the prostate showing a hypoechoic lesion (arrow) suspicious for cancer **(a)**. Its nature is proven by ultrasound-guided biopsy **(b)**. (Courtesy of Professor R. Oyen, Department of Radiology.)

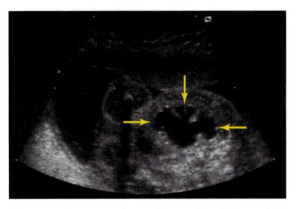

**Figure 6.47** A transverse ultrasound image of the abdomen of this fetus shows a fluid-filled and dilated collecting system of the left kidney (arrows) resulting from a renal outflow obstruction. (Courtesy of Dr. I. Witters, Department of Obstetrics and Gynecology, and Professor M. H. Smet, Department of Radiology.)

the ultrasound scanner and must not exceed a certain threshold.

- In areas of low local density resulting from a negative pressure (rarefaction regions), microscopic gas bubbles can be formed. When the pressure increases, these bubbles collapse. This can cause tissue damage. A mechanical index based on the peak negative pressure is shown by the system and must be kept under a specified threshold.

In diagnostic imaging both effects are avoided as much as possible. However, they can also be exploited

for therapy. Heating can be used for *ultrasound surgery* to burn malignant tissue. Cavitation is the basis for lithotripsers, which destroy kidney or bladder stones by means of high-pressure ultrasound.

## Future expectations

From a technical point of view 3D systems with full 2D-array transducers and real time 3D velocity and strain imaging will become available. Increased resolution and contrast-to-noise ratio can be expected for all imaging modalities. In ultrasound imaging, several technical improvements will contribute to a better image quality, such as new silicon based transducer technology and real time phase aberration correction. Miniaturization of the transducers and the electronics of high-end ultrasound devices is also a continuing trend, making them useful for screening and diagnosis outside the practitioner's office and for wireless telemedicine.

Because the microstructure of tissue is defined by the tissue type (e.g., heart muscle) and status (e.g., ischemic or infarcted) and because this microstructure is closely related to the way ultrasonic waves are scattered, backscattered signals contain information on the tissue type, status, or both. Some initial methods of tissue characterization based on backscatter have become commercially available and sooner or later this technique may be introduced into standard clinical practice.

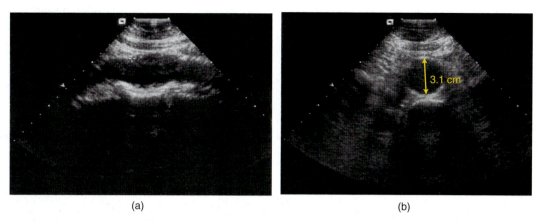

(a)   (b)

**Figure 6.48** Sagittal and transversal views of the abdominal aorta showing an aneurysm (3.1 cm versus a normal size of 1.5–2.0 cm). (Courtesy of Dr. D. Bielen, Department of Radiology.)

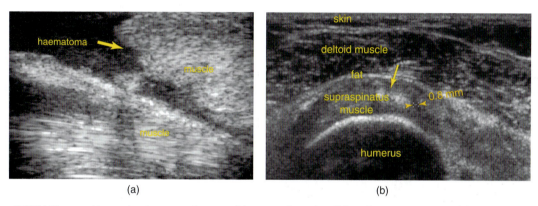

(a)   (b)

**Figure 6.49 (a)** Ultrasound image showing a complete tear of the pectoral muscle with large hematoma, contracted during a power training session. (Courtesy of Dr. P. Brys, Department of Radiology.) **(b)** Ultrasound image showing an unsharply defined hyperreflective zone because of a calcification (arrow) and a linear anechoic gap because of a partial thickness tear of 0.8 mm wide of the supraspinatus muscle. (Courtesy of Dr. E. Geusens, Department of Radiology.)

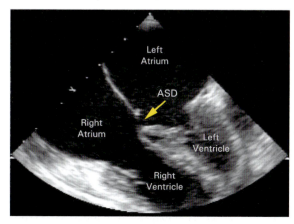

**Figure 6.50** Transesophageal echocardiographic (TEE) image showing an atrial septal defect (ASD). (Courtesy of the Department of Cardiology.)

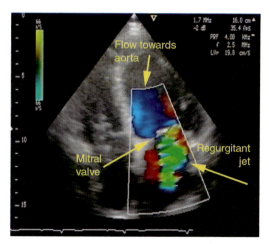

**Figure 6.51** Doppler color flow image of a patient with mitral regurgitation in the left atrium. The bright green color corresponds to high velocities in mixed directions because of very turbulent flow leaking through a small hole in the mitral valve. (Courtesy of the Department of Cardiology.)

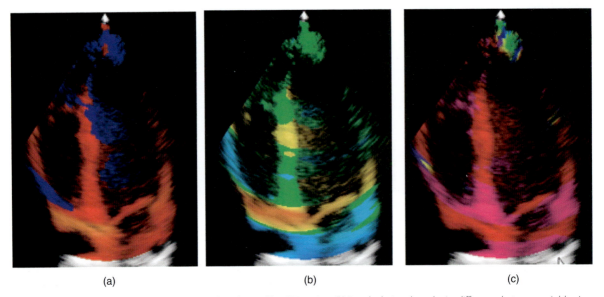

| (a) | (b) | (c) |

**Figure 6.52 (a)** Tissue velocity, represented by color, obtained by CF imaging. **(b)** By calculating the velocity difference between neighboring points, a strain rate image is obtained. **(c)** The strain is calculated as the cumulative strain rate over time. (Courtesy of the Department of Cardiology.)

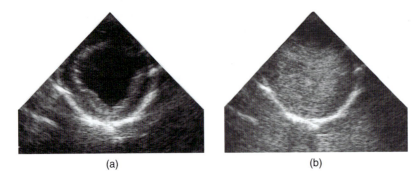

| (a) | (b) |

**Figure 6.53** B-mode gray scale image of the left ventricle of the heart in a short-axis view before **(a)** and during **(b)** pervenous injection of a contrast agent. (Courtesy of the Department of Cardiology.)

Further progress can also be expected in contrast echography and its therapeutic application. In practice, air quickly dissolves in blood, and the contrast obtained disappears almost immediately. To prevent this, the gas can be encapsulated in a thin shell, which decreases the amount of scattering but stabilizes the bubbles for several hours, depending on the material of the gas and the shell. Recently, attempts have been made to load the encapsulated shells with drugs with the intention that the ultrasonic pressure will tear the shell and yield a local drug delivery.

Very promising is the use of microbubbles with targeting ligands that bind specific receptors. This technique, known as *targeted contrast-enhanced ultrasound*, has a great potential for ultrasound molecular imaging (see Chapter 5, p. 126) and targeted drug and gene delivery.

# Medical image analysis

## Introduction

Advances in medical imaging technology have made it possible routinely to acquire high-resolution, three-dimensional images of human anatomy and function using a variety of imaging modalities. Today the number of acquired 2D images per exam varies from 150 images for screening up to 700 to 3000 for the diagnosis of complex cases. This large amount of images per case together with the growing importance of medical imaging in clinical practice, have continuously increased the workload of the radiologist, which explains the need for computer-assisted medical image analysis. Furthermore there is a quest for objective, quantitative information from medical images. In radiotherapy for instance, outlines of the irradiation volume and the neighboring organs at risk are delineated in 3D images and used to calculate a suitable radiation therapy. In neurology, degenerative diseases of the brain, such as multiple sclerosis, Alzheimer's, or schizophrenia, are studied by measuring brain shape and tissue changes in MR images. In cardiology, the health condition of the heart is assessed by studying the dynamics, the perfusion, and tissue characteristics of the heart muscle as revealed by MR or ultrasound images, and so forth.

Traditionally, medical images are interpreted by visual inspection of the 2D images displayed slice by slice. Such radiological protocol is necessarily *subjective*, as it is based on the perception by a human observer and is usually restricted to mere *qualitative* statements and judgments. Moreover, the traditional 2D display of 3D images allows immediate inspection of anatomical structures in the *two dimensions* of the image plane only, whereas the third dimension has to be reconstructed mentally by the radiologist by looking at adjacent image slices.

Today, most medical imaging modalities generate digital images, which can be easily manipulated by computers. The use of 3D image processing and visualization techniques makes direct inspection of the scene in *three dimensions* feasible and greatly facilitates the extraction of *quantitative* information from the images. For example, when a radiologist delineates the contour of a lesion of interest using the computer mouse, the outlined volume can be determined immediately and exactly. By measuring the size of the same lesion in a second similar image acquired at a later stage, a change of the lesion volume can easily be assessed. However, the outcome may be affected by inter- and intra-user variability in the lesion delineation or by the contrast–brightness settings on the screen. Appropriate computing strategies explained in this chapter can be applied to automate the measurement process so that highly *objective* and reproducible results are obtained. In brain research for instance, automated procedures for image analysis that are capable of accurately and reliably measuring brain morphology in vivo from MR images offer new possibilities for detecting and quantifying abnormal brain development by comparing measurements in a group of patients with measurements in a population of normal controls.

Because of the rapid technical advances in medical imaging technology and the introduction of new clinical applications, medical image analysis has become a highly active research field. Improvements in image quality, changing clinical requirements, advances in computer hardware, and algorithmic progress in medical image processing all have a direct impact on the state of the art in medical image analysis. Within the limited space of this book, it is not possible to discuss all ongoing developments. Therefore, we restrict this chapter to methods that are being used in clinical practice. We first discuss the possibilities and limitations of interactive analysis in which the delineation of structures is done manually by the clinician. Next, the challenges of automated analysis are introduced, and the basic computational strategies in clinical practice are explained and illustrated.

## Manual analysis

The most difficult subtask for a computer is the delineation of tissue. This is known as *image segmentation*. In principle, however, this can be performed by the clinician on the computer screen provided that the necessary hardware and software infrastructure is available. Medical images are often multidimensional, have a large dynamic range, are produced on different imaging modalities in the hospital, and make high demands upon the software for visualization and human–computer interaction.

- *Hardware requirements* The memory required to store 3D image data is quite large. A high-resolution MR image of the brain, for instance, may consist of more than 200 slices of $512 \times 512$ pixels each, i.e., more than 50 million voxels in total. Because the intensity of each pixel in digital medical images is represented by 2 bytes, this corresponds to more than 100 MB. High-resolution CT images, as used for instance for bone surgery planning, may be as large as 1000 images of $512 \times 512$ pixels each, which requires more than 250 million pixels or 500 MB storage capacity per study. Even 2D digital radiography already requires $2000 \times 2000$ pixels or 8 MB per image. In clinical studies that involve the analysis of time sequences or multiple scans of many subjects, the amount of data to be processed can easily exceed 10 GB. It is clear that storage and visualization of such large datasets imply large disk capacity and computer memory and that even simple image operations, such as navigation, zooming, and reslicing, require fast computer hardware.

  Medical image analysis usually requires a network environment involving multiple computers that communicate information with each other. Typically, the images are reconstructed on the scanner's computer and are transferred to a medical image archive. In a modern hospital, a so-called "Picture Archiving and Communication System" (PACS) connects all the digital imaging modalities via a communication network. The images are stored in a standard format [23] in a (central or decentralized) archive from where they can be retrieved for display and analysis on any suitable workstation. Without a PACS, the cumbersome transfer of images is often an insurmountable obstacle in the daily routine.

- *Display requirements* While 8 bits or 1 byte per pixel is usually sufficient in digital photography, most medical images need 12 bits per pixel (represented by 2 bytes in the computer memory). When displaying such images on the computer screen an appropriate gray value transformation is needed to obtain the necessary brightness and contrast in the region of interest. However, changing the brightness–contrast settings affects the appearance of an object on the screen. Especially when the intensity changes gradually from the object to its background, small changes in the brightness–contrast settings may result in significant displacements of the apparent position of the object boundary. This means that the perceived size of a lesion varies with the display parameters, which is an obvious problem for manual delineation. It is therefore common in radiological practice to define standard display protocols for each particular investigation, such as a "lung window" and a "bone window" for CT images of the thorax. However, even then the brightness–contrast of the monitor together with the external light conditions may affect the assessment of the size of an object. Standardization of viewing conditions is therefore recommended.

- *Software requirements* Interactive image analysis requires extensive tools for 3D image navigation, visualization, and human–computer interaction. This includes drawing facilities to delineate object contours in gray scale images. All of these functional requirements put high demands on software tools for medical image analysis.

Even if the necessary computer facilities are available, manual delineation of tissue in 3D images can be very tedious and time consuming and is therefore often not feasible in clinical practice. Moreover, manual analysis is highly subjective because it relies on the observer's perception. This results in intra- and inter-observer variability in the measurements (Figure 7.1). Automated analysis is the only way to overcome this problem. Note, however, that manual intervention is often still required to correct errors of the automated algorithms.

## Automated analysis

Different strategies for image analysis exist. However, few of them are suited for medical applications. The

[23] Digital imaging and communications in medicine (DICOM) version 3.0. ACR-NEMA Standards Publication No. 300-1999, 1999.

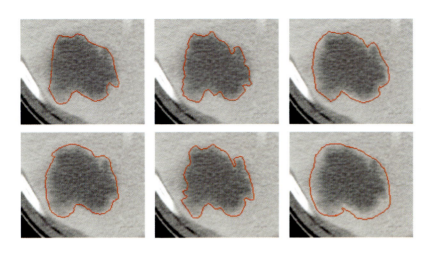

**Figure 7.1** Impression of intra- and inter-observer variability of manual delineations of a lesion in a CT image of the liver. Three trained observers (two radiologists and one radiotherapist) delineated this lesion twice with an interval of about one week (upper row and bottom row, respectively). The area delineated varies up to 10% per observer, and the difference between observers amounts to more than 20%. (Courtesy of the Departments of Radiology and Radiotherapy.)

reason is that both the medical image data and the model or prototype (i.e., the a priori description of the features to be analyzed), are typically quite complex.

- *Complexity of the image data* Despite the ever-improving quality of the images generated by the various medical imaging modalities, the information captured by medical images is not always unambiguous because of technological and physical limitations of the imaging process, yielding inadequate resolution, insufficient SNR, or artifacts. For some applications involving accurate quantification of small objects with complex shapes, the resolution of the imaging modality is still insufficient. Furthermore, clinical imaging protocols often specify a lower imaging quality than is technically achievable, for example, to limit the patient radiation dose in CT or to constrain the acquisition time in MRI. Three-dimensional tomographic images that consist of a series of 2D slices often have a higher resolution within each slice (e.g., pixel size $\approx 1$ mm$^2$) than perpendicular to the slice (e.g., slice distance $\approx 5$ mm). Hence, the location of the boundary of a globular object, for example, can be determined accurately at places where it is cut more or less orthogonally by the image slices, but is vague at places where it is more or less parallel to the slices. In the latter case, the voxels near the object boundary contain both object tissue and tissue of the surrounding area, yielding an unsharp boundary. This is the so-called linear *partial volume effect* or linear PVE (see also the nonlinear PVE described in Chapter 3, p. 51).

Fast imaging sequences, such as those used for functional or diffusion images in MRI, have a low SNR and need statistical methods to distinguish the areas with significant activation. Artifacts such as geometric distortions (see Figure 4.34) and intensity inhomogeneity (see Figure 4.35) have a negative effect on the accuracy of quantitative measurements.

- *Complexity of the model or prototype* Medical image analysis involves the analysis of a large variety of different structures or features in a large range of different applications. The objects of interest in medical image analysis can be anatomical structures (e.g., spine, brain cortex, coronary arteries), but also pathological tissue (e.g., tumor, myocardial infarction, inflammation, edema), functional areas (e.g., motor cortex, glucose metabolism), or artificial objects (e.g., implants, electrodes, catheter tips) and typically show important *biologic variability between subjects*. Modeling or prototyping, that is, describing the object based on the available prior knowledge, must cope with this large variability in appearance, which is not an easy task. One possibility is to impose only generic constraints that are general enough to include each possible instance of a particular object's appearance, such as boundary continuity or smoothness. Another useful modeling approach that also takes the appearance variability into account is obtained by statistical analysis of a set of instances of the same object in different subjects. This object is then represented by an average expected shape and photometry and some of its typical modes of variation that best

**161**

characterize the variability in the set of appearances from which the model was constructed. If the training set is representative of the true biologic variability, the model provides a complete and concise description for each individual.

However, modeling object variability can further be complicated by the *complexity of the shape of the anatomy*, such as for the gyri and sulci of the brain and the cerebral and coronary blood vessels. The topological variability of the coronary blood vessels, for instance, can be illustrated by the following rule [24]: "When the sinus node artery is a branch of the left coronary, which happens in 41% of the cases, this vessel usually (4 times out of 5) originates from the initial portion of the circumflex." Hence, these complex shapes or shape constraints cannot easily be described by a mathematical function. Likewise, statistical modeling suffers from the excessive shape variability. To establish the desired model, these structures should rather be considered as a set of components that must be assembled or hierarchically related.

Finally, for *pathological objects* such as tumors, for which each instance is different from all others, no such shape models can be constructed at all. The lack of prior shape knowledge makes accurate automated segmentation of pathological objects highly complicated.

In medical practice a wide variety of different imaging modalities is at the disposal of the clinician, such as digital radiography, CT, MRI, ultrasound, PET, and SPECT as discussed in the previous chapters. Different imaging modalities often capture complementary information. The same modality can also be used to assess the status of a certain pathology over time. Many applications benefit from the ability to combine information derived from multimodal or multitemporal acquisitions.

- *Multimodal analysis* A typical example of multimodal analysis is the combination of functional information about the brain derived from PET or fMRI images with anatomical information provided by MRI. In radiotherapy treatment planning, CT is required for dose calculations, whereas the target volume and the surrounding organs can often be defined more accurately using MRI

because of its better soft tissue discrimination (see Figure 7.2).

- *Multitemporal analysis* In longitudinal studies multiple images of the same modality and the same patient acquired at different moments are analyzed in order to detect and measure changes over time because of an evolving process or a therapeutical intervention. In multiple sclerosis, for instance, comparison of MR images of the brain over time allows the neurologist to assess the appearance and disappearance of white matter lesions (Figure 7.3). Whether a surgical implant has been inserted at the position planned on the preoperative images can be assessed by comparison with postoperatively acquired images.

An essential prerequisite for the analysis of multimodal or multitemporal images is that they be aligned. This mostly requires a 3D geometric operation, known as *image registration*, *image matching*, or *image fusion*. The registration may be done interactively by the radiologist assisted by visualization software that supplies visual feedback of the quality of the registration. Although such a subjective approach may be sufficient to support clinical decisions in some applications, a more objective and mathematically correct registration procedure is often needed.

Automatic image matching may be simplified if external markers are attached to the patient. If these markers are clearly visible in the images, the problem of image fusion is reduced to point matching, which is quite simple (see Chapter 8, p. 211) and is often used in surgical applications. However, the application of such markers is time consuming, unpleasant for the patient, and often more or less invasive. Moreover, registration based on external markers is inaccurate if the structures of interest move with respect to the markers.

An alternative method to match images automatically is to employ the image content itself. If the geometric operation is restricted to a translation, rotation, scaling and skew, or shear (see Chapter 1, p. 7), the registration is called affine or rigid. Many applications require a rigid registration even if the internal structures deform between two acquisitions, such as in follow-up studies of evolving processes like multiple sclerosis (MS) in the brain. Quite often, however, in case of impeding deformations induced by breathing, bladder filling, or posture, for example, nonrigid registration is needed. From a mathematical point of view, a distinction must be made between rigid and nonrigid image fusion as well as between unimodal or

[24] G. G. Gensini. *Coronary Arteriography*. Mount Kisco, NY: Futura Publishing Company, Inc., 1975.

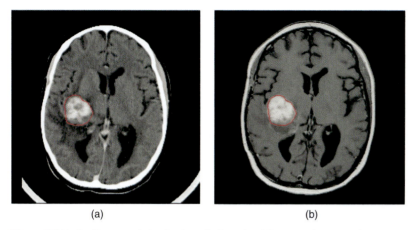

(a)  (b)

**Figure 7.2** Medical image analysis often benefits from the ability to combine complementary information provided by multimodal images, as is illustrated here in the case of radiotherapy planning. **(a)** CT slice of the brain of a patient with a brain tumor. **(b)** MR image of the same patient that was reformatted after 3D registration of CT with MRI so that pixels at the same position in both images are anatomically identical. Although CT is needed for dose calculations, the lesion boundary can be located more accurately using MRI. After registration, the lesion was delineated in the MR image and the outline transferred to the CT image. (Courtesy of the Departments of Radiology and Radiotherapy.)

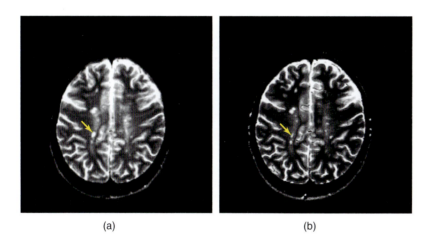

(a)  (b)

**Figure 7.3** In medical image analysis, it is often necessary to combine image information acquired at different moments in time. This example shows two $T_2$-weighted MR images of the same multiple sclerosis (MS) patient acquired with a time interval of one year. Image **(b)** was resliced after proper registration with image **(a)** to compensate for differences in patient positioning in the scanner. After registration, corresponding pixels in both images refer to the same anatomical location in the patient and can straightforwardly be compared. This way the evolution of MS lesions over time can be accurately inspected (arrow).

multimodal image matching. It is interesting but, for the computer vision expert, not so surprising that the computational strategies for image analysis can also be used to solve this registration problem. For this reason, the strategies for image registration and image analysis are discussed simultaneously in this chapter.

## Computational strategies for automated medical image analysis

*General problem statement* A prerequisite of automatic image analysis is to have a suitable prototype or model available. Such a model is a description of the prior knowledge about the photometry and the geometry. Photometric properties are, for example, the expected object intensity, contrast and texture. Geometric features are, for example, the expected position, size, shape, motion and deformation. The problem then is to find the best model instance that describes the image data. This is typically solved by optimizing a suitable objective function that includes measures to express how likely the model instance a priori is and how similar the model instance and the data are. Hence, the basic tasks in computer based image analysis are (1) representing and describing the prototype or model, and (2) finding a suitable objective function and optimizing it.

Different objective functions may need different optimization strategies. In some cases a closed-form solution is available. In general, however, search

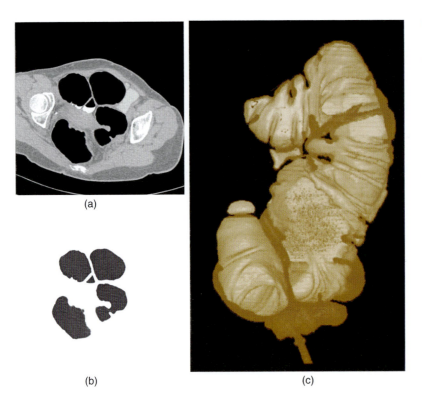

(a)

(b)

(c)

**Figure 7.4** Segmentation of an empty colon in a CT image of the abdomen for virtual endoscopy. **(a)** Original CT image through the colon. **(b)** A 3D region growing procedure initiated from a seed point in the colon extracts all contiguous pixels with CT intensity similar to air while excluding nonconnected pixels with similar intensity such as the background. Segmented regions that are not connected on this slice are effectively connected in 3D. **(c)** 3D rendering of the segmented colon. (Courtesy of Dr. G. Kiss, Medical Imaging Research Center.)

algorithms are needed, such as relaxation, dynamic programming, and gradient descent. Typically, proper initialization of the model is required for the optimization in order to allow convergence to the global optimum. If the number of free parameters is large, the search may become computationally expensive. In that case, heuristics are often applied to limit the search space and reduce the computation time at the possible risk of finding a nonoptimal solution. In the remainder of this chapter the emphasis is on the modeling and the definition of the objective function. The optimization methods are considered beyond the scope of this textbook. For details about optimization theory we refer to [3].

## Low-level methods

The simplest methods rely entirely on local image operators and a heuristic grouping of pixels with similar local photometric characteristics. Hence, these methods do not incorporate a specific model of the

photometry or geometry and are therefore considered *low level*. They consist of the following steps. First, a local image operator may be applied, yielding a new image in which the local features are emphasized. Examples of local image operators are given in Chapter 1 p. 8. Second, pixels with similar local photometric characteristics are grouped. Typical examples of low-level methods are region growing and edge detection.

- *Region growing* This partitions an image into regions by grouping adjacent pixels with similar gray values, thus creating boundaries between contrasting regions (Figure 7.4). It is often initiated by indicating so-called seed points, which grow by iteratively merging adjacent pixels with similar gray values. Gray value similarity is assessed with simple measures that compare the gray values of neighboring regions. Two adjacent regions are merged if, for example, their mean values differ less than a specified value. In medical imaging, the assumptions on which region growing is based are usually violated. Object intensity is often not homogeneous because of noise and artifacts (see, e.g., Figure 4.35), and adjacent structures may not have sharp boundaries because of

[3] J. Nocedal and S. Wright. *Numerical Optimization*, Volume XXII of *Springer Series in Operations Research and Financial Engineering*. Springer, second edition, 2006.

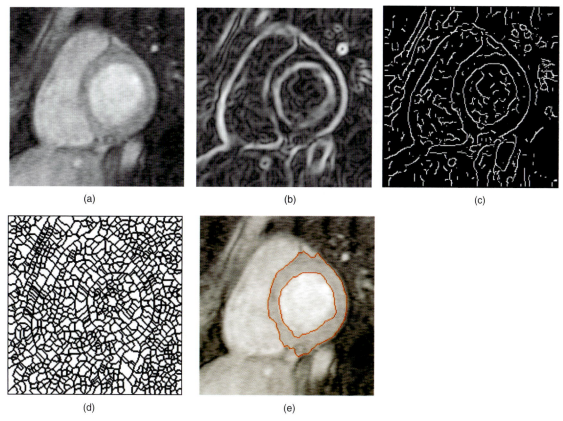

(a)      (b)      (c)

(d)      (e)

**Figure 7.5** Delineation of the myocardial wall in an MR image of the heart by edge detection. **(a)** Original image. **(b)** Gradient magnitude image. **(c)** Edges detected as local maxima of the gradient magnitude. **(d)** Edges converted into closed contours by considering the gradient magnitude image as a topographic relief and computing watershed lines. This typically results in oversegmentation of the image into a large number of small regions. **(e)** By interactively merging adjacent regions with similar intensity, only relevant boundaries corresponding to prominent edges such as the epicardial and endocardial borders remain.

poor contrast or insufficient resolution. When applied to medical images region growing typically results in regions that are either too small or too large.

- *Edge detection* This is basically similar to region growing, but instead of grouping pixels, boundary points are linked or tracked. Boundaries are found by first applying a local differential operator, such as the gradient or Laplacian (see Chapter 1, p. 9), and subsequently linking those pixels that are most sensitive to this operator. In the ideal case of images with high contrast and without noise, the physical object boundary is found. Medical image data, however, are typically complex. Consequently, the output of a local differential operator does not always reflect the expected meaningful edges, causing an automatic edge linking procedure to get lost (Figure 7.5).

Despite the heuristic nature and the poor performance of these low-level approaches, they are very popular in most commercial image analysis tools. The reason is that these approaches are simple to understand and to implement, and they are very generic, as they do not assume specific knowledge about the objects to be analyzed. In the case of simple image data, these methods can also be used initially to segment the image into subparts that are subsequently organized into larger patterns corresponding to meaningful objects. Hence, low-level methods are often the starting point for more sophisticated, model-based methods [25]. For complex image data, such as medical images, however, their usefulness is quite limited. They will not be discussed further in this chapter.

[25] P. Suetens, P. Fua, and A. J. Hanson. Computational strategies for object recognition. *ACM Computing Surveys*, 24(1): 5–61, 1992.

# Model-based methods

Effective image analysis methods must incorporate prior knowledge of the photometry and/or geometry of the considered structures. The nature of the geometric and photometric properties can be physical, statistical and can be tissue dependent as well. Such methods rely on a built-in conceptual model for the objects they are looking for based on characteristic features or patterns. Furthermore, these model-based methods must be able to cope with complex image data. This strongly limits the number of possible problem-solving strategies. In the remainder of this chapter the basic model-based methods for medical images are discussed. The following categories are distinguished:

- *Pixel classification* This category assigns pixels to the most likely class based on a model of the photometry for each class. The a priori class probability may be position dependent, which is represented in a so-called statistical atlas. Unlike in the next two categories, the size and shape of this geometric model as well as its position with respect to the image are fixed and known.

- *Geometric model matching using a transformation matrix* These strategies assume that the geometric variability of the appearance of the model can be represented by a general geometric transformation matrix (using homogeneous coordinates, see Chapter 1, p. 7), such as a translation, rotation, scaling, shear, affine transformation and perspective projection. The shape can be represented explicitly as a set of points, a curve or a surface, or implicitly as a picture or image itself.

  Photometric properties are, for example, a particular pattern, a probability distribution, or a measure of the color, gradient, texture or any other feature along or inside the contour.

  Given the model and the image data, the goal then is to find the best model instance that describes these image data. This is typically solved by optimizing a measure that expresses the similarity between the model instance and the image data.

- *Flexible geometric model matching* In many cases, the model needs to be more flexible to take the variability in appearance into account. Flexible geometric models can be represented as constraints or penalties on the geometric properties of a deformable curve or on a deformable picture or image itself. Examples of geometric properties are smoothness, curvature, rectilinearity, parallelism, symmetry, elasticity and rigidity.

  Fitting a flexible geometric model to the image data then consists of finding the best model instance that describes the image data. This problem can be solved by optimizing a suitable objective function that includes measures to express how likely the model instance is a priori and how similar the model instance and the data are.

## Pixel classification

Pixel classification is a special case of *feature vector classification*. The feature vector strategy is well established and has proved its usefulness in many industrial applications. It has been described extensively in the literature [26, 27]. In this approach, objects are modeled as vectors of characteristic features, such as mean gray value or color, area, perimeter, compactness, and so forth. Obviously, these features can only be calculated if the considered objects have been delineated in the image. This segmentation process is typically based on low-level operations and is therefore restricted to simple image data. There is one exception. Pixels can be considered as the smallest possible objects and do not need to be outlined. Pixel features can simply be calculated or are directly available as a single value, such as the gray value, or, more generally, as a vector, such as the red-green-blue (RGB) values in color images or $(\rho, T_1, T_2)$ in MRI. Partly because of this simplicity, pixel classification is very popular in medical image analysis. Based on their feature vector, pixels can then be assigned, for example, to a vegetation type in aerial images or a particular tissue type in medical images.

If the set of features is well chosen, pixels of the same type have similar feature vectors that contrast with the feature vectors of pixels of a different type. If the feature vectors are represented in a multidimensional feature space, the classification strategy then consists of partitioning the feature space into a number of *classes* (i.e., nonoverlapping regions that separate the different pixel types). An unclassified pixel then receives the label of its class in the feature space.

[26] R. O. Duda and P. E. Hart. *Pattern Classification and Scene Analysis.* New York: John Wiley & Sons, 1973.

[27] J. T. Tou and R. C. Gonzales. *Pattern Recognition Principles.* Reading, MA: Addison-Wesley, 1974.

The boundaries between the regions in the feature space are constructed by means of a decision criterion that is based on prior knowledge or assumptions about the different classes. A variety of decision criteria exists. Most popular in medical imaging are thresholding and statistical classification.

## Thresholding

The simplest and most straightforward pixel classification strategy is thresholding (see Figure 1.7(b)). It is particularly useful for images with a bimodal histogram (see Figure 1.8). The threshold value partitions the image into two classes, which typically correspond to object pixels and background pixels. More than one threshold value can also be used to model one or more different classes, each corresponding to a distinctive interval in the histogram.

Thresholding can also be extended to pixels that are characterized by a feature vector instead of a single value. A 2D feature space, for example, is then partitioned into a number of rectangular regions, each of which corresponds to a different class. Obviously, a strong limitation is that the decision boundaries are parallel or orthogonal lines or, in the general case, parallel or orthogonal hyperplanes. Few structures in medical images satisfy this assumption, which explains the limited success of this strategy despite its wide usage. An important positive exception is the segmentation of bony structures in CT images. Because bone is much denser than soft tissue, its CT values are significantly higher, and a simple threshold operation is usually sufficient to separate bone from its surrounding structures (see Figure 7.6).

## Statistical pixel classification

Statistical pixel classification uses a statistical model for the different classes. Pixels are then assigned to the most likely class. The shape of the decision boundaries in feature space is defined by the transitions where one class becomes more likely than another. Often the intensity variations within a given tissue class $c_j$ (e.g., white matter, gray matter, cerebrospinal fluid, and so forth in the case of brain tissue classification) are assumed to have a Gaussian distribution as a result of noise and small tissue inhomogeneities, i.e.,

$$p(I_k \mid \phi_k = c_j; \mu_j, \sigma_j) = \frac{1}{\sqrt{2\pi}\sigma_j} \cdot \exp\left(-\frac{(I_k - \mu_j)^2}{2\sigma_j^2}\right),$$

(7.1)

where $I_k$ is the intensity and $\phi_k$ the tissue label of pixel $k$. $\mu_j$ and $\sigma_j$ are the unknown mean and standard deviation of class $c_j$.

### Supervised learning

The values of $\mu_j$ and $\sigma_j$ for each class can be learned from a representative set of pixel samples for which the class they belong to is known. This can, for example, be done by manually outlining several regions of pixels, each corresponding to a different class. This process is known as *supervised learning*. After this training

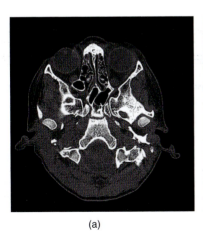
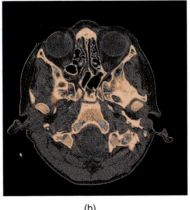
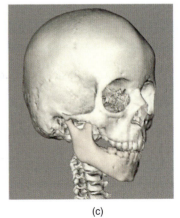

(a)  (b)  (c)

**Figure 7.6** Segmentation of the skull and the mandibula in CT images using thresholding. **(a)** Original CT image of the head. **(b)** Result with a threshold value of 276 Hounsfield units. The segmented bony structures are represented in color. **(c)** 3D rendering of the skull shows a congenital growth deficiency of the mandibula in this 8-year-old patient. This information was used preoperatively to plan a repositioning of the mandibula. (Courtesy of Nobel Biocare.)

phase, unclassified pixels are assigned to the class $c_j$ with the highest probability $p(\phi_k = c_j | I_k)$. Assuming that this probability does not depend on neighboring class assignments $\phi_i$, $i \neq k$, it can be calculated using Bayes' rule:

$$p(\phi_k = c_j \mid I_k) = \frac{p(I_k \mid \phi_k = c_j) p(\phi_k = c_j)}{\sum_{i=1}^{M} p(I_k \mid \phi_k = c_i) p(\phi_k = c_i)},$$

$$(7.2)$$

where the likelihood $p(I_k \mid \phi_k = c_j)$ is the Gaussian class intensity model defined in Eq. (7.1) and $p(\phi_k = c_j)$ the prior probability that pixel $k$ belongs to class $c_j$. Note that $p(\phi_k = c_j)$ can be different for each pixel and is assumed to be known. If no such prior information is available, all classes are typically assumed to be equally likely in each pixel (i.e., $\forall k, j: p(\phi_k = c_j) = 1/M$).

Equation (7.2) computes a classification of the pixels in the form of object class probability maps $p(\phi_k = c_j | I_k)$ with values ranging from 0 to 1 such that $\sum_i p(\phi_k = c_i | I_k) = 1$. The pixels are then assigned to the most probable class $c_j$, i.e., the one with the maximal posterior probability $p(\phi_k = c_j | I_k)$. This way the image is segmented into the different classes. It is also possible to represent the a posteriori probabilities $p(\phi_k = c_j | I_k)$ as gray values in each pixel, yielding a so-called *fuzzy segmentation* or classification.

Note that maximizing the a posteriori probability $p(\phi_k = c_j | I_k)$ is in principle not the same as maximizing the likelihood $p(I_k | \phi_k = c_j)$. The former finds the most probable model instance or class that describes the image data, while the latter finds the model instance or class that best explains the data whatever the prior probability of that model instance is. Only if the prior $p(\phi_k = c_j)$ is uniform for all classes, i.e., $p(\phi_k = c_j) = 1/M$, will maximizing the posterior probability also maximize the likelihood.

The problem of statistical pixel classification can be stated more generally as finding the maximum of $p(\Phi|I)$ with $\Phi = \{\phi_k; k = 1, \ldots, N\}$ and $I = \{I_k; k = 1, \ldots, N\}$. According to Bayes' rule

$$p(\Phi|I) = \frac{p(I \mid \Phi) \cdot p(\Phi)}{p(I)}, \qquad (7.3)$$

where $p(I \mid \Phi)$ is the conditional probability or likelihood and $p(\Phi)$ the prior probability. When maximizing $p(\Phi|I)$, the probability $p(I)$ is constant and can be ignored. Hence,

$$\arg \max_{\Phi} p(\Phi|I) = \arg \max_{\Phi} (p(I \mid \Phi) \cdot p(\Phi)). \quad (7.4)$$

Because the logarithm is monotonically increasing, maximizing $\ln p(\Phi|I)$ corresponds to maximizing $p(\Phi|I)$:

$$\arg \max_{\Phi} \ln p(\Phi|I) = \arg \max_{\Phi} (\ln p(I \mid \Phi) + \ln p(\Phi)).$$

$$(7.5)$$

If a uniform prior distribution $p(\Phi)$ can be assumed, the parameters $\Phi$ with the highest probability are found by maximizing the log-likelihood, i.e.,

$$\arg \max_{\Phi} \ln p(\Phi|I) = \arg \max_{\Phi} (\ln p(I \mid \Phi)). \quad (7.6)$$

If the tissue labels of neighboring pixels are independent, $p(I|\Phi)$ can be written as

$$p(I|\Phi) = \prod_k p(I_k \mid \phi_k). \qquad (7.7)$$

Using Eq. (7.1) yields

$$p(I|\Phi) = \frac{1}{\sqrt{2\pi} \prod_k \sigma_k} \cdot \exp\left(-\frac{1}{2} \sum_k \frac{(I_k - \mu_k)^2}{\sigma_k^2}\right)$$

$$(7.8)$$

and

$$\arg \max_{\Phi} (\ln p(I \mid \Phi)) = \arg \min_{\Phi} \sum_k \frac{(I_k - \mu_k)^2}{\sigma_k^2}.$$

$$(7.9)$$

Hence, each pixel $k$ is assigned to the tissue class $c_j$ for which $(I_k - \mu_k)^2/\sigma_k^2$ is minimal. Note that a uniform prior distribution $p(\Phi)$ was assumed. Instead, prior knowledge about the spatial distribution of the various tissue classes in the image can be derived from a statistical atlas and used in Eq. (7.5) (see Figure 7.7).

If multispectral MR data or multimodal image data are available, the model for each class can be extended to a multivariate distribution with vector mean $\mu_j$ and covariance matrix $S_j$. For the $n$-dimensional case the likelihood $p(I|\Phi)$ then becomes (compare with Eq. (7.8))

$$p(I|\Phi) = \frac{1}{(2\pi)^{n/2}\sqrt{|S|}} \cdot \exp\left(-\frac{1}{2}(I - \mu)^{\mathrm{T}} S^{-1}(I - \mu)\right)$$

$$(7.10)$$

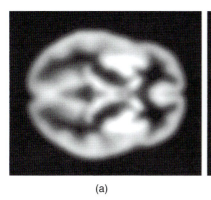 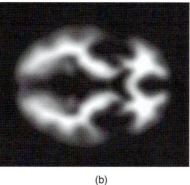

(a)　　　　　　　　　　　　　　　(b)

**Figure 7.7** Statistical images of **(a)** the gray brain matter and **(b)** the white brain matter. The intensity in each pixel is proportional to its prior probability $p(\phi_k = c_j)$ of belonging to that particular tissue class.

and the most likely tissue labels (compare with Eq. (7.9))

$$\arg \max_{\Phi} (\ln p(I\,|\Phi)) = \arg \min_{\Phi} ((I - \mu)^{\mathrm{T}} S^{-1} (I - \mu)).$$
$$(7.11)$$

## Unsupervised learning

The training phase in supervised learning typically requires user interaction, which is too cumbersome in clinical practice. For a fully automated procedure, the values of the mean $\mu_j$ and standard deviation $\sigma_j$ can, for example, be considered as unknowns in the optimization process. This is called *unsupervised learning*. Let $\Theta = \{\mu_j, \sigma_j; j = 1, \ldots, M\}$ be the unknown mean and standard deviation of the tissue classes $C = \{c_j; j = 1, \ldots, M\}$. The goal is to find $\{\Phi, \Theta\}$ with the highest probability given the data $I$, i.e., $\arg \max_{\Phi,\Theta} p(\Phi, \Theta | I)$. According to Bayes' rule

$$p(\Phi, \Theta | I) = \frac{p(I, \Phi | \Theta) \cdot p(\Theta)}{p(I)}. \qquad (7.12)$$

When maximizing $p(\Phi, \Theta | I)$, the probability $p(I)$ is constant and can be ignored. If the prior probability $p(\Theta)$ is uniform, we obtain

$$\arg \max_{\Phi,\Theta} p(\Phi, \Theta | I) = \arg \max_{\Phi,\Theta} p(I, \Phi | \Theta) \qquad (7.13)$$

and

$$\arg \max_{\Phi,\Theta} \ln p(\Phi, \Theta | I) = \arg \max_{\Phi,\Theta} \ln p(I, \Phi | \Theta).$$
$$(7.14)$$

Maximizing the log-likelihood $\ln p(I, \Phi | \Theta)$ can be solved iteratively with the expectation-maximization (EM) algorithm, but its theory is beyond the scope of this textbook. Figure 7.8 shows an example.

## Model extensions

- In order to account for the partial volume effect, mixture classes can be introduced whose intensities are a weighted sum of the intensities of the pure tissue classes.

- A rejection class that collects all pixels that cannot be classified into one of the modeled classes can be included to cope with pathological areas, such as MS lesions (see Figure 7.28 below).

- The intensities in real MR data can be modulated by slowly varying intensity inhomogeneities (see Figure 4.35). It can be shown that this bias field can be taken into account in the Gaussian intensity model.

- Tissue labels of neighboring pixels are not necessarily independent. For example, neighboring pixels can be expected to belong to the same class. Employing this contextual knowledge yields a smooth label image. Similarly, local geometric knowledge can be incorporated in pixel classification. Consider for example the problem of blood vessel classification, in which for each pixel the probability that it belongs to a vessel needs to be calculated. Blood vessels are smooth tubular structures. If the labels of neighboring pixels were independent it would be sufficient to apply a local image operator sensitive to bar-like primitives to obtain a label image in which the gray value is proportional to the likelihood that the pixel belongs to a tubular structure. However, tubular structures of neighboring pixels have a similar orientation. This requirement should also be taken into account. Because the classification of a pixel depends on the labels of its neighboring pixels, iterative optimization is typically needed to find the global optimum. Although these examples show

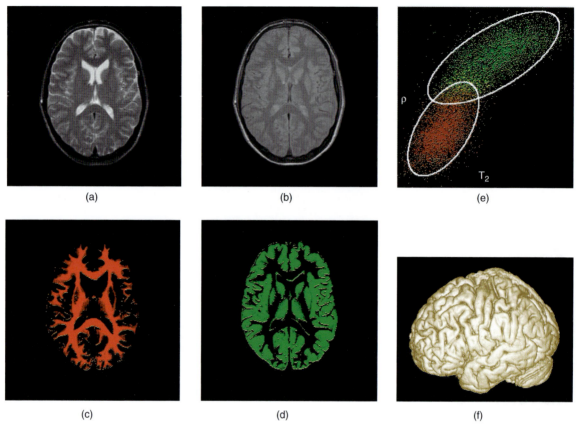

**Figure 7.8** Brain tissue segmentation in multispectral MR images using unsupervised pixel classification. (**a** and **b**) Original $T_2$- and $\rho$-weighted MR images. (**c** and **d**) Classification of white and gray matter represented in red and green, respectively. (**e**) The probabilities for each point, shown in (c) and (d), are represented in a scatter plot as a function of $\rho$ and $T_2$ together with the 0.99 percentile contours of the Gaussian class intensity model that was fitted using the EM algorithm. (**f**) 3D representation of the cortex obtained by volume rendering of the gray matter segmentation (d). (Courtesy of K. Van Leemput, Medical Imaging Research Center.)

that limited spatial context can be included in pixel classification, they should rather be considered as special cases of flexible geometric model matching using local properties (see p. 175 below).

In some applications, more sophisticated intensity models are needed. In perfusion studies, for example, a time-dependent model for the contrast or tracer accumulation in tissue is fitted to the observed intensity changes. Another example is the statistical analysis of fMRI data. In Figure 7.9, the intensity variation in a time series of fMRI images acquired during brain stimulation is modeled as a linear combination of time-dependent functions that represent the stimulation course in the experiment and the low-frequency signal drift over time. A statistical test is then applied in each voxel to calculate the statistical significance of the photometric response to the applied stimulus in that voxel.

Regions of voxels with a high significance are classified as functional areas that respond to the stimulus.

## Geometric model matching using a transformation matrix

Unlike the strategies used for pixel classification, the strategies described in this and the next section incorporate geometric variability in the model, which make them potentially more powerful. In this section the shape variability of the object to be recognized is limited and represented by a general geometric transformation matrix (using homogeneous coordinates, see Chapter 1, p. 7), such as a translation, rotation, scaling, shear, affine transformation and perspective projection. If more geometric variability is required, flexible geometric models are needed (see p. 175 below). The shape itself can be represented

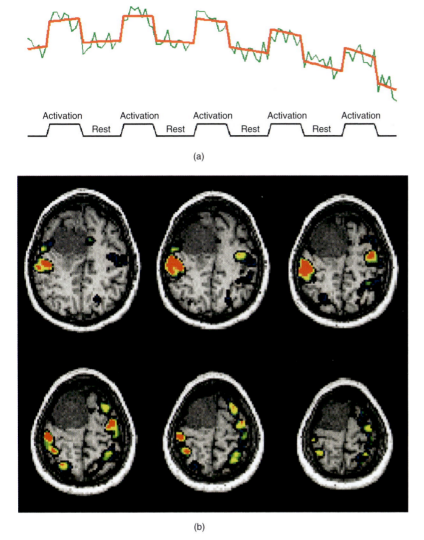

(a)

(b)

**Figure 7.9** Statistical modeling of fMRI signals. **(a)** The fMRI signal in each voxel (green noisy line) is represented (red line) as a linear combination of functions that reflect the activation stimuli ("activation–rest" step signal) and the low-frequency signal drift. Clusters of voxels with a significant response to the applied stimulus are classified as brain activation areas. **(b)** Activation areas during a finger-tapping experiment in a patient with a large extra-axial lesion in the right frontal lobe. Three bilateral functional areas are visible, which correspond to the premotor cortex (anterior), the sensory motor cortex (middle), and the proprioceptive superior parietal region (posterior). Note how the lesion displaced these areas in the right hemisphere by comparing them with the same functional areas in the left hemisphere. (Courtesy of Dr. S. Sunaert, Department of Radiology.)

explicitly as a set of points, a curve or a surface, or implicitly as a picture or image itself.

The photometric properties can be any measure (e.g., homogeneity) or description (e.g., average and statistical variation) of the color, gradient, texture or any other feature along the boundary or inside the object.

Rigid shape structures are naturally uncommon in medical images, and more flexible models are mostly needed. Among the few exceptions are a set of artificial markers or landmarks with known rigid topology, or a prosthetic implant with known rigid geometry. Quite often, multimodal or multitemporal images of the same patient must be aligned for comparison, a process known as *image registration*, *image matching*, or *image fusion*. One image can then be considered as the model that has to be matched with the other image. Rigid image registration has a large variety of clinical applications and has become very popular in medical imaging. The algorithms, discussed below, can be implemented on the graphics processing unit (GPU) of the computer, yielding a nearly real time performance. The idea of using an image as a model can be extended to multiple images represented by an average image and some typical modes of variation that characterize the variability of the appearance. For this kind of modeling a learning or training phase is a prerequisite.

Once the model is available, a model instance must be found that best describes the image data. This

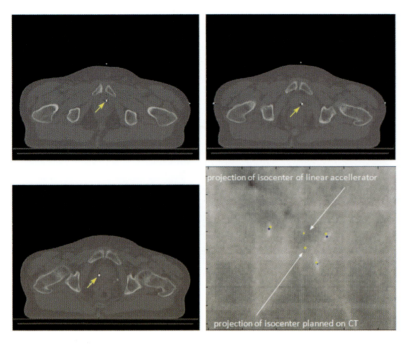

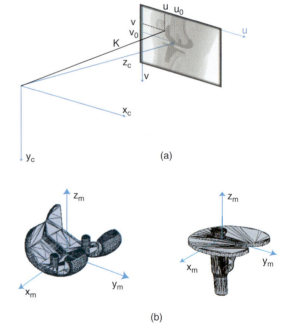

**Figure 7.10** Marker-based 3D-to-2D registration for radiotherapy of prostate tumors. Gold markers were inserted in the prostate and are visible in the CT images before and the 2D portal image (bottom right image) during the treatment. Registration was performed by minimizing the root mean square error of the markers projected in the portal image (yellow) and their observed portal image positions (blue). The isocenter of the linear accelerator, i.e. the rotation point of the irradiation source, is then shifted towards the isocenter as calculated during the planning.

is typically performed by optimizing a measure that reflects the similarity between the model instance and the image data while satisfying the model constraints. The similarity measure can be expressed in terms of a total penalty, cost or energy that should be minimized, or the likelihood that should be maximized. Below some well-known matching strategies are discussed for explicit and implicit shape representation respectively.

## Shape matching

### Point matching

In some cases artificial markers or anatomical landmarks can be used. For example, in image guided interventions preoperative planning data must be matched with the intraoperative instruments. If the coordinates of three or more points in the 3D preoperative and 3D intraoperative space are known, the geometric transformation, consisting of a rotation and translation, can be calculated by simple 3D-to-3D point matching. More details are given in Chapter 8, Eqs. (8.12) through (8.15). Sometimes the point coordinates are only known in a 2D projection space, such as shown in Figure 7.10. In this case the geometric transformation is not only a rotation and translation, but also includes a perspective projection. The projective transformation is discussed in more detail in

**Figure 7.11** 2D projection radiograph of a knee prosthesis (top) and computer simulations of the 3D shape of the femoral and tibial prosthetic implants (bottom).

Chapter 8, Eqs. (8.16) through (8.20). To find the best match between the two sets of points a measure such as the sum of squared differences between corresponding points must be optimized.

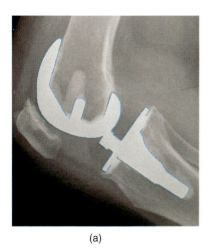
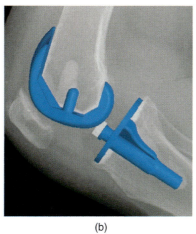

(a)  (b)

**Figure 7.12** **(a)** Edge image of the prosthesis obtained by segmentation (edge detection) of the radiographic image. **(b)** Projection of the prosthesis onto its corresponding image after 3D-to-2D matching.

## Contour matching

Figure 7.11 shows an example of a prosthetic knee implant that consists of two subparts, a femoral and tibial part, whose relative 3D poses have to be calculated from a 2D projection radiograph. The contours of the prosthesis are easily segmented in the radiographic image due to the high contrast between the prosthetic implant and its neighborhood (Figure 7.12(a)). The objective then is to find the best geometric transformation between the 3D model surface and the 2D edge image using a suitable optimization strategy, for example by minimizing the sum of squared differences between the outer contour of the projected model shape and the edges found in the radiographic image (Figure 7.12(b)).

An efficient method to match rigid curves is the *Hough transform* [28]. It detects curves whose shape can be described as an analytic function with a set of parameters, such as the slope and intercept of a straight line. The method was generalized to detect arbitrary shape templates represented as a list of contiguous pixels.

## Image registration

### Correlation

The simplest class of metrics quantifies similarities between two images by correlation measures (see Chapter 1, p. 8). They assume that the gray values in both images are similar. To detect photometric similarities in both images, it is natural to use the raw image data. When other object features are more indicative, however, the raw image can be processed first, for example, by performing a low-level operation such as edge filtering or line filtering.

### Mutual information

For images that are characterized by pronounced mutual intensity differences, such as $T_1$- and $T_2$-weighted images or CT and PET images, the correlation approach is not appropriate. The strategy for matching two such images is to maximize their *mutual information*.

Image fusion by maximization of mutual information assumes that the statistical dependence between the intensities $a$ and $b$ of corresponding voxels in images $A$ and $B$ or the information that one image contains about the other is maximal at registration. Mutual information $I(A, B)$ is a basic concept in information theory [29] that is computed from the histograms $p(a)$ and $p(b)$ and from the joint histogram $p(a, b)$ of the images:

$$I(A, B) = \sum_{a,b} p(a, b) \log_2 \frac{p(a, b)}{p(a).p(b)}. \qquad (7.15)$$

If the intensities are completely independent, $p(a, b) = p(a).p(b)$ and $I(A, B) = 0$. However, if the intensities are one-to-one related, then $p(a, b) = p(a) = p(b)$ and $I(A, B)$ is maximal.

[28] J. Illingworth and J. V. Kittler. A survey of the Hough transform. *Computer Vision Graphics and Image Processing*, 44(1): 87–116, October 1988.

[29] T. M. Cover and J. A. Thomas. *Elements of Information Theory.* New York: John Wiley & Sons, 1991.

Registration of both images is performed iteratively. During the matching procedure, samples taken from one image with intensities $a_i$ are geometrically transformed into the other image using the current transformation parameters, and the corresponding intensities $b_i$ are obtained by interpolation (see Chapter 1, p. 7). The joint histogram for the current registration position is then constructed by binning the intensity pairs $(a_i, b_i)$. Next, the mutual information is computed, and the transformation parameters are updated using an iterative optimization strategy in order to maximize $I(A, B)$.

Because this approach does not rely on the absolute value of the intensities but on their co-occurrences, and because no limiting assumptions are imposed on the photometric relationship between both images, maximization of mutual information is a powerful method that has been applied successfully to a wide range of different applications of image registration (Figure 7.13).

## Eigenfaces

The idea of using an image as a model can be extended to multiple images represented by an average image and some typical modes of variation that characterize the variability of the appearance. This is the so-called *eigenfaces* technique [30], initially applied to images of human faces for face modeling and face recognition. For this kind of modeling a learning or training phase is a prerequisite. Using *principal component analysis* (PCA, more mathematical details are given on p. 180) the image model can be represented as

$$I = \bar{I} + \sum_i c_i \cdot I_i, \tag{7.16}$$

where $\bar{I}$ is the average intensity image of the training set and $I_i$ the eigenvectors, i.e., the principal modes of variation, determined by statistical analysis of the intensities in the set of training images. Each eigenvector $I_i$ has a corresponding eigenvalue $\lambda_i$, which is the variance of parameter $c_i$ in the set of training images. If, for example, the values of the parameters $c_i$ are Gaussian distributed, then 99.7% of the training samples can be described by Eq. (7.16) if $c_i$ is restricted to

$$-3\sqrt{\lambda_i} \le c_i \le 3\sqrt{\lambda_i}. \tag{7.17}$$

Because $\lambda_1 \ge \lambda_2 \ge \cdots$, the foremost modes of variation explain most of the variability in the training set. By constraining the model to include only the $v$ most important modes of variation, i.e., $\lambda_1, \lambda_2, \ldots, \lambda_v$, the complexity of the model can be reduced without significant restriction of its descriptive power.

By varying the coefficients $c_i$, the intensity pattern of a model instance can be tuned to the intensities of a given image. The goal is then to find the best model instance in the image data by applying a suitable geometric operation while varying the parameters $c_i$. If the parameters $c_i$ have a normal distribution, the model instance with the highest probability is the one that maximizes

$$\prod_{i=1}^{v} p(c_i) = \frac{1}{\prod_{i=1}^{v} \sqrt{2\pi\lambda_i}} \cdot \exp\left(-\frac{1}{2}\sum_{i=1}^{v} \frac{c_i^2}{\lambda_i}\right). \tag{7.18}$$

Because the exponential function is monotonically decreasing as a function of $c_i^2$, maximizing $\prod p(c_i)$ yields the same result as minimizing $\sum c_i^2/\lambda_i$:

$$\arg\max_{c_i} \prod_{i=1}^{v} p(c_i) = \arg\min_{c_i} \sum_{i=1}^{v} \frac{c_i^2}{\lambda_i}. \tag{7.19}$$

Figure 7.14 shows an example. A drawback of this approach is that it is negatively affected by pose or shape differences between different images in the training set from which the intensity model is constructed. Proper geometric and photometric normalization of the training images is therefore required to maximize the discriminative power of the eigenface model.

## Statistical atlas

On p. 168, in the section on statistical pixel classification, it was mentioned that prior knowledge about the spatial distribution of the various tissue classes in the image can be derived from a statistical atlas $p(\Phi)$ (Figure 7.7), while the goal was to maximize $p(\Phi | I)$ (Eq. (7.4)), i.e.,

$$\arg\max_{\Phi} p(\Phi|I) = \arg\max_{\Phi}(p(I|\Phi) \cdot p(\Phi)) \tag{7.20}$$

or similarly (see Eq. (7.5))

$$\arg\max_{\Phi} \ln p(\Phi|I) = \arg\max_{\Phi}(\ln p(I|\Phi) + \ln p(\Phi)), \tag{7.21}$$

[30] M. Turk and A. P. Pentland. Eigenfaces for recognition. *Journal of Cognitive Neuroscience*, 3(1): 71–96, 1991.

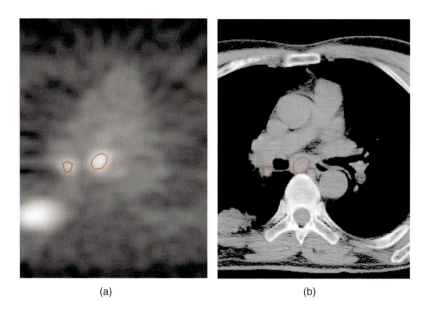

**Figure 7.13** Diagnosis of metastatic lymph nodes in the mediastinum in a lung cancer patient using image fusion. **(a)** Detection of metastatic lymph nodes is performed most easily with PET, but anatomical localization is difficult because of the lack of anatomical landmarks. **(b)** CT on the other hand, clearly shows the anatomy but does not differentiate the affected lymph nodes. After registration of the PET and CT images, the lesions, delineated in the PET scans (a), were displayed in the CT images (b). (Courtesy of the Department of Nuclear Medicine.)

(a)  (b)

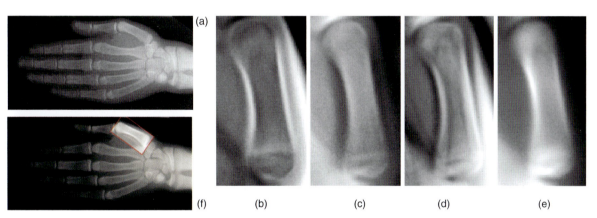

(a)

(f)  (b)  (c)  (d)  (e)

**Figure 7.14** Object recognition by template matching using the eigenfaces approach. **(a)** Radiographic image of the hand. **(b)** Template of the first metacarpal bone constructed by averaging a set of similar training images. **(c–e)** The three most prominent modes of variation as determined by statistical analysis of the intensity variation in the training set. The eigenface model is the sum of the average template (b) and a linear combination of the modes (c), (d), and (e). **(f)** Result of fitting the eigenface model to the image (a). This result provides a proper initialization of the pose parameters of a flexible contour model used to delineate accurately the contour of the bone (see Figure 7.18 below). (Courtesy of G. Behiels, Medical Imaging Research Center.)

which was to be solved without any geometric uncertainty. However, if the position and scale of the atlas are unknown, the affine transformation parameters have to be taken into account as additional unknowns in the optimization process.

## Flexible geometric model matching

Flexible geometric models can be represented as geometric constraints or penalties on a deformable curve or on a deformable picture or image itself. Examples

are constraints or penalties on the smoothness, curvature, rectilinearity, parallelism, symmetry, rigidity and elasticity. These geometric models offer flexibility to the geometry and are more suitable for modeling biological variability than the geometric models of the previous section, where the flexibility was limited to a transformation matrix.

The model properties can be specified as physical or biomechanical characteristics, or as statistical distributions obtained from a representative set of

**175**

images during a training phase. Furthermore, they can have a global nature (e.g., global elasticity) or a local nature (e.g., local curvature) and they can be tissue dependent, which has an important influence on the behavior of the shape and on the complexity of the optimization method. The more flexibility is offered the more computationally expensive the search may become and the higher the probability that the optimization may converge to a local instead of the global minimum. A proper initialization of the model is therefore typically required.

As in the previous section, fitting a flexible geometric model to the image data consists of finding the best model instance that describes the image data. This problem can be solved by optimizing a suitable objective function while satisfying the model constraints. This function includes measures to express how likely the model instance is a priori and how similar the model instance and the data are. The measure can be expressed in terms of a total penalty, cost or energy that should be minimized, or a probability that should be maximized. Typically the objective function consists of two components, which can easily be explained using Bayes' rule. If the optimization aims to find the model instance $\Phi$ that maximizes the posterior probability of the model instance $\Phi$ given the image data $I$, Bayes' rule states

$$p(\Phi|I) = \frac{p(I\,|\Phi) \cdot p(\Phi)}{p(I)}. \qquad (7.22)$$

When maximizing $p(\Phi|I)$, the probability $p(I)$ is constant and can be ignored. Hence

$$\arg\max_{\Phi} p(\Phi|I) = \arg\max_{\Phi}(p(I\,|\Phi) \cdot p(\Phi)) \qquad (7.23)$$

and

$$\arg\max_{\Phi} \ln p(\Phi|I) = \arg\max_{\Phi}(\ln p(I\,|\Phi) + \ln p(\Phi)). \qquad (7.24)$$

The log-likelihood $\ln p(I\,|\Phi)$ expresses how well the model instance $\Phi$ fits the image data $I$ and the term $\ln p(\Phi)$ reflects how likely the model instance $\Phi$ is a priori.

Instead of using probabilities it is common practice to write the similarity criterion as an energy function. In mathematics the Gibbs measure gives the probability of a system being in state $X$ with associated

energy $E(X)$:

$$p(X) = \frac{e^{-\beta E(X)}}{\sum_X e^{-\beta E(X)}}, \qquad (7.25)$$

where $\beta$ is a free parameter. Assume, for example, that $p(X)$ is a multivariate distribution with vector mean $\mu$ and covariance matrix $S$, i.e., for the $n$-dimensional case,

$$p(X) = \frac{1}{(2\pi)^{n/2}\sqrt{|S|}} \cdot \exp\left(-\frac{1}{2}(X-\mu)^{\mathsf{T}}S^{-1}(X-\mu)\right). \qquad (7.26)$$

The corresponding energy according to Eq. (7.25) then is

$$E(X) = \frac{1}{2}(X-\mu)^{\mathsf{T}}S^{-1}(X-\mu). \qquad (7.27)$$

If the elements $x_i$ of $X$ are independent and have zero mean and standard deviation $\sigma_i$, Eq. (7.26) becomes

$$\prod_i p(x_i) = \frac{1}{\sqrt{2\pi}\prod_i \sigma_i} \cdot \exp\left(-\frac{1}{2}\sum_i \frac{x_i^2}{\sigma_i^2}\right) \qquad (7.28)$$

and the corresponding energy is

$$E(X) = \frac{1}{2}\sum_i \frac{x_i^2}{\sigma_i^2}. \qquad (7.29)$$

Using Eq. (7.25), Eq. (7.24) can be rewritten as

$$\arg\min_{\Phi} E(\Phi|I) = \arg\min_{\Phi}(E(I\,|\Phi) + E(\Phi)) \qquad (7.30)$$

or

$$\arg\min_{\Phi} E_{\text{total}} = \arg\min_{\Phi}(E_{\text{ext}} + E_{\text{int}}). \qquad (7.31)$$

The term $E_{\text{ext}}$ is called the external energy, which increases with the dissimilarity between the model instance and the image data, and $E_{\text{int}}$ is called the internal energy, which reflects how unlikely the appearance of the model instance is a priori.

In practice the internal and external energy functions are typically not derived from their corresponding probabilities. Instead, they are defined using heuristic criteria about the expected model appearance. A normalization factor $\gamma$ is usually introduced to weight the contribution of both energy terms:

$$\arg\min_{\Phi} E_{\text{total}} = \arg\min_{\Phi}(E_{\text{ext}} + \gamma E_{\text{int}}). \qquad (7.32)$$

For example, $\gamma$ can be tuned to yield the optimal result for a set of training samples.

Below some examples of well-known matching strategies for flexible geometric models are discussed, for both explicit and implicit shape representation. A further subdivision is made between physical/biomechanical and statistical properties.

## Shape matching
### Physical/biomechanical properties
#### Global properties
In this strategy a curve or surface, such as the boundary of an object, deforms from a given initial shape to an optimal shape. Shape properties yield an internal energy $E_{int}$ and include boundary smoothness and curvature, rectilinearity, parallelism, and radial symmetry. The photometric properties, yielding an external energy $E_{ext}$, attract the contour to relevant image features, such as high image gradients. The curve can also be attracted toward particular places imposed by neighboring objects or components or specified interactively by the user. The photometric properties can also take the area enclosed by the curve into account and, for example, force the curve to circumscribe homogeneous regions.

Generally, the objective function has no closed-form solution and iterative techniques are needed to solve the optimization problem. During the iterative optimization process, the flexible curve typically behaves like a "snake" [31] (Figure 7.15).

The objective function can be written as a weighted sum of an internal and an external energy:

$$E_{total} = E_{ext} + \gamma E_{int}. \qquad (7.33)$$

If $v(s) = \{x(s), y(s)\}, s \in [0,1]$, is the continuous parameterization of the contour, these energy terms can for example be defined as

$$E_{int} = \int_0^1 \frac{\alpha}{2} \cdot \left|\frac{dv}{ds}\right|^2 + \frac{\beta}{2} \cdot \left|\frac{d^2v}{ds^2}\right|^2 ds \qquad (7.34)$$

$$E_{ext} = \int_0^1 -|\nabla I(v)|^2 ds. \qquad (7.35)$$

Minimizing the first-order term in the internal energy function $E_{int}$ keeps the elasticity of the contour under

[31] M. Kass, A. Witkin, and D. Terzopoulos. Snakes: active contour models. *International Journal of Computer Vision*, 1(4): 321–331, September 1988.

control, and the second-order term controls its flexibility. The parameters $\alpha$ and $\beta$ are material properties, to be specified by the user. Minimizing the external energy term $E_{ext}$ attracts the contour to high-intensity gradients $\nabla I(v)$, which correspond to edge points in the image. Fitting the deformable model to the image then implies finding the contour $v^*$ for which $E_{total}(v)$ is minimal:

$$v^* = \arg \min_v E_{total}(v). \qquad (7.36)$$

The optimization problem can be solved iteratively, for example by gradient descent. This means that the snake is stepwise displaced in the direction of the descending gradient of the objective function, which finally leads to a minimum of this function. A necessary condition is that the initial contour lies sufficiently close to the optimal one. Nevertheless, the snake can still get stuck in a local optimum. A possible solution in that case is to pull the snake out of its entrapped position interactively and restart the optimization process.

Many variants of the preceding strategy have been developed. They differ by the choice of the shape representation, the definition of the external energy, and the optimization method used.

- Alternative contour parameterizations are based on splines or Fourier descriptors. As compared with simple polygons, they have a smaller number of degrees of freedom and an intrinsic built-in smoothness. Models with distributed parameters, such as polygons and splines, facilitate the modeling of local detail, while models with global parameters, such as Fourier descriptors, are more suited for modeling global shape. An interesting feature of splines is that global smoothness is maintained when displacing individual points, which makes them well suited for interactive editing. The concept of 2D deformable contours has also been extended to 3D deformable surfaces by replacing the contour $v(s)$ by the surface

$$S(u,v) = \{x(u,v), y(u,v), z(u,v)\}$$

defined on the 2D grid $(u,v)$.

- To reduce the risk that the snake is trapped in a weak local minimum far away from the global one, additional external energy terms can be included, such as a global inflating balloon energy that can be counterbalanced only by strong image gradients.

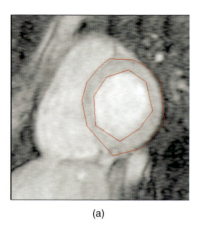 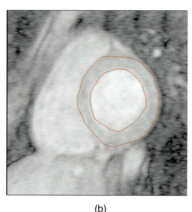

(a)                                                         (b)

**Figure 7.15** Delineation of the myocardial wall of the left ventricle in short axis cross-sectional MR images using "snakes." **(a)** The heart wall was roughly outlined by the user to initiate the deformation process. **(b)** The snake is attracted to high image gradients and is forced to be smooth.

- Optimization strategies other than gradient descent have also been used for deformable models, such as genetic algorithms and simulated annealing. Optimization strategies are considered beyond the scope of this textbook. See [3] for details about optimization theory.

### Local properties

This strategy assumes that the model can be represented as a trajectory or path of contiguous pixels and that the objective function can be expressed in terms of *local* properties along the path.

In contour tracking for instance, a high gradient value in each path pixel is desired. For blood vessel delineation, trajectory points are expected to lie on the centerline of a tube-like structure. For fiber tracking (Figure 7.16) neighboring trajectory points have an anisotropic diffusion whose main directions are in line. This kind of property yields an external energy $E_{\text{ext}}$.

Additional local properties, focusing on the shape of the trajectory, can be added and yield the internal energy $E_{\text{int}}$. For example, smoothness can be expressed by charging local changes in the direction of the trajectory course. Parallelism to a specified curve can be forced by penalizing orientation differences between both trajectories.

An energy $E_{\text{total}}(\mathbf{r}_i) = E_{\text{ext}}(\mathbf{r}_i) + \gamma E_{\text{int}}(\mathbf{r}_i)$, assigned to each pixel $\mathbf{r}_i$ in the image, expresses how unlikely it is that this pixel belongs to the trajectory. In contour tracking, for example, a suitable choice for the external energy $E_{\text{ext}}(\mathbf{r}_i)$ is $(-|\nabla I(\mathbf{r}_i)|)$. To force parallelism, for example, the internal energy $E_{\text{int}}(\mathbf{r}_i)$ can be defined as $|d(\mathbf{r}_i) - d(\mathbf{r}_{i-1})|$, where $d$ is the distance to the specified curve.

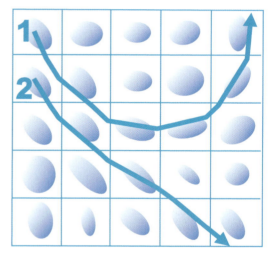

**Figure 7.16** Schematic representation of fiber tracking. In each voxel the diffusion is represented by an ellipsoid (see Chapter 4, p. 88 for more details about MR diffusion tensor imaging). Along each fiber trajectory, neighboring points have an anisotropic diffusion whose main directions are in line.

The energy $E_{\text{total}}(P)$ of a path

$$P = \{a = \mathbf{r}_0, \mathbf{r}_1, \mathbf{r}_2, \ldots, \mathbf{r}_{n-1}, \mathbf{r}_n = b\}$$

from $a$ to $b$ is defined as the sum of the local energy along its trajectory:

$$E_{\text{total}}(P) = \sum_{i=1}^{n} (E_{\text{ext}}(\mathbf{r}_i) + \gamma E_{\text{int}}(\mathbf{r}_i))$$

$$= \sum_{i=1}^{n} (-|\nabla I(\mathbf{r}_i)| + \gamma |d(\mathbf{r}_i) - d(\mathbf{r}_{i-1})|).$$

(7.37)

**178**

The optimal path $P^*$ between $a$ and $b$ is then found by minimizing this energy function over the set $\mathcal{P}$ of all paths that connect $a$ to $b$:

$$P^* = \arg\min_{\mathcal{P}} E_{\text{total}}(P). \qquad (7.38)$$

The number of possible paths in an image is very large, and blind search can be computationally expensive. Fortunately, this optimization problem can be solved efficiently with the so-called $F^*$-algorithm, which uses the principle of *dynamic programming*. Dynamic programming is based on the observation that the minimal energy path from $a$ to $b$ and passing through $c$ is the union of the minimal energy path from $a$ to $c$ and from $c$ to $b$. Hence, from all the trajectories that arrive at point $c$ during the search, it is sufficient to keep the least expensive. This is typically implemented by constructing a minimal energy matrix with elements $E_{\text{total}}(c)$ for all pixels in a region of interest that includes start point $a$ and target point $b$. The energy $E_{\text{total}}(c)$ of the minimal energy path from $a$

to $c$ is computed iteratively by initializing the energy of all pixels $c$ to infinity ($E_{\text{total}}^{(0)}(c) = \infty$), except for pixel $a$ whose initial energy is zero ($E_{\text{total}}^{(0)}(a) = 0$), and updating these values at iteration $(m+1)$ as follows:

$$E_{\text{total}}^{(m+1)}(c)$$
$$= \min\left\{E_{\text{total}}^{(m)}(c), \min_{k \in N(c)}\left\{E_{\text{total}}^{(m)}(k) + E_k(c)\right\}\right\},$$
$$(7.39)$$

where $N(c)$ denotes the neighboring pixels $k$ of $c$ and $E_k(c)$ the energy to go from pixel $k$ to pixel $c$. The updating rule (7.39) is applied repeatedly to all pixels $c$ until $\forall c \; E_{\text{total}}^{(m)}(c) = E_{\text{total}}^{(m+1)}(c) = E_{\text{total}}(c)$, where $E_{\text{total}}(c)$ is the minimal energy from $a$ to $c$. The minimal energy path from $a$ to $b$ can simply be traced in the minimal energy matrix with elements $E_{\text{total}}(c)$ as the path of steepest descent from $b$ to $a$.

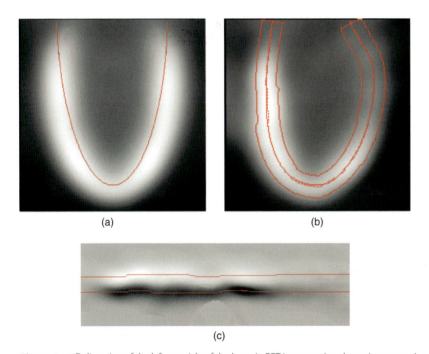

(a)

(b)

(c)

**Figure 7.17** Delineation of the left ventricle of the heart in PET images using dynamic programing. **(a)** An initial estimate of the centerline is determined first by fitting an elliptic curve to the average intensity of a number of regularly spaced cross-section images through the long axis of the ventricle. This can be done interactively or automatically. **(b)** Dynamic programming is then applied in a resampled region around the centerline in each cross-section image. Two paths, nearly parallel to the centerline, were found, one with maximal positive and one with maximal negative gradient values. These paths correspond to the inner and outer ventricular boundaries, respectively. **(c)** An efficient implementation was obtained by first resampling the image in a small band along the centerline. Next, the elliptic centerline is updated and the procedure is repeated iteratively a few times until it converges. Because of the shape model, the method can cope with low-contrast regions, such as the infarcted area in the upper right part of the image. (Courtesy of Professor J. Nuyts, Department of Nuclear Medicine.)

The $F^*$-algorithm is particularly suited to delineate curves in the neighborhood of a specified shape (see, e.g., Figure 7.17). This strategy is therefore very appropriate for semiautomated, user-guided delineation. The user can, for example, manually trace a contour using the mouse, while the corresponding optimal boundary contour will follow in real time.

## Statistical shape properties

### Global properties

The deformable curve models discussed above employ physical or biomechanical shape constraints, such as smoothness and elasticity. The models discussed in this section, in the literature known as *active shape models* [32] or *active appearance models* [33], are constructed by learning the shape or appearance of one specific object type from a representative set of examples. This way, the number of degrees of freedom of the model is significantly reduced, but the model retains the necessary flexibility to cope with the normal shape variability between different instances of this object type. A shape model is built by examining the statistics of the coordinates of corresponding points in a training set of shapes. Each shape is described by $n$ labeled points and corresponding points in different shape instances have the same label. The model and image template are first aligned using the eigenfaces method (see p. 174) to correct for differences in pose. This way, $m$ contours $\{v_i, i = 1, 2, \ldots, m\}$ in the same reference frame are obtained. Each contour can be written as a column vector of coordinates $(x_{ik}, y_{ik})$, that is, $\mathbf{v}_i = [x_{i1}\ y_{i1}\ x_{i2}\ y_{i2} \cdots x_{in}\ y_{in}]^{\mathrm{T}}$.

The shape variations $\mathbf{v}_i - \bar{\mathbf{v}}$, where $\bar{\mathbf{v}}$ is the mean shape and defined as

$$\bar{\mathbf{v}} = \frac{1}{m} \sum_{i=1}^{m} \mathbf{v}_i, \tag{7.40}$$

can be represented in a $2n$-dimensional feature space whose axes correspond to the $2n$ labeled points along the contour. The variations on different labels are not necessarily uncorrelated. To work in an uncorrelated feature space, the theory of *principal component analysis* (PCA) can be applied as follows. The shape

variability in the training set is represented by the $2n \times 2n$ covariance matrix $S$ of shape distortions $\mathbf{v}_i - \bar{\mathbf{v}}$ of all the shapes in the set

$$S = \frac{1}{m} \sum_{i=1}^{m} (\mathbf{v}_i - \bar{\mathbf{v}}) \cdot (\mathbf{v}_i - \bar{\mathbf{v}})^{\mathrm{T}}. \tag{7.41}$$

This matrix can also be written as

$$S = Q \cdot \Lambda \cdot Q^{\mathrm{T}}, \tag{7.42}$$

where $Q = [\mathbf{r}_1\ \mathbf{r}_2 \cdots \mathbf{r}_{2n}]$ is the $2n \times 2n$ unitary matrix of eigenvectors $\mathbf{r}_k$ of $S$, and $\Lambda$ is the diagonal matrix of corresponding eigenvalues $\lambda_k$ (with $\lambda_1 \geq \lambda_2 \geq \cdots$). The new axes $\mathbf{r}_k$ in feature space correspond to the new modes of variation, which are mutually uncorrelated and are characteristic for the shape diversity in the training set. $\sqrt{\lambda_k}$ is the standard deviation along $\mathbf{r}_k$ of all the shapes in the learning set.

The shape model can then be written as

$$\mathbf{v} = \bar{\mathbf{v}} + \sum_{k}^{2n} c_k \cdot \mathbf{r}_k. \tag{7.43}$$

Each eigenvector $\mathbf{r}_k$ has a corresponding eigenvalue $\lambda_k$, which is the variance of parameter $c_k$ in the set of training shapes. Because $\lambda_1 \geq \lambda_2 \geq \cdots$, the foremost modes of variation explain most of the variability in the training set. By constraining the model to include only the $v$ most important modes of variation that explain most of the variability in the training set, the number of degrees of freedom of the model can be significantly reduced without affecting much of its descriptive power. Any contour instance $\mathbf{v}^*$ can then be written as

$$\mathbf{v}^* = \bar{\mathbf{v}} + \sum_{k}^{v} c_k \cdot \mathbf{r}_k. \tag{7.44}$$

By varying the coefficients $c_k$, the shape of a model instance can be modified.

If the parameters $c_k$ have a normal distribution, the internal energy is (see Eqs. (7.29) and (7.19))

$$E_{\mathrm{int}} = \frac{1}{2} \sum_{k=1}^{v} \frac{c_k^2}{\lambda_k}. \tag{7.45}$$

[32] T. F. Cootes, C. J. Taylor, D. H. Cooper, and J. Graham. Active shape models: Their training and application. *Computer Vision and Image Understanding*, 61(1): 38–59, 1995.

[33] T. F. Cootes, G. J. Edwards, and C. J. Taylor. Active appearance models. *IEEE Transactions on Medical Imaging*, 23(6): 681–685, 2001.

The external energy can for example be defined heuristically as in Eq. (7.35):

$$E_{ext} = \int_0^1 -|\nabla I(\mathbf{v})|^2 ds. \qquad (7.46)$$

An alternative is, for example, to maximize the similarity with a statistical model of the image intensities perpendicular to each characteristic contour point.

Finally the goal is to find the parameters $c_k$ by minimizing the weighted sum of the external and internal energies, i.e., $E_{ext} + \gamma E_{int}$. Figure 7.18 shows an example.

A drawback of the method is that a training phase is needed for each new object type. This usually involves a manual delineation of a sufficient number of representative shapes and the identification of corresponding points in the training set. This can be tedious and time consuming but needs to be done carefully, as differences in point coordinates resulting from inconsistencies in the labeling cannot be discriminated from true shape variability. The matching procedure further assumes that the initialization is sufficiently accurate for convergence to the correct optimum. The initial pose can be specified interactively or obtained through a separate procedure, such as the *eigenfaces* approach, discussed on p. 174.

*Local properties*

As stated before, this strategy assumes that the model can be represented as a trajectory or path of contiguous pixels and that the objective function can be expressed in terms of *local* properties along the path. While before these properties had a physical or biomechanical meaning, in this section the local geometric and photometric properties are obtained by learning the local shape and appearance from a training set. Figure 7.19(a) shows an example of a thoracic radiograph in which a radiologist delineated the lung boundary by indicating a set of characteristic points, which are connected by straight lines. Repeating this procedure for a representative set of images yields a training set of contours, characterized by the local photometry around each point and by the direction between neighbors.

The local photometry around each labeled point can be modeled studying a small window around this point and applying the theory of eigenfaces (see Figure 7.14). After applying PCA this yields the following local external energy for each labeled point $l_i$ (see Eqs. (7.19) and (7.45))

$$E_{ext}(l_i) = \frac{1}{2} \sum_{k=1}^{v} \frac{c_k^{i\,2}}{\lambda_k}, \qquad (7.47)$$

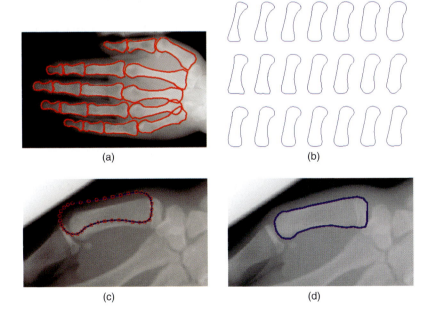

(a)

(b)

(c)

(d)

**Figure 7.18** Active shape model for delineation of the finger bones in radiographic images. The result can be used to compare the shape of the bones to their normal shape in order to calculate the bone age of the patient. **(a)** Manual delineation of the bones. **(b)** Three principal modes of variation for the first metacarpal bone in a database of manually segmented training images. **(c)** The mean shape is put on top of a new image to initiate the optimization process. **(d)** Result of the optimization. While fitting the active shape model, the contour is displaced iteratively to match the intensity appearance observed in the training images with that along the contour. (Courtesy of G. Behiels, Medical Imaging Research Center.)

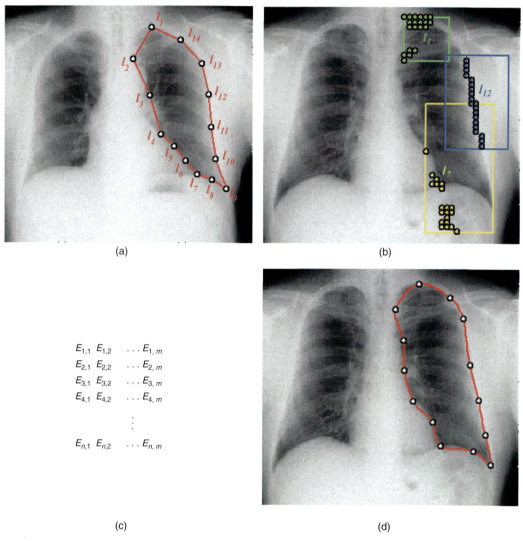

$$
\begin{array}{llll}
E_{1,1} & E_{1,2} & \cdots & E_{1,\,m} \\
E_{2,1} & E_{2,2} & \cdots & E_{2,\,m} \\
E_{3,1} & E_{3,2} & \cdots & E_{3,\,m} \\
E_{4,1} & E_{4,2} & \cdots & E_{4,\,m} \\
& & \vdots & \\
E_{n,1} & E_{n,2} & \cdots & E_{n,\,m}
\end{array}
$$

(a)  (b)  (c)  (d)

**Figure 7.19** Illustration of lung segmentation using local statistical properties and the principle of dynamic programming. **(a)** Result of manual delineation of the lung boundary as a set of characteristic labeled points, connected by straight lines. Repeating this procedure for a representative set of images yields a training set of contours whose local properties are calculated and processed into a statistical model (see text). **(b)** For each label $l_i$ a predefined search area limits the number of candidates for this label. In each search area the $m$ best candidate labels are retained based on their local energy $E_{ext}(l_i)$. In this picture three such search areas and their corresponding candidates are shown. **(c)** For each candidate $j = 1, \ldots, m$ of each label $l_i$ its local energy $E_{i,j}$ is put in a matrix. The trajectory that traverses the matrix from the top to the bottom row, with minimal total energy, is found using dynamic programming. The energy to connect two neighboring matrix elements in the path is given by the local internal energy $E_{int}(l_i, l_{i+1})$. **(d)** Lung contour through the optimal set of landmarks. The piecewise linear contour, obtained by connecting the optimal landmarks by straight lines, is entered in the $F^*$-algorithm, which traces a contour in the neighborhood of the straight lines that fits the high image gradients more accurately. This result can then be used to calculate thoracic measurements such as the cardiothoracic ratio.

assuming that the parameters $c_k$ have a normal distribution. Further assuming photometric independence between the labeled points $l_i$, the total external energy is the summation along the contour of the local external energies:

$$E_{\text{ext}} = \sum_i \sum_{k=1}^{\nu} \left( \frac{1}{2} \frac{c_k^{i\,2}}{\lambda_k} \right). \tag{7.48}$$

The local geometry can be trained by learning the distribution of each orientation vector $\theta_i$ between neighboring labels. Assume that this is a multivariate normal distribution with vector mean $\mu_i$ and covariance matrix $S_i$, then the internal energy $E_{\text{int}}$ to connect point $l_i$ with its neighbor $l_{i+1}$ can be written as (see Eq. (7.27))

$$E_{\text{int}}(l_i, l_{i+1}) = \frac{1}{2} (\theta_i - \mu_i)^{\text{T}} S_i^{-1} (\theta_i - \mu_i). \tag{7.49}$$

Assuming independence between the subsequent orientation vectors, the total internal energy is the summation of the local internal energy along the curve:

$$E_{\text{int}} = \sum_i E_{\text{int}}(l_i, l_{i+1})$$

$$= \sum_i \frac{1}{2} (\theta_i - \mu_i)^{\text{T}} S_i^{-1} (\theta_i - \mu_i). \tag{7.50}$$

Finding the solution with the highest probability corresponds to minimizing the sum of the total internal and external energy:

$$E_{\text{total}} = \frac{1}{2} \sum_i \left( (\theta_i - \mu_i)^{\text{T}} S_i^{-1} (\theta_i - \mu_i) + \sum_{k=1}^{\nu} \frac{c_k^{i\,2}}{\lambda_k} \right). \tag{7.51}$$

Because all the energy terms are locally defined, the principle of dynamic programming can be applied to find the solution with minimal total energy, which is also the solution with the highest probability. Note that Eq. (7.51) does not contain a heuristic parameter $\gamma$. However, this expression is correct only if all the assumptions are satisfied, i.e., normal and independent distributions. In practice this condition may not hold and the internal and external energy terms may not be equally weighted, which favors the introduction of a normalization factor $\gamma$ again (see Eq. (7.32)).

Figure 7.19 illustrates the subsequent steps of the algorithm for lung segmentation in projection radiographs.

# Image registration

A flexible shape can be represented *implicitly* as a picture or image itself with *deformation* properties. Hence, an image is interpreted by fitting it to this iconic representation.

Any pictorial representation or label image can be used as the prototype. In the case of a statistical atlas for example (Figure 7.7), the affine geometry (see p. 175), can be extended to arbitrary deformations. Equation (7.5) can then still be used, i.e.,

$$\arg \max_{\Phi} \ln p(\Phi|I) = \arg \max_{\Phi} (\ln p(I|\Phi) + \ln p(\Phi)). \tag{7.52}$$

However, the prior knowledge $p(\Phi)$ is now the probability of the flexibly deformed statistical atlas instance. This expression can also be rewritten as (see Eq. (7.31))

$$\arg \min_{\Phi} E_{\text{total}} = \arg \min_{\Phi} (E_{\text{ext}} + E_{\text{int}}) \tag{7.53}$$

where the internal energy is defined by the deformed statistical atlas, i.e. by the given tissue class probabilities (see Figure 7.7) together with the probability of the displacement field, including pose and size.

The prototype can also be an image of the same patient taken at a different time or with a different acquisition system. Comparing both images is known as *nonrigid image fusion*.

Deformations can be defined in different ways. They should have a sufficient degree of freedom and robustness in order to cope with the biologic variability and pathological abnormalities. Below are some examples.

## Physical/biomechanical properties
### Tissue independent deformations
Examples of biomechanical deformation properties are rigidity, elasticity and compressibility (a measure of the relative volume change). Figure 7.20 illustrates an example of longitudinal registration of breast MRI images. In this study breast tissue is considered as incompressible elastic tissue. Furthermore, the stress $\sigma$ and strain $\epsilon$ are assumed to be linearly proportional without distinction between muscles, skin, fatty tissue and glandular tissue (Figure 7.21). Note that even then there is no agreement in the literature on the value of the degree of elasticity. In these conditions the internal energy $E_{\text{int}}$ to deform a tissue volume $V$ can be

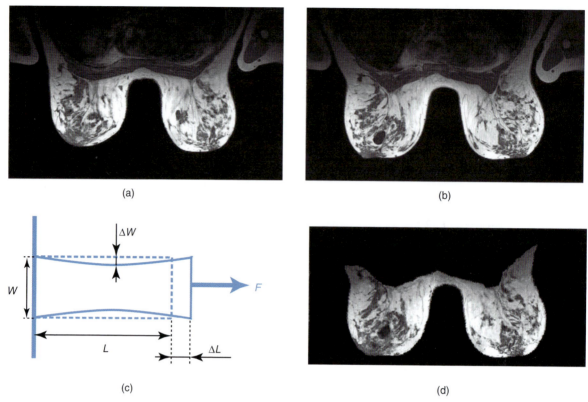

**Figure 7.20** **(a)** and **(b)** Breast MRI of the same patient acquired at different moments. **(c)** Schematic representation of stress and strain. A force $F$ is acting on a bar with length $L$ and area $A$. The axial stress is $\sigma_{axial} = F/A$, the axial strain is $\epsilon_{axial} = \Delta L/L$ and the lateral strain is $\epsilon_{lateral} = \Delta W/W$. **(d)** Image (a) after nonrigid registration using a linear stress–strain relationship.

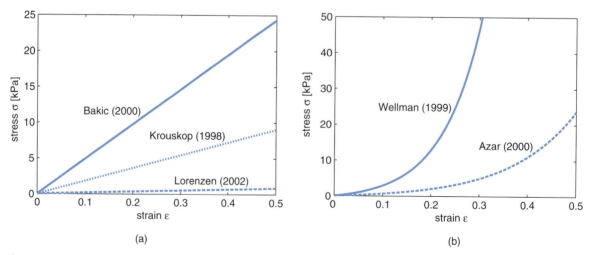

**Figure 7.21** Different relationships between stress and strain in breast tissue are found in the literature. **(a)** Some studies show a linear relationship, i.e., $\sigma = E \cdot \epsilon$ where Young's modulus $E$ is constant. **(b)** Other studies show a nonlinear relationship. At a high stress the tissue stiffens. Note that more complex models also include viscoelasticity, growth and necrosis.

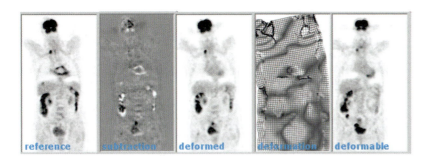

**Figure 7.22** Image registration in a longitudinal PET study. One of the two images is deformed and fit to the reference image using different deformation properties for bone and soft tissue. The subtraction image and the deformation field are also shown. Courtesy of Professor J. Nuyts. Department of Nuclear Medicine

reference  subtraction  deformed  deformation  deformable

defined as

$$E_{int} = \frac{1}{2} \int_V \sigma \, \epsilon \, dV. \qquad (7.54)$$

The external energy is a measure for the dissimilarity between the image data and the prototype. In the case of multimodal or multitemporal image fusion the mutual information between images $A$ and $B$, which reflects the statistical dependence between both images, is a popular measure, i.e.,

$$E_{ext} = -I(A, B). \qquad (7.55)$$

During the optimization the deformation can, for example, be represented by a mathematical function, such as a spline, which is a piecewise polynomial curve with an implicit smooth behavior. An alternative, but computationally much more demanding, approach is to consider the deformable image as a fluid medium with certain viscoelastic properties and to solve the differential equations for viscoelastic motion as in fluid dynamics. In this case, it can be shown that optimizing the objective function is identical to solving the Navier–Stokes equation. Figure 8.16 (Chapter 8) shows another example of nonrigid registration with a heuristic definition of the rigidity and compressibility of the tissue. Precontrast CT images of the blood vessels of head and neck are matched with postcontrast CT images. This way the image deformation due to patient movement between the two CT scans, can be eliminated.

### Tissue dependent deformations

Until now in this section we have seen that the model can be either a specific or statistical deformable image, or an object description in the form of a deformable shape or label image (atlas). In the first case matching is known as multitemporal or multimodality intra-patient *image fusion* and in the second case as *image segmentation* yielding tissue delineation. However, from a methodological point of view we have not made any difference between the two processes. Consequently, nothing prevents us from building a model that consists of a combination of, for example, a deformable label image (atlas) and an explicit shape description. Segmentation and image fusion are then performed simultaneously. Note, however, that the objective function as well as the optimization strategy may become quite complex. Nevertheless, segmentation may sometimes be required to perform image fusion. This is the case if the deformation properties are tissue dependent. The complexity of solving the problem may be drastically reduced if the segmentation and image fusion can be performed sequentially. Figure 7.22 shows an example of subtraction of two whole-body PET bone scans of the same patient taken at different times. Bone appears dark in the images due to a high tracer uptake. Segmentation of bone and soft tissue is then performed simply by thresholding. Next, the internal energy $E_{int}$ can be defined as (see Figure 7.23)

$$E_{int} = \Sigma \, w_{ij} f(L_{ij} - L_{ij}^0), \qquad (7.56)$$

where $w_{ij}$ is the stiffness of the rod $L_{ij}^0$, which connects pixel $i$ with its neighbor $j$. $L_{ij}^0$ is deformed into the rod $L_{ij}$, yielding the deformation vector $(L_{ij} - L_{ij}^0)$. The stiffness $w_{ij}$ is large for bone and small for soft tissue. The external energy can be defined, for example, as in the previous examples

$$E_{ext} = -I(A, B). \qquad (7.57)$$

### Statistical deformation properties

On p. 180, methods for statistical shape properties (see Figure 7.18) were described. These methods can also

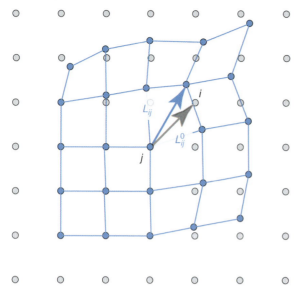

**Figure 7.23** Schematic representation of a deformation field where $L_{ij}^0$ is deformed into $L_{ij}$.

be applied to model image *deformation*. In Figure 7.18, for example, a statistical shape model was built by examining the statistics of the coordinates of corresponding points in a training set of curves. In the case of image deformation the elements of the vectors $v_i$ are the coordinates $(x_{ik}, y_{ik})$ of a number of landmarks in the image. If two images per patient are available in the training set, the deformation between the two images can be described as $\Delta v_i$ with coordinates $(\Delta x_{ik}, \Delta y_{ik})$. Using principal component analysis (PCA) any deformation $\Delta v$ can then be written as

$$\Delta v = \overline{\Delta v} + \sum_k^v c_k \cdot r_k. \qquad (7.58)$$

As compared to Eq. (7.44) only the deformation is expressed here, not the shape. If the deformation does not show any bias, then $\overline{\Delta v} \approx 0$. If the parameters $c_k$ have a normal distribution, the internal energy is (see Eq. (7.45))

$$E_{\text{int}} = \frac{1}{2} \sum_{k=1}^v \frac{c_k^2}{\lambda_k}. \qquad (7.59)$$

In the case of image fusion, the external energy can be defined again as

$$E_{\text{ext}} = -I(A, B). \qquad (7.60)$$

Using, for example, an interpolating spline through the landmarks, one image can be deformed into another while minimizing the total energy. Figure 7.24 shows the chosen landmarks in 2D chest radiographs and examples of their deformation along the principal modes of variation. They define a deformation model that can be applied to temporal subtraction as shown in Figure 7.25.

Again, nothing prevents us from combining a deformation model with an explicit statistical shape description (see, e.g., Figure 7.19) to analyze and register subsequent images in a dynamic or time sequence. Segmentation and image fusion are then performed simultaneously. Examples of this integrated approach have been described in the scientific literature, but this approach is still the subject of fundamental research and immature for clinical use.

## Validation

A general problem in medical image analysis is that validation of the algorithms requires a ground truth or golden standard to which the outcome of the analysis can be compared. In vivo measurements in humans cannot be used in principle to obtain such a ground truth. In vivo measurements in animals are limited by ethical concerns. The lack of an in vivo ground truth has resulted in three alternative methods for validating accuracy, that is, the use of software simulations, phantoms, and cadaver studies. If possible, they are all used one after the other and in this order.

- **Software simulations** Artificial images can be generated with programs that simulate the acquisition process of the imaging modality (Figure 7.26). This way, the ground truth is known exactly. Validation is highly flexible because the influence of acquisition parameters, imaging artifacts, and various appearances of the acquired structures can all be investigated independently or together. Numerous validation tests can be performed with little effort. A drawback of software simulations, however, is that they require substantial modeling and computer power and are usually approximate, as in practice a software simulator cannot adequately take all factors into account that influence the imaging process.

- **Phantoms** Because of the limitations of software simulations, assessment of new algorithms

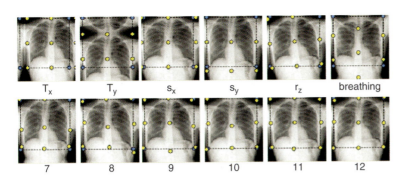

**Figure 7.24** 2D chest radiographs deformed along the axes of the principal modes of variation of nine landmarks. In this example the nine landmarks are defined as equidistant grid points on the bounding rectangle of the lungs.

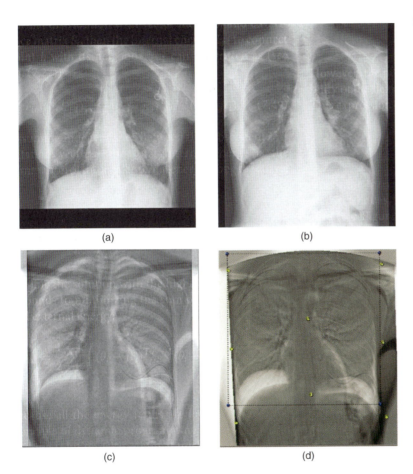

**Figure 7.25** (a,b) 2D chest radiographs of the same patient taken at different times. (c) Straightforward subtraction of images (a) and (b). (d) Subtraction after nonrigid registration using a statistical deformation model. Note that a perfect subtraction is not possible due to the nature of 2D radiographs, which are projection images.

is also recommended by means of anthropomorphic phantoms (Figure 7.27) whose geometry and material properties are known accurately and are comparable to the in vivo properties. Because the images are generated by the imaging modality, phantom tests are in general more realistic than simulations. On the other hand, they are labor intensive and do not offer the flexibility of software simulations.

- **Cadaver studies** After software simulations and phantom tests, cadaver studies may be considered. The analysis results can then be compared to the postmortem structures in the body. This validation method best resembles the in vivo

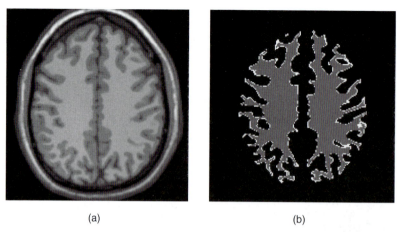

(a)　　　　　　　　　　(b)

**Figure 7.26** Evaluation of MR tissue segmentation by pixel classification (see p. 167 and Figure 7.8) in artificial images. **(a)** Simulated $T_1$-weighted MR image of the brain obtained by simulating both the MR imaging process and a brain with known geometry and tissue distribution. **(b)** Comparison between the white matter segmentation computed from (a) and the ground truth used to generate (a). Misclassified pixels (bright) are primarily located at the interface between white and gray matter and can be attributed to the partial volume artifact. By changing the parameters of the MR simulator the performance of the segmentation algorithm can be tested in a wide range of controlled conditions. (Courtesy of Dr. K. Van Leemput, Medical Imaging Research Center, and Bruce Pike and Alan Evans, McConnell Brain Imaging Centre, Montreal Neurological Institute, McGill University, Montreal, Canada.)

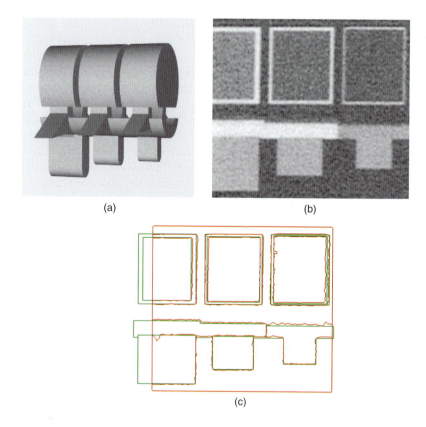

**Figure 7.27** Validation of image segmentation using a phantom with known geometry. **(a)** Mathematical model of an anthropomorphic spine phantom. **(b)** CT image of the phantom. **(c)** The mathematical model was registered with the CT images of the phantom. The position of the image contours segmented by edge detection can be compared with their true location as specified by the geometry of the model. (Courtesy of Professor J. Van Cleynenbreugel, Medical Imaging Research Center.)

(a)　　　　　　　　　　(b)

(c)

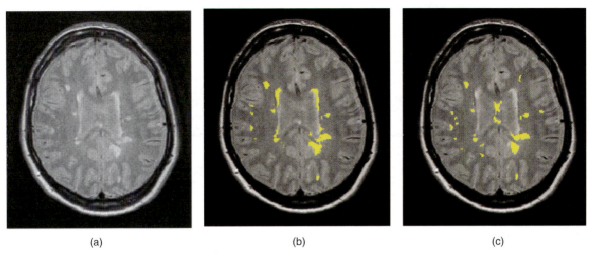

(a)                    (b)                    (c)

**Figure 7.28** Validation of automated MS lesion segmentation by comparison with manual analysis. (a) $\rho$-weighted MR image of an MS patient showing the typical MS lesions as hyperintense blobs inside white matter. (b) Lesions detected using automated pixel classification (see p. 167). (c) Lesions delineated by a trained radiologist. When comparing both segmentations the intra- and inter-observer variability in the expert segmentation has to be taken into account. (Courtesy of K. Van Leemput, Medical Imaging Research Center.)

situation. However, the tissue characteristics of a cadaver generally differ from those of a living person. Hence, care must be taken when interpreting the results. As compared with phantoms tests, the internal shape and geometry are typically known with less accuracy and the practical organization is more cumbersome. Note also that cadaver studies are not suited to assessing dynamic processes in the body.

Because of the lack of an indisputable ground truth, an alternative popular strategy used to assess the algorithmic accuracy is to compare the outcome of the algorithm with the solution generated by the established method used in daily clinical practice. Common practice is validation by comparison with the results obtained from manual analysis by one or more human experts (Figure 7.28). The results of such a validation should be critically reviewed because manual analysis is highly subjective and variable (see Figure 7.1).

## Future expectations

Today, the use of computer-aided image analysis is often too time consuming. Faster computers, easy to use computer programs, and fast and easy digital image transfer will change this. Programs for image registration and quantification will be smoothly integrated in a PACS environment and used in daily routine. Improved imaging modalities and adapted image acquisition schemes will offer a higher SNR and a better differential diagnosis capability, this way simplifying the automatic analysis method.

From an algorithmic point of view, more accurate and profound modeling can be expected. These models will be partly based on statistical processing of static and dynamic images of large normal and pathological population studies. This will yield a variety of digital atlases for automated quantitative analysis and more reliable methods for nonrigid registration.

# Visualization for diagnosis and therapy

## Introduction

Medical images are typically generated as 2D projection images or sequences, as in radiography, or as stacks of 2D image slices, as in tomographic imaging. To use them for diagnostic or interventional purposes, the image data can be visualized as such, but they can also be shown as resliced images or as three-dimensional (3D) images. This chapter discusses the clinically relevant visualization methods.

Medical images are used not only for diagnostic purposes, but also often serve as the basis for a therapeutic or surgical intervention during which the instruments are guided by and navigate through the image content. Images can be obtained prior to and during surgery. Preoperative images, such as CT, MRI, and PET, can be used for accurate planning and can be acquired with the available diagnostic imaging modalities. However, the planning has to be accurately applied to the patient in the operating room. This requires a method to register geometrically the preoperative images and planning data with the surgical instruments. A computer can assist in both this planning and the registration, a process known as *computer assisted intervention*.

To plan or simulate an intervention, preoperative images are imported in a 3D graphics computer workstation and manipulated as real 3D volumes. Planning is surgery specific and typically consists of defining linear or curved trajectories to access a lesion, to position an implant, to simulate ablations and resections, or to reposition resected tissue.

Stereotactic* brain surgery played a pioneering role in the development of computer assisted interventions. It is based on the principle that a predefined area in the brain can be approached by a surgical instrument, such as an electrode or a biopsy needle, through a small burr hole in the skull. In order to realize this, a *stereotactic frame* (see Figure 8.1) with inherent coordinate system was developed and fixed to the brain. Images, planned trajectories, and instruments are all defined in this coordinate space. The first frame was built in 1908 by Horsley, a physician, and Clarke, an engineer. This instrument allowed them to reach a predefined area in the brain of a monkey (*Macacus rhesus*) with an electrode guided through a small burr hole in the skull. To define the target location, a brain atlas was used. It consisted of a collection of topographic maps with sketches of sagittal and frontal intersections of a standard *Macacus rhesus* brain. The stereotactic frame was designed to transfer the 3D coordinate system of the atlas to the monkey mechanically, using anatomical landmarks on the skull, such as the external auditory canals and the inferior orbital rim.

The stereotactic frame quickly became an important instrument for neurophysiologists and neuroanatomists in order to approach a desired target in the brain of a living animal with little damage to vital brain tissue. In this early stage, the stereotactic approach did not use images in which the target point could be localized. Instead, the target was defined in an atlas and was transferred to the operating space by means of external landmarks on a skull. However, the large intersubject variability of the relative positions of deep intracerebral targets with respect to external skull landmarks, particularly in humans, prevented accurate use of this technique without proper images of the subject's brain.

With the use of radiographic images, intracerebral landmarks became available by means of ventriculography.[†] In 1947, the first image-guided stereotactic intervention was applied to a human by Spiegel and Wycis. Since then, much emphasis has been placed on the topography of deep brain structures and

---

* The term *stereotaxy* is derived from the Greek words *stereos* and *taxis* and can be translated as "three-dimensional (3D) ordering."

† Radiography of the ventricles filled with a contrast dye.

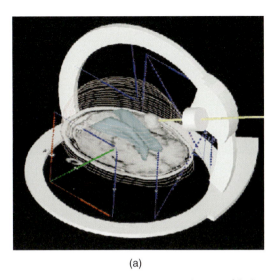

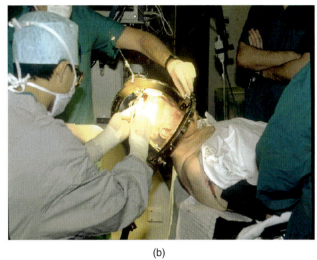

(a)                                                       (b)

**Figure 8.1** The stereotactic arc is mounted on top of the base ring. **(a)** Arc setup during the software planning. **(b)** Intraoperative view with instrument holder and biopsy needle in the planned position. The stereotactic arc shown here is the BRW system of Radionics.

on techniques to guide a probe through predefined human brain structures.

In its early years (1950–1970) stereotactic surgery was used primarily to treat functional disorders, such as certain persistent pain syndromes. During such interventions, selective cerebral pathways of nuclei were stimulated or destroyed. Such target structures were invisible, however, with the imaging modalities (X-rays, ultrasound) of that period. The nearest internal brain structures that could be visualized in a radiographic image were the ventricles. The target point was then localized in an atlas of the brain with respect to two anatomical reference points (i.e., the commissura anterior (CA) and the commissura posterior (CP)), which are characteristic points on the third ventricle and visible in the radiographic images as well. This way, the planning performed in an atlas plate could easily be transferred to ventriculograms of the patient. Because the ventriculograms were taken in stereotactic conditions (i.e., while the patient was fixed into the stereotactic frame), the relationship between the target point in the radiographic images and the stimulating electrode could be calculated.

Soon after the introduction of CT in 1974 as a diagnostic modality, methods were developed to localize a target point in a CT image volume and to approach it stereotactically with millimeter precision. New stereotactic instruments became commercially available for CT, PET, and MRI-guided neurosurgery. Since the 1980s image-guided procedures have vastly expanded in orthopedics and traumatology. Like the brain, the

skeleton can be assumed to be a rigid structure, which is a necessary condition for the use of preoperative images. Planning bone surgery requires software for complex user interaction, whereas in brain surgery the planning typically consists of the definition of one or more straight trajectories.

The use of preoperative images requires that the tissue to be treated be rigid. Except for the brain and skeleton, this condition is not the case for most other anatomical structures. For soft tissue treatment, interventional imaging is the obvious solution.

This chapter is built up as follows.

- It starts with a comprehensive overview of image visualization methods for diagnosis and therapy. The images delivered by the acquisition systems can be resliced into multiplanar reformatted images (MPR) and curved slices; multimodal or multitemporal image data can be visualized as co-registered images; and stacks of 2D slices can be rendered as 3D surfaces or as 3D volumes.

- 3D rendering yields depth perception by several contributing factors, such as perspective projection, hidden surface removal and light reflections. Object motion, head movement parallax* and stereo vision offer additional depth cues. By integrating them an immersive visualization technique is obtained, known as *virtual reality*.

---

* Parallax is the perceptual change of the 3D scene when the viewer moves.

- Ways to interact with 3D images, useful for preoperative planning as well as for education and training, are subsequently discussed.

- The next section explains how the surgical instruments can navigate through these images and preoperative planning data. To exploit the preoperative images during surgery and execute the planning on the patient, their geometrical relationship with the surgical instruments has to be established and maintained.

- Intraoperative images can also be integrated with preoperative images and planning and other virtual data into a single image. This visualization technique, which combines virtual and real-world elements, is known as *augmented reality*.

## 2D visualization

Typically 3D medical image data are stacks of 2D images. Radiologists and nuclear medicine physicians are trained to provide their diagnosis based on these 2D images. These images show the anatomy or function of thin slices through the body and are mostly acquired directly from the imaging system. The orientation of these slices is defined by the constraints of the imaging modality. However, it is quite easy to calculate slices of a different orientation from the

original stack of images by simple interpolation. This reslicing process is known as *multiplanar reformatting (MPR)*. Curved slices are also useful but less common than planar reslices. Figure 8.2 shows such a curved slice through one of the main coronary arteries.

Due to the recent advances in multimodal acquisition systems (e.g., PET-CT) and image registration software, corresponding multimodal or multitemporal images can be visualized together. Figure 8.3 shows an example of a longitudinal study displayed in synchronized windows. After nonlinear registration of two 3D CT data sets of the same patient, taken at a different times, corresponding spatial positions in both data sets are known and can be shown simultaneously when the user points to one of them either in the recent or in the reference data set.

## 3D rendering

3D rendering is the process of creating realistic computer-generated images of a 3D scene. Photorealism is obtained by simulating the interaction of light coming from one or more light sources with the illuminated 3D scene (Figure 8.4). The illumination can be ambient, i.e., coming equally from all directions, or directional, i.e., coming from point sources or from more extended sources. When the

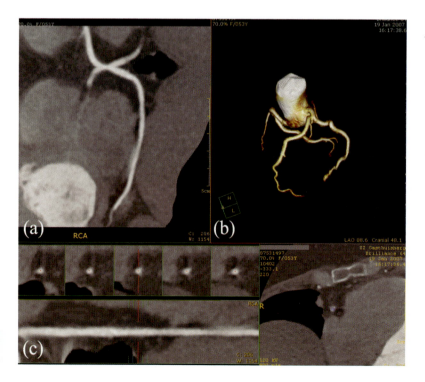

**Figure 8.2** Analysis of the coronary arteries. The computer automatically delineates the main arteries, the myocard and heart chambers and a 3D image of the delineated structures can be shown **(b)**. The centerline of the main coronary arteries is automatically found and a curved slice through each of these arteries can be shown **(a)**. The centerline can be stretched and reslices along or perpendicular to the centerline of the blood vessel can then be visualized **(c)**.

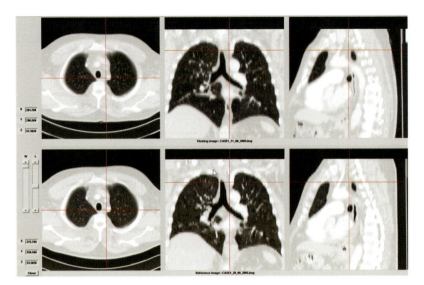

**Figure 8.3** This user interface shows corresponding thoracic 2D slices of the same patient over time after nonrigid registration. When navigating through one of the image stacks and pointing to a position with the cursor, the corresponding position in the co-registered images is shown.

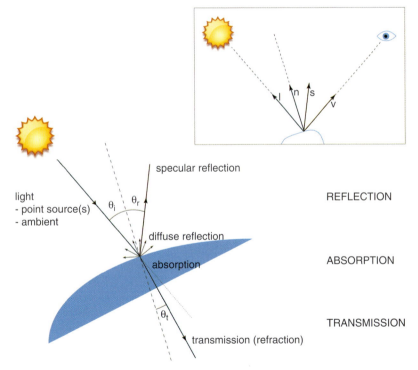

**Figure 8.4** Schematic representation of the interaction of light with material.

light hits an object, part of the incident intensity is *absorbed*, another part is *reflected* and the remainder is *transmitted*.

- The energy of absorbed light photons is partly transformed into heat. The remainder is scattered. Part of the scattered light photons escape from the material again and contribute to the reflected

or transmitted signal. Note that the amount of absorption is frequency dependent.

- The reflected light defines the color of the object. It is typically subdivided into a specular and a diffuse component, or a combination of both. Specular reflection occurs at flat transitions between two media. In the specular direction the reflected photons are in phase and the diffraction pattern yields

**193**

an intense signal that falls off sharply away from this direction. Diffuse reflection is due to light scattered back in many directions. The amount of diffuse and specular reflection depends on the material properties of the object. Dull materials disperse the light equally in all directions while shiny surfaces reflect the light directionally.

- Objects pervious to light are transparent (e.g., eye lens, some liquids, air) or translucent (e.g., human skin). Theoretically the transmitted rays in a transparent object are refracted slightly, but this property is often neglected for medical 3D visualization. In translucent objects the incident light is scattered through the material, giving it a specific smooth appearance.

Note that not only the material properties are responsible for the appearance of the object but also the position and orientation of the object with respect to the light sources and the viewer. The more oblique the surface is to the light direction, the smaller the incident intensity. The specular reflection depends on the angles of the normal to the surface with both the incident light and the view direction (see Figure 8.4).

As a rule of thumb, the greater the photographic realism the more computationally expensive the 3D rendering process is. Multiple reflections and refractions, for example, require secondary light rays and ray trees, which increase the computation time drastically. Recursive ray tracing and radiosity methods are able to cope with the interchange of light between objects. However, these methods are beyond the scope of this textbook. For diagnostic and therapeutic visualization, simplified nonphysically based models of illumination and shading are mostly employed. Accuracy and real time interaction are given priority at the cost of photorealism. As we will see below (Figure 8.25), the use of properties like specularity and shadowing may even deteriorate the interpretation of an image.

Three-dimensional medical images are acquired as 3D matrices of voxels. Two different approaches can be distinguished to render them. The most straightforward method from a computer graphics point of view is to extract objects from the 3D data and render their surfaces. This way the same 3D rendering software can be used as employed in graphics for entertainment. Surface rendering has a long-standing tradition in computer science and graphics packages are redundantly available. A problem, however, is that object segmentation is often not straightforward, as

we have discussed in Chapter 7. An alternative is to consider all the voxels as separate objects and render them all. This technique is known as *volume rendering*. More details about surface and volume rendering are discussed below.

# Surface rendering

Visualizing surfaces extracted from volumetric image data requires object segmentation. As we have seen in Chapter 7 this is not a trivial task except for high-contrast structures such as bony structures in CT images. Nevertheless 3D surface visualization has become common practice today in medical imaging. Figure 8.5 shows an example.

A 3D surface is described by its geometry and its reflection and transmission properties, including its intrinsic color pattern or texture.

### Surface geometry

A surface of a segmented object can be represented in different ways. Chapter 7 offers several potential representations, such as a set of voxels, a polygon or a spline. In computer graphics it is common practice, however, to represent the surface as a *triangular mesh*. This popularity can be explained by the availability of standard software libraries that are based on this type of surface description. In medical image analysis this kind of representation is rather unusual.

Different methods exist to calculate a triangular mesh. A classical approach consists of joining segmented planar contours in adjacent image slices by triangles, a process known as *tiling* (Figure 8.6). This method is quite useful for thick slices. It avoids staircase artifacts arising from large shifts between corresponding contour segments in adjacent slices. Today, 3D scanners provide nearly isotropic voxels, which reduces the practical value of tiling contours.

Another class of methods considers the image data as a 3D lattice where the voxels constitute the lattice points, lying inside or outside the object. A popular approach is the so-called *marching cubes* algorithm. It cleaves each elementary lattice or cell of eight voxels (see Figure 8.7(a)) into internal and external object parts. Each cutting surface consists of one or more triangles. It can easily be shown that there are only fifteen unique cleaving configurations, including their rotated and symmetrical shapes (Figure 8.7(b)).

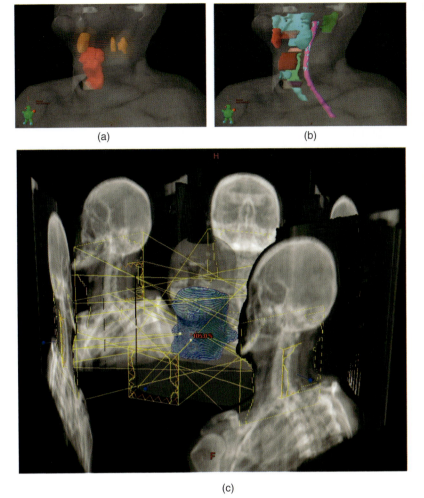

(a)

(b)

(c)

**Figure 8.5** Intensity modulated radiotherapy (IMRT) is a highly conformal treatment technique routinely used in certain cancers, such as head and neck cancer. It allows the delivery of complex dose distributions to the patient by modulating the radiation beam intensity. Three-dimensional representations are common practice during treatment planning for IMRT. **(a)** Delineated tumor and malignant nodal tissue. **(b)** Organs at risk including the salivary glands, swallowing structures and spinal cord, which should be avoided during irradiation. **(c)** IMRT treatment plan with the corresponding dose distribution for this patient. This plan maximizes the dose to the target (a) and minimizes the dose to the organs at risk (b). Courtesy of the Department of Radiotherapy

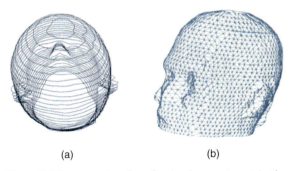

(a)

(b)

**Figure 8.6** Representation of a surface by planar contours joined by tiling.

## Illumination and shading

### Illumination

Surfaces can be illuminated by ambient light, coming equally from all directions, and one or more directional point sources. More extended sources can be considered as a set of point sources. Light is reflected and transmitted at the surface of the objects in the scene. The reflection of light can be diffuse for dull surfaces, specular for shiny surfaces, or a combination of both for glossy surfaces.

- *Ambient light* If $I_a$ is the intensity component of the ambient light, the reflected intensity in any direction from surface point $\mathbf{r}$ can be written as

$$I(\mathbf{r}) = k_a(\mathbf{r})\, I_a, \qquad (8.1)$$

where $k_a(\mathbf{r})$ is the ambient reflection coefficient, a property of the material.

- *Diffuse and specular reflection* Diffuse reflection coming from a point source with intensity $I_p$ can be expressed as

$$I(\mathbf{r}) = (\mathbf{l} \cdot \mathbf{n}(\mathbf{r}))\, k_d(\mathbf{r})\, I_p. \qquad (8.2)$$

**195**

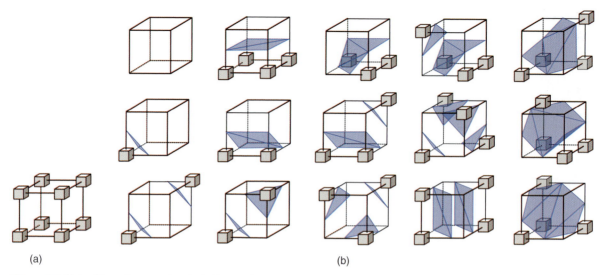

(a)                                                                        (b)

**Figure 8.7** **(a)** A cell is an elementary hexahedral lattice of eight voxels. **(b)** The *marching cubes* algorithm assigns each cell to one of the fifteen unique cleaving configurations. Each cleaving surface consists of one or more triangles.

l is the direction to the light source and can be assumed to be independent of r if the point source is sufficiently distant from the surface. n(r) is the surface normal in surface point r. $k_d(r)$ is the material dependent diffuse reflection coefficient. It represents the color of the surface* and is often the same as the ambient light coefficient $k_a(r)$.

Perfect specular reflection or mirroring has been explained in Chapter 6, p. 134 for ultrasound waves. Light can be treated similarly. According to Snell's law, the angle of incidence $\theta_i$ equals the angle of reflection $\theta_r$ (see Figure 6.8). However, most shiny objects are imperfect reflectors because their surface is not perfectly smooth. Their specular reflection is visible as a highlight observable within a small angle around the direction of perfect reflection, s. It can be approximated by

$$I(r) = (s(r) \cdot v)^n k_s(r) I_p. \qquad (8.3)$$

In this equation $I(r)$ is the intensity from specular reflection in the direction of the viewer, v; $k_s(r)$ is the material dependent specular reflection coefficient, and $n$ the specular reflection exponent, which is infinite for a perfect reflector (usually between 1 and 200).

The effect of ambient light and multiple point sources $m$ can be approximated by adding the individual contributions, expressed by Eqs. (8.1), (8.2) and (8.3). Taking into account that the intensities and reflection coefficients for light spectra can depend on the wavelength $\lambda$, yields

$$I_\lambda(r) = k_{a,\lambda}(r) I_{a,\lambda} + \sum_{i=1}^{m} \left( (l_i \cdot n(r)) k_{d,\lambda}(r) \right.$$
$$\left. + (s_i(r) \cdot v)^n k_{s,\lambda}(r) \right) I_{p_i,\lambda}. \qquad (8.4)$$

- The specular reflection coefficient, $k_{s,\lambda}(r)$, is often independent of the wavelength $\lambda$ and the position r, that is, $k_{s,\lambda}(r) = k_s$. This means that the color of the reflected light is the same as that of the incident light and that the specularity of the object is constant along its surface.

- The ambient reflection coefficient, $k_{a,\lambda}(r)$, is often the same as the diffuse reflection coefficient, $k_{d,\lambda}(r)$.

- The diffuse reflection coefficient, $k_{d,\lambda}(r)$, is position dependent, but independent of the light direction and view direction. Consequently, it can be precalculated. In computer graphics it is still common practice to store $k_{d,\lambda}(r)$ as a color image, called *texture map*. Each surface point r can then be transformed or mapped onto the texture map to retrieve its

* The color of a surface is the color reflected from it when it is illuminated by white light.

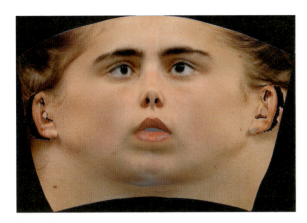

**Figure 8.8** Cylindrical texture map of a face. It can be used to color the 3D facial tissue segmented from a volumetric CT scan (see Figure 8.32). By folding the texture map into a cylinder that surrounds the 3D surface, each surface point can be projected or mapped onto the texture map, this way defining the correspondence between both coordinate systems.

intrinsic color. Figures 8.8 and 8.9 show two examples.

- *Transparency* Transparent objects transmit part of the incident light intensity, expressed by a transmission coefficient $k_t$, which varies from 0 for a completely opaque material to 1 for a totally transparent material. Assume a nonrefractive transparent surface with transmission coefficient $k_{t_1,\lambda}$ and a second surface behind it in the view direction. The total reflected intensity in the direction of the viewer can then be written as

$$I_\lambda(\mathbf{r}) = I_{1,\lambda}(\mathbf{r}) + k_{t_1,\lambda}(\mathbf{r})\, I_{2,\lambda}(\mathbf{r}), \qquad (8.5)$$

where $I_{1,\lambda}(\mathbf{r})$ and $I_{2,\lambda}(\mathbf{r})$ are obtained with Eq. (8.4). If several transparent objects lie behind each other, Eq. (8.4) can be used recursively from back to front.

- *Depth cueing* Distant objects have a lower intensity than objects closer to the viewer due to atmospheric attenuation. If the distance $z$ to the viewer varies

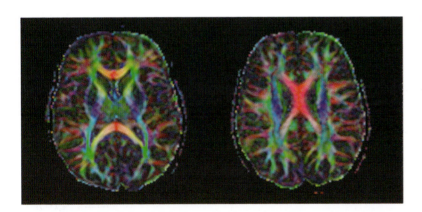

**Figure 8.9** Textured diffusion tensor image (DTI). The hue represents the main direction and the brightness the fractional anisotropy of the diffusion (see Chapter 4, p. 89). In this example a tumor is surrounded by the fibers of the motor cortex. The mapping between the 3D texture map and 3D rendered surface is trivial because both use the same 3D coordinate system. Courtesy of Professor S. Sunaert, Department of Radiology.

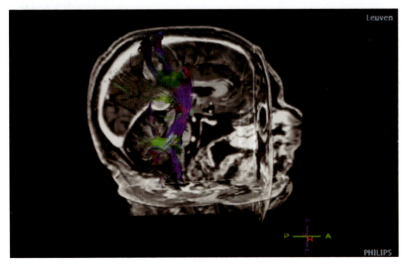

in the scene from $z_{min}$, i.e., closest to the viewer, to $z_{max}$, i.e., most distant from the viewer, and due to atmospheric conditions the intensity can decrease from $I$ at $z_{min}$ to $I_{low}$ at $z_{max}$, the updated, attenuated intensity $I_{att}(z)$ can be approximated by

$$I_{att}(z) = \frac{z_{max} - z}{z_{max} - z_{min}} I + \frac{z - z_{min}}{z_{max} - z_{min}} I_{low}. \quad (8.6)$$

### Shading

Triangular and other polygonal meshes are usually approximations of curved surfaces. Shading each planar surface emphasizes this polygonal appearance due to brightness discontinuities at the boundaries between adjacent facets. Gouraud shading and Phong shading, named after their inventors, are two popular methods used to obtain smoother transitions. In both methods the vertex normals are first calculated by averaging the normals of the polygons that share this vertex.

Gouraud shading then calculates the reflected intensity in each vertex by using for example Eq. (8.4). Next, the vertex intensities are interpolated to calculate the intensities in between.

Phong shading on the other hand first calculates the surface normals in each point by interpolating the vertex normals. Using these normals the reflected intensities are subsequently calculated. Although Phong shading is computationally more expensive than Gouraud shading, it yields superior images.

## Volume rendering

Surface rendering requires segmentation, which is typically not obvious. A straightforward alternative to overcome this problem is to think of voxels as being separate objects with simply a color and a transparency (or opacity). Besides its position a voxel obviously has no other geometric properties and neither is a texture map needed. Theoretically, each voxel can then be visualized with a similar illumination model as used for surface rendering.

Volume rendering looks quite attractive for visualizing 3D image data. This is true if the 3D matrix is sparse and naturally largely transparent. If the 3D matrix is highly populated with meaningful information, it has to be decided which voxels will be made invisible by assigning them a high transparency. Actually this comes down again to image segmentation.

One of the early, but clinically still relevant, examples of volume rendering is the *maximum intensity projection* (MIP), already explained in Chapter 4, p. 87. For each projection line only the voxel with the maximum gray value (typically the brightest) along that line is visualized. The other voxels along the projection line are considered to be totally transparent. This method is well suited to visualizing sparse structures, such as blood vessels in MRA (Figure 8.10), pulmonary bronchi in CT and hot spots in PET. A disadvantage is that keeping only the voxels with the maximum intensity along each projection line can be considered as a heuristic inaccurate way of segmentation. The remaining voxels do not necessarily belong to meaningful objects and, vice versa, meaningful voxels may have become invisible. Another, minor disadvantage is that in a pure MIP 3D perception can only be obtained by motion or stereoscopy. A single static MIP does not contain any depth cue.

Instead of keeping the brightest voxel along each projection line, it is of course also possible to keep the darkest voxel. This visualization mode, called *minimum intensity projection* (mIP), is less popular but does have some clinical relevance in cases of hyperintense structures, such as lung emphysema.

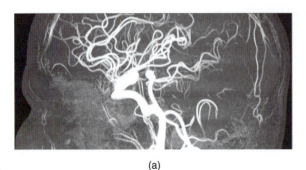
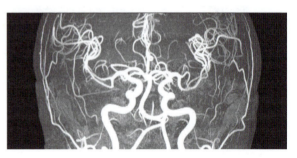

(a)                                             (b)

**Figure 8.10** Maximum intensity projection (MIP) ((a) sagittal and (b) frontal view) of the cerebral blood vessels obtained by 3D time-of-flight MRA.

Today computers have become fast enough to calculate more natural 3D representations with improved depth perception. The current methods can be classified into two classes. The first category considers voxels with identical gray values as identical objects. Segmentation is not needed here, which is one of the advantages of this kind of volume rendering as compared to surface rendering. However, the applications are rather limited. The second category is more powerful but needs segmented objects again. Both methods are now discussed in detail.

### Position independent transfer functions

This method assigns an opacity and a color to each gray value using gray value transformations (Figure 8.11).

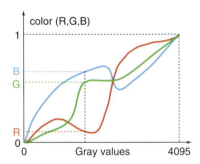

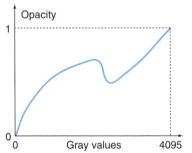

**Figure 8.11**
Gray value transformations for opacity and color.

An advantage of this kind of volume rendering is that it does not necessarily require a segmentation as was the case for surface rendering. A disadvantage is that the handling of the transformation functions requires a high degree of interaction. Note that three transformation curves are needed for color, i.e., for red, green and blue. In Chapter 1, p. 1 we have seen that it is also possible to use hue, saturation and brightness (Figure 1.2) instead of red, green and blue.

Figures 8.12 and 8.13 show a practical example of volume rendering of a 3D cardiac ultrasound image using gray value transformations. Ultrasound imaging typically yields sparse matrices because of the high reflection at the boundaries of neighboring structures. Consequently the 3D images are naturally highly transparent, which improves the perception of deep structures. A similar result can be simulated in images coming from other modalities by calculating the spatial gradient, yielding high voxel values at the boundaries and low values in the majority of the voxels. Instead of using pure gradient images, a weighted mixture of the original gray value data and gradient information is often used to enhance edges and silhouettes. Edge enhancement can be obtained, for example, by simply using the magnitude of the gradient, that is,

$$I'(\mathbf{r}) = I(\mathbf{r}) + \gamma \, \|\nabla(\mathbf{r})\|, \tag{8.7}$$

where $I(\mathbf{r})$ is the original gray value, $I'(\mathbf{r})$ the enhanced gray value in voxel $\mathbf{r}$, and $\gamma$ a user defined positive value. Alternatives for edge enhancement are for example unsharp masking and multiscale image enhancement (see Chapter 1). Instead of enhancing all the edges, only the silhouette can be enhanced, giving the object a glass-like effect. This can be achieved by emphasizing only the object boundaries whose

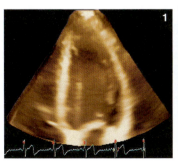

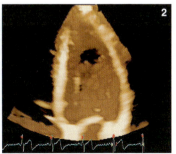

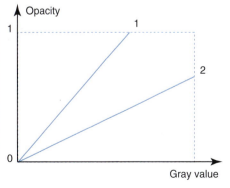

**Figure 8.12** Volume rendering of 3D cardiac ultrasound image using different opacity transformations. (Courtesy of the Department of Cardiology.)

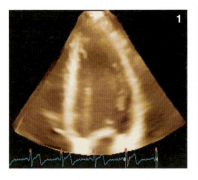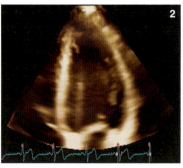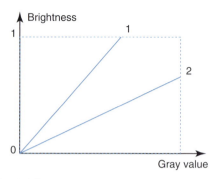

**Figure 8.13** Volume rendering of 3D cardiac ultrasound image. The images were obtained with different brightness transformations. (Courtesy of the Department of Cardiology.)

gradient points away from the view direction, for example

$$I'(\mathbf{r}) = I(\mathbf{r}) + \gamma \, \|\nabla(\mathbf{r}) \times \mathbf{v}\|, \qquad (8.8)$$

v being the normalized direction towards the viewer.

The above transfer functions yield a shading effect of ambient light, which reflects equally in all directions. 3D perception in volume rendering is often improved by adding illumination models that are similar to those used in surface rendering. The surface normal is then approximated by calculating the normalized gradient. However, if transfer functions are used in combination with additional illumination models, the interpretation of colors and gray values may become confusing. Indeed, the transfer functions replace each original gray value by an opacity and color, this way giving opacities and colors a specific meaning related to the meaning of the gray values. By adding illumination models, however, the opacity and/or color are modified and no longer depend only on the transfer functions but also on the other rendering modes. Improving the 3D perception should therefore be applied with caution and must not be performed at the cost of diagnostic certainty. Figure 8.26 in the next section shows an example. This problem can be avoided if clearly distinguishable colors are assigned to the different illumination contributions. For example, in Figure 8.14 the transfer functions use only the brightness scale while the depth is encoded by the hue and saturation. Artificial colors are employed for depth cueing. The color $I$ (i.e., hue and saturation) changes gradually with depth from one color $I(z_{\min}) = I_1$ to another $I(z_{\max}) = I_2$, that is,

$$I(z) = \frac{z_{\max} - z}{z_{\max} - z_{\min}} I_1 + \frac{z - z_{\min}}{z_{\max} - z_{\min}} I_2. \qquad (8.9)$$

Highlighting surface orientation, obtained by diffuse illumination, can also be obtained by color encoding as follows

$$I(\mathbf{r}) = \frac{1}{2}\left(1 + \frac{\mathbf{l} \cdot \nabla(\mathbf{r})}{\|\nabla(\mathbf{r})\|}\right) I_1 + \frac{1}{2}\left(1 - \frac{\mathbf{l} \cdot \nabla(\mathbf{r})}{\|\nabla(\mathbf{r})\|}\right) I_2, \qquad (8.10)$$

where $\nabla(\mathbf{r})$ is the spatial gradient in voxel r and l is the normalized direction to the light source.

### Thresholding

Figure 8.15 shows a special case of volume rendering using gray value transformations. The gray value scale is subdivided into different intervals, each corresponding to a different structure. Each interval is subject to different gray value transformations for opacity and color, which can be specified independently by the user. Of course, this approach is useful only if the considered structures can be segmented by simple thresholding which is rarely the case. Figure 8.16 shows an example in which the bony structures and the blood vessels, injected with contrast dye, can be selected independently to assign them a different color and opacity. This is a clinically useful application for the assessment of the carotid arteries in case of a stroke, as shown by the calcified stenosis in Figure 8.17.

Note however that this method assumes that different tissues have separated gray level intervals, which is not actually the case for bone and blood filled with contrast dye. Their gray value ranges in CT images strongly overlap. To overcome this problem, the CT numbers of bone are inverted (see Figure 8.18), which requires a prior segmentation of bone and contrast filled blood vessels. Instead of applying this somewhat unnatural operation the problem could also be solved

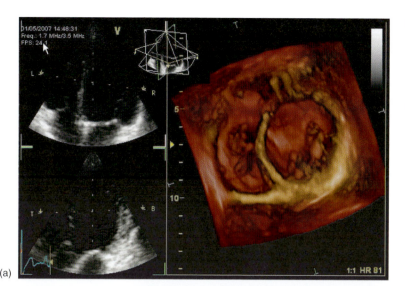

(a)

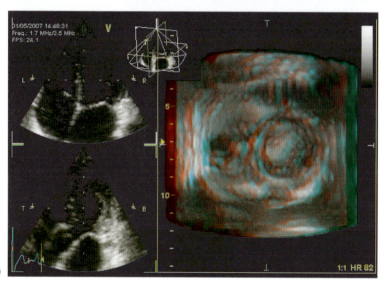

(b)

**Figure 8.14** Volume rendering of 3D cardiac ultrasound image with color used to improve the depth impression. This is possible because the gray value transformation itself does not employ color. **(a)** Artificial depth cueing is obtained by changing color with depth. **(b)** Stereoscopic red-green image. (Courtesy of the Department of Cardiology.)

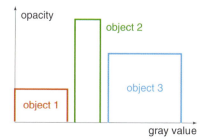

**Figure 8.15** The gray value scale is segmented into different intervals, each of which is assumed to correspond to a different structure. Each interval can then independently be assigned an opacity and color transformation.

if position dependent gray value transformations were used. This method is discussed in the next section.

Volume rendering of the blood vessels, using the method explained in this section, clearly yields a more realistic appearance than a maximum intensity projection (MIP) (see Figure 8.19). A static MIP does not contain any depth cue. Nevertheless the MIP has proved its usefulness in clinical practice. Figures 8.20 and 8.21 show two examples of its clinical relevance.

An interesting feature of volume rendering is that the image segmentation does not have to be a binary decision process. In Chapter 7, p. 168 we have already seen that a posteriori probabilities can be represented as gray values, yielding a so-called *fuzzy segmentation*.

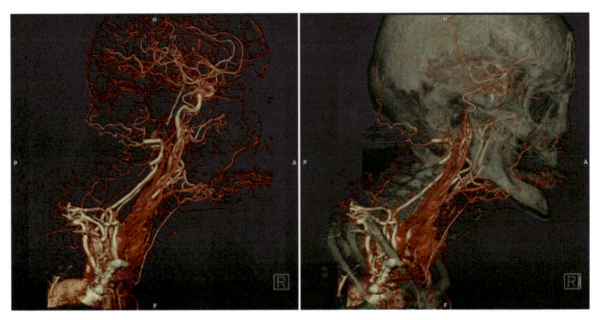

**Figure 8.16** Volume rendering of subtraction CT angiography (CTA). Bone and blood vessels can be treated independently. In the left image the bone is removed, while it is shown as a transparent object in the right image. Due to nonlinear patient movement between postcontrast and precontrast imaging, the subtraction is not straightforward. To solve this problem, nonrigid image registration was applied.

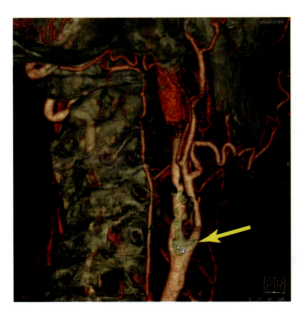

**Figure 8.17** Assessment of the carotid arteries in case of a stroke. By adding the bony structures to the image of the blood vessels, it becomes apparent that the stenosis is due to a calcified plaque.

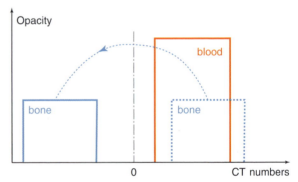

**Figure 8.18** The gray values of bone are inverted. This way the gray value ranges of bone and blood filled with contrast dye do not overlap anymore.

These probabilities can then be rendered by an opacity and color. A fuzzy segmentation is a way to cope with the unsharp boundaries due to the limited spatial resolution of the acquisition system. Because of these unsharp edges a binary segmentation has difficulties locating the exact position of the object surface. This may for example yield holes in a 3D rendering of a CT image of the thin nasal bones. Figure 8.22 shows how volume rendering can cope with this problem. In the CT slice the red pixels are potential boundary pixels of the skull. Their gray values are smaller than those of the white skull pixels because of the unsharpness of the point spread function of the acquisition system. The smaller the gray value the less likely that bone is contained within a voxel. The opacity transformation

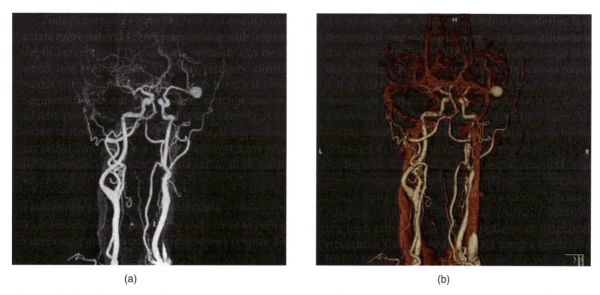

**Figure 8.19** CTA with aneurysm. **(a)** A static maximum intensity projection (MIP) image does not contain any depth information. **(b)** 3D rendering using depth cues.

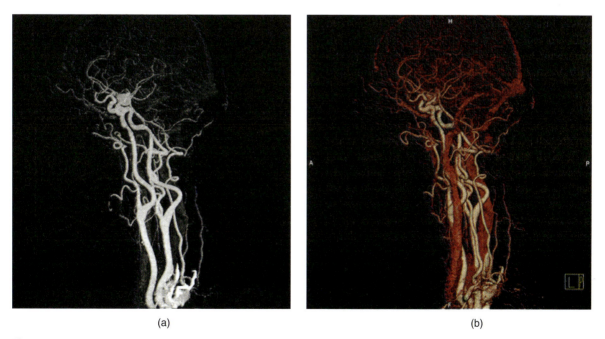

**Figure 8.20** Aneurysm in CTA. **(a)** In the MIP the aneurysm remains visible from all viewing directions. **(b)** The right image offers depth perception, but the aneurysm disappears behind the left hemisphere.

curve in Figure 8.22 shows how the lower gray values in the red area are assigned a smaller opacity. The less likely it is that bone is contained within a voxel, the more transparently the voxel is rendered, giving the outer bone layer its translucent smooth appearance (Figure 8.23).

### Position dependent transfer functions

A disadvantage of the method described in the previous section is that different objects within the same gray value range are treated identically. Position dependent rendering solves this problem. This is illustrated in Figures 8.24 and 8.25, which show a

**203**

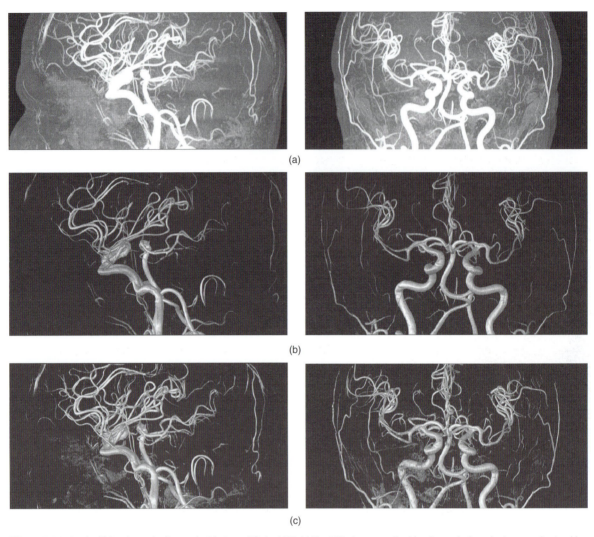

(a)

(b)

(c)

**Figure 8.21** Cerebral blood vessels obtained with time-of-flight MRA. **(a)** The MIP shows smaller blood vessels than the images obtained by more realistic rendering **(b,c)**. The reason is that in **(b,c)** transfer functions are used with a *global* threshold between background and visible structures. Decreasing this segmentation threshold as in **(c)**, does not reveal the smallest vessels because other brain tissue shows up and prevents the perception of less intense blood vessels.

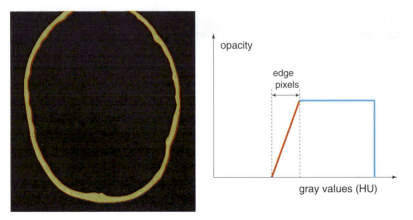

**Figure 8.22** CT slice of segmented skull. The red pixels are considered to be edge pixels and have a lower gray value due to the limited spatial resolution. The opacity transformation curve makes these voxels partially transparent.

probabilistic brain atlas. In the 3D image different colors are assigned to different brain structures and the opacity of a voxel is linearly proportional to the classification probability. The 3D scene is exposed to ambient light and no other illumination models were used.

Additional illumination models like point light sources and specularity must be used carefully and should not mislead the diagnosis. Figure 8.26 shows an example of how different the 3D brain atlas image may look when applying different rendering modes. The color and brightness depend not only on the classification probability but also on the lighting and viewing conditions. Note that, even if only ambient light is used, the interpretation of color and brightness may not be straightforward because each view is a projection image in which color and brightness values are integrated along the projection lines.

## Virtual reality

When rendering a 3D scene as explained above, the depth impression can be obtained from several contributing factors, such as perspective projection, hidden-surface removal, directional light with diffuse and specular reflection and shadowing, dimming of distant objects, and surface texturing using a repetitive pattern that decreases with depth. This three-dimensional perception can be further improved using additional depth cues, such as stereopsis (stereo vision), object motion and head movement parallax. Figure 8.27 shows one of the earliest integrated stereoscopic images of the cerebral blood vessels obtained with traditional X-ray angiography, a tumor segmented from CT images, and a simulated biopsy needle. The stereoscopic depth perception is obtained with red-green glasses. Several alternatives to red-green images exist, such as LCD shutter glasses and displays with filter arrays (see Figure 8.28).

Object motion can be used if a true 3D image is available, as obtained with MRA. A 3D impression is

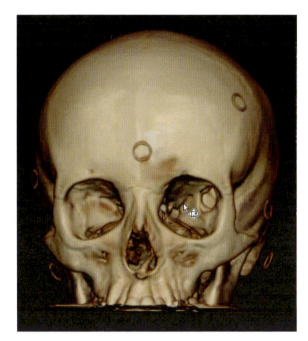

**Figure 8.23** 3D rendered skull showing the partially transparent voxels at the boundary in red color. Note that the fiducial markers (see Figure 8.37 below), used for stereotactic surgery, are also visible because their gray values lie in the same interval as the bony edge pixels.

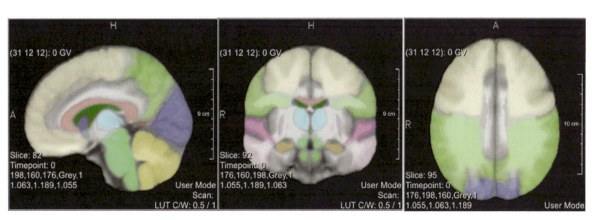

**Figure 8.24** Statistical atlas. 2D sagittal, coronal and axial probabilistic atlas slices are shown in which the pixel color represents the most likely brain structure and the pixel brightness represents the corresponding probability. This atlas was used to produce the 3D images shown in Figure 8.25.

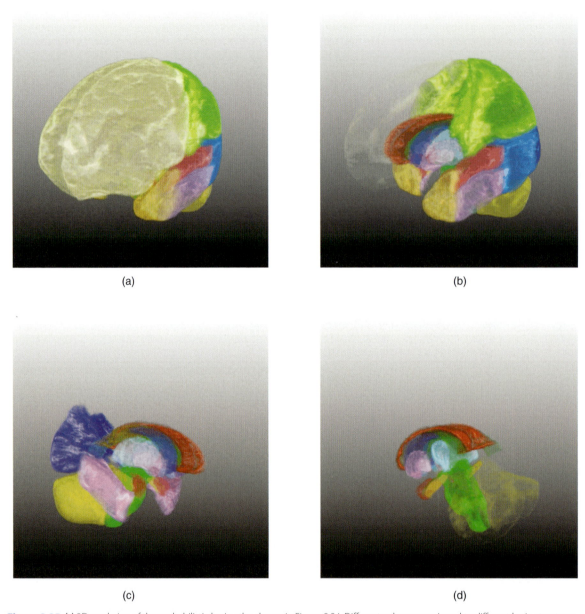

(a)

(b)

(c)

(d)

**Figure 8.25** **(a)** 3D rendering of the probabilistic brain atlas shown in Figure 8.24. Different colors are assigned to different brain structures and the opacity of a voxel is linearly proportional to its classification probability. **(b,c,d)** The opacity can also be used to hide external structures, so that central brain structures can be perceived more easily.

obtained by calculating views from consecutive orientations around the brain and displaying them as subsequent frames of a digital video.

Combining the principles of stereoscopy, object motion, and head movement parallax yields the most realistic 3D impression.

Figure 8.29 illustrates one of the early realizations of these principles. Head movement parallax can be

obtained by attaching a sensor to the viewer in order to measure the position and rotation of the head and to show the expected view of the 3D scene. Today, this immersive visualization technique is known as *virtual reality* and the whole system is miniaturized into a *head mounted display* (HMD), a helmet with two small integrated screens in front of the eyes. However, this system is not commonly used in clinical routine.

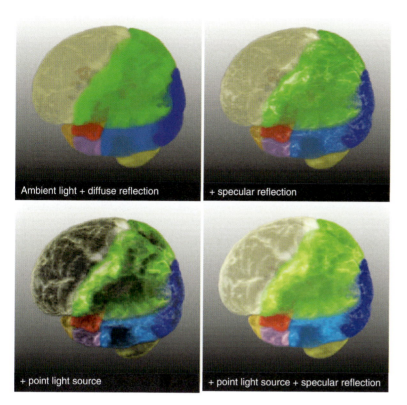

**Figure 8.26** Different 3D images of the same probabilistic brain atlas using ambient light and a point light source with diffuse and specular reflection as additional illumination models. Because the images are projection images the meaning of color and brightness is not obvious in static views. Adding depth cues enhances the 3D perception but may further complicate the diagnosis.

Ambient light + diffuse reflection

+ specular reflection

+ point light source

+ point light source + specular reflection

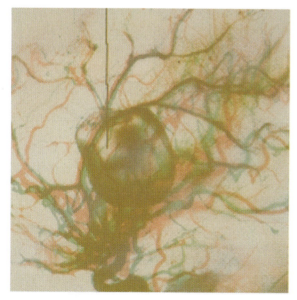

**Figure 8.27** Angiogram of the cerebral blood vessels, CT view of a tumor, and simulated biopsy trajectory integrated into one stereoscopic red-green image. Its 3D impression can be obtained with red-green glasses.

## User interaction

In the early days user interaction was limited to the calculation of multiplanar reformatted images (MPR) (see p. 192) of the brain to plan a probe trajectory for stereotactic neurosurgery. An accurate analysis of the complete trajectory in the images, for example, is clinically important in order not to damage any critical structures. For this reason, it is quite useful to reslice the image data along a plane, defined by the surgeon, that contains the probe trajectory (see Figure 8.30). Today, planning systems for bone interventions include tools for cutting curved surfaces and for bone repositioning. An example of cutting and repositioning during the planning of a maxillofacial intervention is given in Figure 8.31. Figure 8.32 shows a simulation of the corresponding changes in facial soft tissue. Figure 8.33 illustrates collision detection during the planning of oral implants. Cutting, repositioning and collision detection are quite easy to implement if surface rendering is used. This kind of interaction is less obvious in combination with volume rendering.

Navigation through the virtual 3D scene is still another type of user interaction, similar to what happens in a flight simulator. Well-known applications

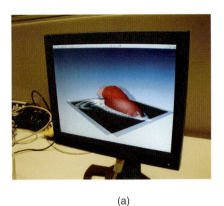

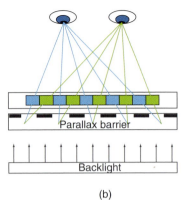

Parallax barrier

Backlight

(a)

(b)

**Figure 8.28** **(a)** Stereoscopic LCD monitor (Sharp Electronics Corporation) with filter arrays. **(b)** The backlight is covered with a so-called parallax barrier, i.e., a vertical grid filter that prevents the perception of odd and even pixel columns by the left and right eye respectively.

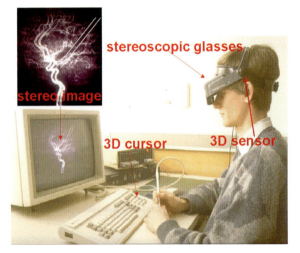

**Figure 8.29** True 3D visualization obtained with stereoscopic glasses and a 3D head sensor to evoke head movement parallax. A 3D cursor allows the viewer to navigate the probe naturally through the blood vessel tree. (Development of Lab. Medical Image Computing, 1989).

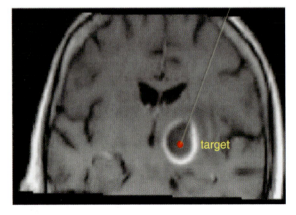

**Figure 8.30** MPR that includes the target and the simulated biopsy needle. The access to the lesion is a straight trajectory.

are virtual bronchoscopy and virtual colonoscopy (see Figure 8.34). The feeling of realism can be even more enhanced by tactile and audio feedback. Figure 8.35 shows four examples of training simulators for practicing medical procedures.

## Intraoperative navigation

The transfer of the image-based planning to the operating theater basically consists of establishing and maintaining the geometrical correspondence between the preoperative images and planning data on the one hand and the patient and instruments during the course of the intervention on the other hand. Such a relationship can be established and maintained by a point sensing device, also called a *navigation system*. This way the actual position of the surgical instruments can be shown in the images together with the preoperatively planned data (Figure 8.36).

The operating principle is based on *point matching*. In theory, it is sufficient to use three noncollinear reference points, either anatomical landmarks or artificial markers, typically attached to the patient's skin. The position of any other point can then be defined uniquely with respect to these three points (Figure 8.37(a)). The assumption is that the coordinates of these points can be accurately defined both in the preoperative images and in the operating room. In practice, however, artificial markers are glued onto the skin (Figure 8.37(b)) and, hence, they are subject to small shifts. To reduce the resulting matching error, more than three reference points are usually used. Similarly, the accuracy of localizing anatomical reference points is limited and the use of more than three anatomical markers is recommended.

The transfer problem can then be solved as follows. The coordinates of at least three fiducial markers $u_i$ are

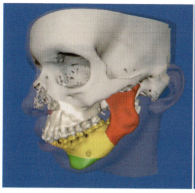
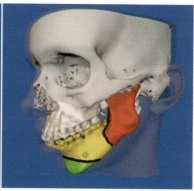

**Figure 8.31** Cutting and repositioning during maxillofacial surgery. The maxillar and mandibular bones are cut and repositioned.

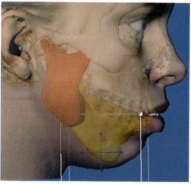
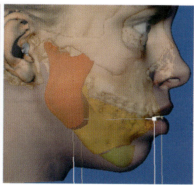

**Figure 8.32** Soft tissue simulation during bone repositioning. Several 2D photos are matched to the 3D soft tissue surface of the CT scan and this way compiled into an integrated 3D photo of the face. The system is able to simulate the effect of the bone replacements on the facial soft tissue.

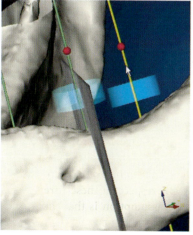
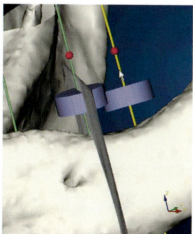

**Figure 8.33** Example of collision detection during oral implant planning. Oral implants are small titanium screws that are inserted in the maxilla and/or mandible. Afterwards, a personalized prosthesis is fixed onto these screws. A cylindrical safety area around each trajectory, initially colored light blue (left), changes to dark blue (right) if both areas overlap.

known in the image space $\mathcal{I}$. These markers must be visible in the surgery space $\mathcal{S}$.

- Find the 3D coordinates of the markers in the surgery space (i.e., in $\mathcal{S}$).
- Calculate the geometric transformation $F : \mathcal{S} \to \mathcal{I}$ based on the coordinates of the markers in both spaces.

## Finding the coordinates in the surgery space

An intraoperative 3D position-sensing device (Figure 8.38) with inherent coordinate space $\mathcal{S}$ can be used to measure the position of any point. When this system is used, the instrumentation (see Figure 8.39) must be equipped with LEDs (light emitting diodes) or with highly reflective markers whose 3D position is

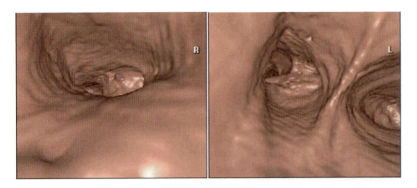

**Figure 8.34** Virtual bronchoscopy showing a fistula (left) and the result of a lung transplant to check the sutures (right).

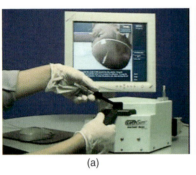

(a)

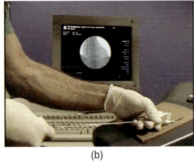

(b)

**Figure 8.35** Four different simulation systems to practice procedures with tactile and audio feedback: **(a)** needle stick procedures, **(b)** cardiac pacing, cardiac catheterization and interventional radiological techniques, **(c)** knot tying and suturing, and **(d)** laparoscopic cholecystectomy.

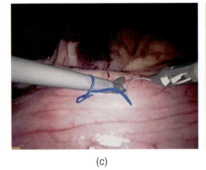

(c)

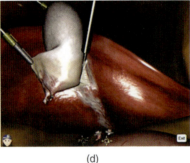

(d)

measured by cameras. The coordinates of the fiducial markers are defined by touching them with a pointer that is also equipped with such LEDs or reflective markers. Figure 8.40 shows a schematic representation of the measuring principle known as triangulation. Given the projections of a 3D point in two camera images, its 3D coordinates can be obtained from the intersection of the projection rays. Assume that both cameras $C_1$ and $C_2$ have identical internal parameters and are separated by a distance $b$ along the $x$-axis of $S$. Assume further that $C_1$ coincides with the origin and that both cameras have optical axes parallel to the $z$-axis and have coplanar image planes $z = f$. The coordinates $(x, y, z)$ of a LED or reflective marker are then calculated as the intersection of the projection

lines through $(u_1, v_1)$ and $(u_2, v_2)$. These two rays can be represented by $(su_1, sv_1, sf)$ and $(b + ru_2, rv_2, rf)$. They intersect if $s = r = b/(u_1 - u_2)$. Hence, the coordinates $(x, y, z)$ are given by

$$x = \frac{b}{u_1 - u_2} u_1$$

$$y = \frac{b}{u_1 - u_2} v_1 \qquad (8.11)$$

$$z = \frac{b}{u_1 - u_2} f.$$

Note that it is assumed that the fiducial markers remain in place as soon as their coordinates in the surgery space $S$ have been measured. In neurosurgery,

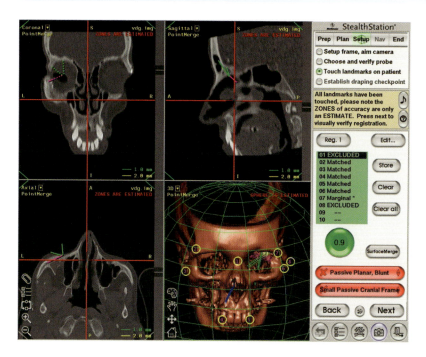

**Figure 8.36** Navigation through CT images during the preparation of the placement of an eye prosthesis. The red cross lines show the position of one of the instruments. Anatomical markers are used to transfer the preoperative images to the coordinate space of the navigation system in the operating room. Courtesy of Professor J. Schoenaers, Department of Stomatology and Maxillofacial Surgery

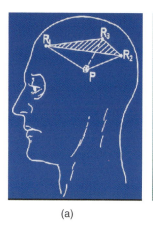

(a)

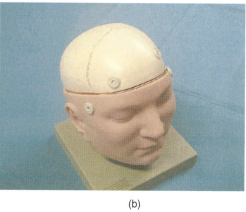

(b)

**Figure 8.37** (a) Any point $P$ can uniquely be defined with respect to three noncollinear reference points $R_1$, $R_2$, and $R_3$. (b) Noninvasive skin markers are attached to the patient prior to preoperative imaging (Reprinted with permission of Radionics.) They are visible in the images and remain in place until the surgery is finished.

for example, the head is still immobilized on the operating table using a so-called Mayfield clamp (see Figure 8.38). For other applications this condition usually does not hold. One way to solve this problem is to attach a LED or marker assembly, called a *dynamic reference frame*, to the moving structure (see for example Figure 8.41), and track it in the same way the surgical instrument is tracked (see Figure 8.39). Obviously, this tracking method is constrained to solid tissue such as bone, which forms one rigid structure with the attached markers. Registration and tracking of soft tissue is a much more difficult problem for which intraoperative imaging is the most elegant solution.

## Calculating the geometric transformation

Once the coordinates of the markers in both the image space $\mathcal{I}$ and the surgery space $\mathcal{S}$ are known, the geometric transformation $F : \mathcal{S} \to \mathcal{I}$ can be calculated. Let $u_i$, $i = 1, \ldots, n$, be the coordinates of the markers in $\mathcal{I}$, and $v_i$, $i = 1, \ldots, n$, the corresponding coordinates in $\mathcal{S}$. The objective is to find $F$ such that $u_i = F(v_i)$, $i = 1, \ldots, n$. This problem is known as *point matching*. As long as there is no geometric deformation between the preoperative and the intraoperative positions of the markers, $F$ is an isometry. In brain surgery, it is therefore assumed that the skin and attached markers do not move with respect to

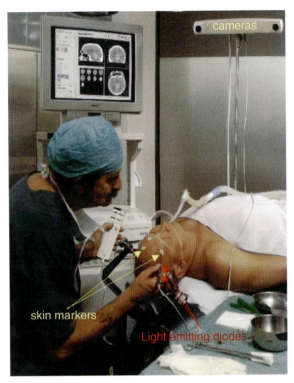

**Figure 8.38** Optical navigation system (with permission of Philips Healthcare.). LEDs are attached to the probe operated by the surgeon.

the brain. Because this is usually not the case in most applications, more than three markers are used, this way improving the accuracy of $F$.

Because $F$ is an isometry, it can be decomposed into a rotation followed by a translation. The problem then consists of finding a $3 \times 3$ rotation matrix $R$ and $3 \times 1$ translation matrix $l$ such that

$$u_i = Rv_i + l, \quad i = 1, \ldots, n. \quad (8.12)$$

Let $u_\mu$ and $v_\mu$ be the centers of mass of the set $u_i$ and the set $v_i$, respectively. Consequently

$$l = u_\mu - Rv_\mu. \quad (8.13)$$

Defining

$$u_i' = u_i - u_\mu$$
$$v_i' = v_i - v_\mu, \quad (8.14)$$

it follows that $R$ must satisfy

$$u_i' = Rv_i', \quad i = 1, \ldots, n. \quad (8.15)$$

The matrix $R$ is a linear transformation and can be determined using numerical linear algebra – for example by "the orthogonal Procrustes problem" [34].

A useful extension of point matching can be obtained with the iterative closest point (ICP) algorithm [35]. It requires a cloud of points, in both the image space and the surgery space, but the one-to-one correspondence between the points is no longer needed. The only restriction is that they belong to the same anatomical surface in both the image and the surgery space. In practice, the skin is segmented in CT or MR images by simple thresholding, yielding a large number $n_\mathcal{I}$ of image points along the skin surface. In the surgery space, $n_\mathcal{S}$ points of the skin surface are measured with a 3D position-sensing device as described above. The major advantage of this transfer method, also known as *surface matching*, is that it does not require fiducial markers anymore. In spine surgery, for example, it is clinically not feasible to attach artificial markers to the spine before the intervention.

Typically, $n_\mathcal{S} \ll n_\mathcal{I}$ (i.e., a few tens against several thousands). Starting from a sufficiently good estimate of the transformation, the principle of the ICP algorithm is to select iteratively a subset of $n_\mathcal{S}$ points in $\mathcal{I}$ and to apply point matching between $\mathcal{I}$ and $\mathcal{S}$. The subset is chosen as the set of $n_\mathcal{S}$ points in $\mathcal{I}$ that are closest to points in $\mathcal{S}$. Next, the geometric transformation $F$ is calculated and applied, yielding a new position of $\mathcal{I}$ with respect to $\mathcal{S}$. This procedure of selecting $n_\mathcal{S}$ points in $\mathcal{I}$ and applying point matching is repeated until it converges according to a certain stop criterion (e.g., root-mean-square error less than a predefined value). A frequent problem with the ICP approach is that it may stick in a local minimum.

Instead of using a navigation system, other procedures have been developed during recent decades to transfer the images and planning data to the operating space. In principle they suffice to perform the intervention exactly as planned. However, navigation with the instruments through the images is then not feasible.

- In stereotactic neurosurgery it has been common practice to use a reference frame fixed onto the

[34] G. Golub and C. van Loan. *Matrix Computations*. London: Johns Hopkins University Press Ltd., third edition, 1996.
[35] P. J. Besl and N. D. McKay. A method for registration of 3-d shapes. *IEEE Transactions on Pattern Analysis and Machine Intelligence*, 14(2): 239–256, 1992.

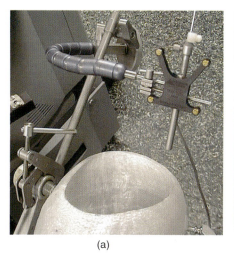
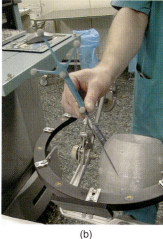

(a)

(b)

**Figure 8.39** The instrumentation used with an optical system is equipped with LEDs **(a)** or highly reflective markers **(b)**. (Courtesy of Medtronic.) Specific LED or marker assemblies must be designed for specific instruments. The instrument holder on the left is supported by a semi-flexible arm that can be immobilized when a proper alignment is obtained.

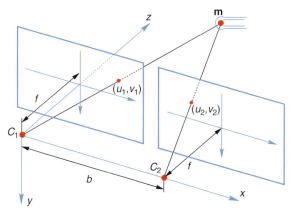

**Figure 8.40** Camera $C_1$, $i = 1, 2$, projects the LED (or marker) **m** onto $(u_i, v_i)$ in its image plane. Knowing the geometry and the intrinsics of the cameras ($b$ and $f$ in this simplified model), the coordinates of **m** can be calculated from $(u_i, v_i)$.

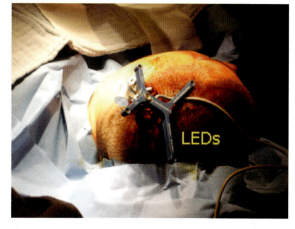

**Figure 8.41** A dynamic reference frame, containing LEDs, is attached to the patient's head during an eye prosthesis placement (see also Figure 8.36). This way the moving head is dynamically tracked and the coordinates of the fiducial markers in the surgery space $\mathcal{S}$ are continuously updated.

patient's head (see Figure 8.1). This frame contains markers that are visible in the preoperative images. This way the images are geometrically related to the frame coordinate system. The frame contains a surgical instrument holder with known frame coordinates. Its position is adjustable to align it with the planned trajectory.

- Several attempts have been made to get rid of the stereotactic frame. Screwing such a frame into the skull is uncomfortable for the patient and inconvenient for the surgeon. A frame may even prevent deep lesions from being reached. Instead, a synthetic nontoxic mold or template can be fabricated (e.g., by stereolithography) that uniquely fits onto

the bone and contains precise information from the planning, such as narrow cylindrical holes to guide the surgical instrument. Figure 8.42 shows the use of a template for oral implant surgery. A drawback of a template is the inflexibility it causes during surgery because the trajectories are irrevocably fixed.

- The spatial relationship between the preoperative image space and the operating space can also be obtained by matching preoperative with intraoperative images. Methods for rigid 3D image fusion have already been discussed in Chapter 7, p. 173. Some cases of matching 3D preoperative CT or

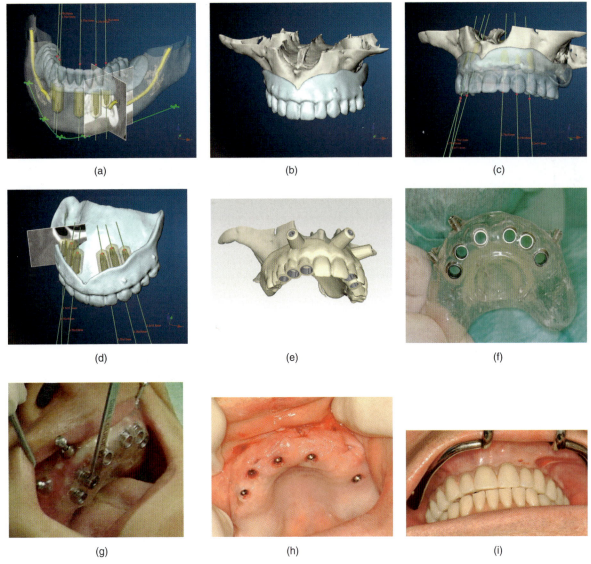

**Figure 8.42** Oral rehabilitation based on implants. **(a)** 3D planning of oral implants to be screwed into the jawbone. A safety zone is drawn around the implant to aid the surgeon in preventing problems such as bone fenestration and nerve damage. The yellow line represents the mandibular canal of the inferior alveolar nerve. **(b)** A removable denture is also scanned and integrated into the 3D images. **(c, d)** The surgeon uses this information to make sure that the oral implants can be covered aesthetically by the teeth of the final fixed prosthesis. **(e)** Using the planning data, a surgical template is digitally designed. It fits on the soft tissues and is secured with anchor pins. **(f)** This patient specific design is manufactured, and **(g)** temporarily fixed to the gum where it serves as a drill guide. **(h)** After insertion of the implants, **(i)** the final prosthesis is fixed. Thanks to digital planning, minimally invasive surgery and immediate restoration is possible. This procedure decreases the failure rate and enhances the patient comfort significantly. (Design and realization by Nobel Biocare.)

MR images with 2D intraoperative radiographs or ultrasound images have also been reported. This kind of 3D-to-2D matching is particularly useful as a means for *augmented reality*, discussed below (p. 216).

## Augmented reality

An *augmented reality* (AR) system generates a composite view that combines a real and a virtual scene. The virtual scene, generated by the computer, augments the real scene with additional image data. In the

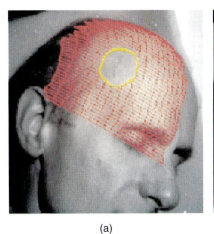
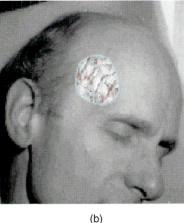

(a) (b)

**Figure 8.43** Augmented reality image showing an intraoperative video image together with **(a)** the planned craniotomy and **(b)** the underlying brain cortex obtained from preoperative images. (Reprinted from [36], with permission of Professor A. Colchester, Kent Institute of Medicine and Health Sciences, UK.)

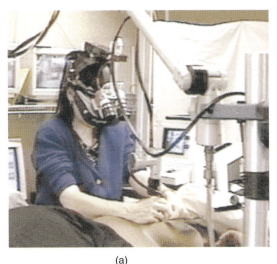
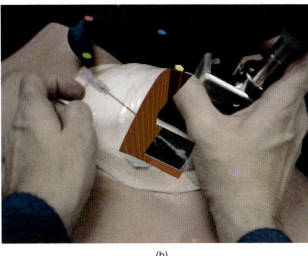

(a) (b)

**Figure 8.44 (a)** A biopsy needle is directed toward a target in a breast under ultrasound image guidance. The physician holds the biopsy needle in one hand and the ultrasound probe in the other and wears a HMD with two small integrated video screens. **(b)** The AR image perceived in the HMD shows an integrated view of the operating field and the ultrasound image at its correct spatial position. (Reprinted with permission of Professor H. Fuchs, University of North Carolina, Chapel Hill, NC.)

context of computer assisted surgery, the real scene is typically an intraoperative 2D video or fluoroscopic sequence, while the virtual scene is obtained from preoperative images, planning and measurements, and is projected onto the intraoperative image.

Figure 8.43 is an example of how intraoperative video images can be integrated with preoperative images and planning data into a single image. Instead of projecting this integrated image on a video screen, it can also be represented in a head mounted display (HMD), which consists of a helmet with two small screens in front of the eyes. The video images

can be abandoned if the HMD has transparent displays. In this case, the surgeon has a real image of the patient together with preoperative images, planning data and possibly other intraoperative images (e.g., ultrasound images, see Figure 8.44). Note that, in order to keep a consistent integrated image, the

[36] A. C. F. Colchester, J. Zhao, K. S. Holton-Tainter, C. J. Henri, N. Maitland, P. T. E. Roberts, C. G. Harris, and R. J. Evans. Development and preliminary evaluation of VISLAN, a surgical planning and guidance system using intra-operative video imaging. *Medical Image Analysis*, 1: 73–90, 1996.

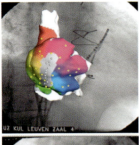

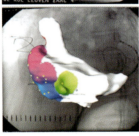

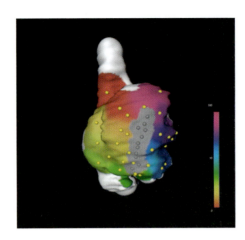

**Figure 8.45** To assist the electrophysiologist during catheter thermoablation of cardiac arrhythmias, a 3D model of the heart is constructed from preoperative CT or MR data. The model is fused with intraoperative fluoroscopic images, such that catheter measurements acquired during the intervention can be mapped onto the model. This allows for 3D visualization of the electrical pathways of the heart, which greatly facilitates the correct interpretation of all available electro-anatomical data.

see-through HMD needs to be tracked when the surgeon's head moves. Head mounted displays are not widely used yet. The question of whether a see-through or video solution should be preferred still remains to be answered. See-through is more natural but has the disadvantage that image slices are more difficult to perceive while looking at the brightly lit operating field.

Another example is electro-anatomical mapping for radiofrequency (RF) catheter ablation to treat cardiac arrhythmias (Figure 8.45). Instead of video images, fluoroscopic images are augmented with a 3D surface rendered image of one or more heart chambers. These images are obtained by segmentation of MRI or CT images. Next, this 3D image is projected onto the 2D fluoroscopic images used during treatment. In these fluoroscopic images, the catheters are visible. At several places along the catheters the time delays of generated pulses are measured. These measured time delays are backprojected onto the 3D surface and represented in color. Based on the obtained color pattern the cardiologist can then identify the arrythmia and perform an ablation.

A basic question in augmented reality is to transfer a point from the 3D preoperative image space $\mathcal{I}$ to the related 3D camera space $\mathcal{C}$ and corresponding 2D intraoperative image space $V$. Assume that the camera can be modeled as a perspective pinhole

camera with its optical center located at $c$ (Figure 8.46). The geometric relation between $\mathcal{I}$ and $\mathcal{C}$ can then be expressed by a rotation $R$ and a translation $l$ as in Eq. (8.12). Once the coordinates of a point $p(x, y, z)$ in $\mathcal{C}$ are known, its projection $(x_p, y_p, f)$ in image $V$, i.e., in the plane $z = f$, can easily be calculated using the following equations (see Figure 8.46):

$$\frac{x}{x_p} = \frac{z}{f}$$
$$\frac{y}{y_p} = \frac{z}{f}. \tag{8.16}$$

This projection can be written in matrix form as follows:

$$\begin{pmatrix} x_p \\ y_p \\ 1 \end{pmatrix} \sim \begin{pmatrix} f & 0 & 0 \\ 0 & f & 0 \\ 0 & 0 & 1 \end{pmatrix} \begin{pmatrix} 1 & 0 & 0 & 0 \\ 0 & 1 & 0 & 0 \\ 0 & 0 & 1 & 0 \end{pmatrix} \begin{pmatrix} x \\ y \\ z \\ 1 \end{pmatrix}. \tag{8.17}$$

Next, a computer image with coordinates $(u, v)$ is acquired from the projection image in the plane $z = f$. This readout process is subject to a scaling, shear and translation, which can be represented as a $3 \times 3$ matrix (see Eq. (1.8)). Hence,

$$\begin{pmatrix} u \\ v \\ 1 \end{pmatrix} = \begin{pmatrix} s_x & k_x & u_0 \\ k_y & s_y & v_0 \\ 0 & 0 & 1 \end{pmatrix} \begin{pmatrix} x_p \\ y_p \\ 1 \end{pmatrix}. \tag{8.18}$$

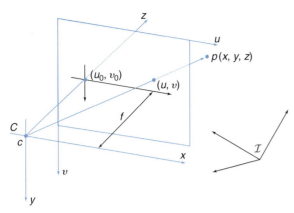

**Figure 8.46** Schematic representation of the 3D preoperative image space $\mathcal{I}$, the 3D camera space $\mathcal{C}$, and the 2D intraoperative image space $V$. The camera is centered at $c$ and projects a point $p(x,y,z)$ onto $(u,v)$ in the 2D intraoperative image.

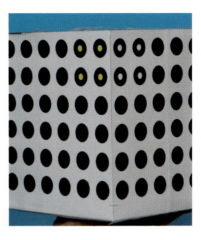

**Figure 8.47**
Object for internal calibration. It contains many markers and its geometry is accurately known. It can be used for the internal calibration of the video or fluoroscopic equipment.

Combining Eq. (8.18) and Eq. (8.17) yields

$$
\begin{pmatrix} u \\ v \\ 1 \end{pmatrix} \sim \begin{pmatrix} s_x & k_x & u_0 \\ k_y & s_y & v_0 \\ 0 & 0 & 1 \end{pmatrix}
$$

$$
\cdot \begin{pmatrix} f & 0 & 0 \\ 0 & f & 0 \\ 0 & 0 & 1 \end{pmatrix} \begin{pmatrix} 1 & 0 & 0 & 0 \\ 0 & 1 & 0 & 0 \\ 0 & 0 & 1 & 0 \end{pmatrix} \begin{pmatrix} x \\ y \\ z \\ 1 \end{pmatrix}. \tag{8.19}
$$

For technical reasons that have to do with the camera readout mechanism, $k_y = 0$. Multiplying the matrices in Eq. (8.19) and substituting $s_x \cdot f$, $s_y \cdot f$ and $k_x \cdot f$ by $f_x$, $f_y$ and $\kappa_x$, respectively, yields

$$
\begin{pmatrix} u \\ v \\ 1 \end{pmatrix} \sim \begin{pmatrix} f_x & \kappa_x & u_0 & 0 \\ 0 & f_y & v_0 & 0 \\ 0 & 0 & 1 & 0 \end{pmatrix} \begin{pmatrix} x \\ y \\ z \\ 1 \end{pmatrix}. \tag{8.20}
$$

The transformation matrix in Eq. (8.20) contains five parameters. When these parameters are known, the camera is said to be calibrated *internally*. The camera is calibrated *externally* if the six degrees of freedom of $l$ and $R$ are known. Together, the whole calibration process thus requires eleven parameters to be defined. This can be done if the patient's body contains sufficient marker points with known preoperative and intraoperative image coordinates. Each such point yields two equations. This means that at least six points are needed to calculate the value of

the eleven parameters. In practice, many more reference points are used in order to improve the accuracy of the solution. Because the calibration accuracy is very sensitive to the accuracy of the coordinates of the reference markers, an alternative procedure consists of an internal calibration with a calibration object whose geometry is accurately known (see for example Figure 8.47). The body markers are then used for the external calibration, i.e., the six translation and rotation parameters. Hence, three such reference points are theoretically sufficient. In practice more markers are helpful to increase the accuracy of the external calibration.

The intraoperative image $V$ can be augmented not only with preoperative images $\mathcal{I}$, but also with data obtained from a navigation system measured in the intraoperative navigation space $\mathcal{S}$.

Co-registration of $\mathcal{S}$ and $V$ can be performed with the same method as explained in this section by replacing the 3D preoperative image space $\mathcal{I}$ by the 3D intraoperative navigation space $\mathcal{S}$ in Figure 8.46. $\mathcal{S}$ and $V$ can also be registered indirectly by transforming $\mathcal{S}$ to $\mathcal{I}$ as explained on p. 211, and $\mathcal{I}$ to $\mathcal{C}$ as explained in this section. Figure 8.48 shows a useful practical example. The intraoperative fluoroscopic image is augmented with a graphical representation of the surgical instrument. The virtual image of the instrument is continuously updated to its changing position by tracking it with an optical navigation system. Because this procedure makes a retake of fluoroscopic images to check the instrument's current position superfluous, it strongly reduces patient irradiation.

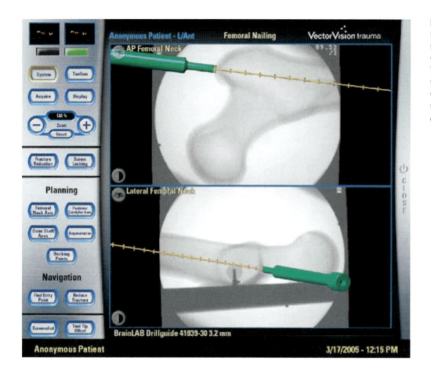

**Figure 8.48** Brainlab's VectorVision trauma system. Intraoperative fluoroscopic images augmented with a virtual image of the surgical instrument. This procedure saves X-ray irradiation to the patient compared to the method in which fluoroscopic images need to be taken to visualize the changing position of the instrument. (Courtesy of Brainlab.)

## Future expectations

Improved and fast visualization goes hand in hand with computer power. Today, personal computers contain powerful graphics processing units (GPU), which are very effective for highly parallel calculations such as available in image fusion and 3D rendering algorithms. This will stimulate the use of challenging visualization methods in clinical practice.

Surface rendering has become standard practice for image guided therapy. Volume rendering is more computationally expensive but offers more flexibility. Its usage will increase, for both diagnostic and therapeutic purposes.

Image-guided surgery allows the surgeon to work more accurately. Consequently, the success rate and the quality of the intervention can be expected to improve. Computer assistance may even modify the operation procedure. Certain interventions, such as in the field of maxillofacial and oral rehabilitation, will largely depend on 3D image based planning. Planning systems will simulate the outcome of the surgery, including soft tissue prediction.

Not only preoperative but also intraoperative imaging, such as CT and MRI, provides assistance to the surgeon. It can be expected that interventional follow up and adjustment based on images will receive increasing attention in the future.

Appendix

# A

# Linear system theory

## Introduction

This appendix summarizes a number of fundamental definitions from linear system and Fourier theory. Only what is relevant for this book is discussed. More information can be found in the specific textbooks on this topic [37, 38, 39].

## Signals

### Definitions and examples

A signal represents the measurable change of some quantity with respect to one or more independent variables such as time or spatial position. Mathematically, a signal can be represented as a function. In medical imaging, the signals are multidimensional. Modern acquisition systems acquire three- (3D) and even four-dimensional (4D) data. The signal can then be written as

$$s = f(\vec{r}, t) = f(x, y, z, t)$$
$$\forall x, y, z, t \in \mathbb{R} \quad \text{and} \quad s \in \mathbb{C}. \quad (A.1)$$

The value of the function is usually real, but it can be complex.

Signals have some particular properties. The most important for this book are defined as follows.
A signal is even if

$$s(-x) = s(x) \qquad \forall x \in \mathbb{R}. \quad (A.2)$$

A signal is odd if

$$s(-x) = -s(x) \qquad \forall x \in \mathbb{R}. \quad (A.3)$$

[37] R. N. Bracewell. *The Fourier Transform and Its Applications*. New York: McGraw-Hill, second edition, 1986.
[38] E. Oran Brigham. *The Fast Fourier Transform and its Applications*. Englewood Cliffs, NJ: Prentice-Hall International, first edition, 1988.
[39] A. Oppenheim, A. Willsky, and H. Nawab. *Signals and Systems*. Upper Saddle River, NJ: Prentice-Hall International, second edition, 1997.

We denote even and odd signals by $s_e(x)$ and $s_o(x)$, respectively. Obviously, the product of two even signals is even, the product of two odd signals is even, and the product of an even and an odd signal is odd. From the definition it is also clear that

$$\int_{-\infty}^{+\infty} s_e(x)\,dx = 2\int_{0}^{+\infty} s_e(x)\,dx \quad (A.4)$$

and

$$\int_{-\infty}^{+\infty} s_o(x)\,dx = 0. \quad (A.5)$$

Any signal can be written as the sum of an even and an odd part:

$$s(x) = \left[\frac{s(x)}{2} + \frac{s(-x)}{2}\right] + \left[\frac{s(x)}{2} - \frac{s(-x)}{2}\right]$$
$$= s_e(x) + s_o(x). \quad (A.6)$$

A signal is periodic if

$$s(x + X) = s(x) \qquad \forall x \in \mathbb{R}. \quad (A.7)$$

The smallest finite $X$ that satisfies this equation is called the period. If no such $X$ exists, the function is aperiodic.

A complex function can be written in Cartesian representation. For 2D signals, we have

$$s(x, y) = u(x, y) + iv(x, y), \quad (A.8)$$

where $u(x, y)$ and $v(x, y)$ are the real part and imaginary part, respectively. A complex function can also be written in polar representation as

$$s(x, y) = |s(x, y)|\,e^{i\phi(x,y)}, \quad (A.9)$$

where

$$|s(x, y)| = \sqrt{u^2(x, y) + v^2(x, y)} \quad (A.10)$$

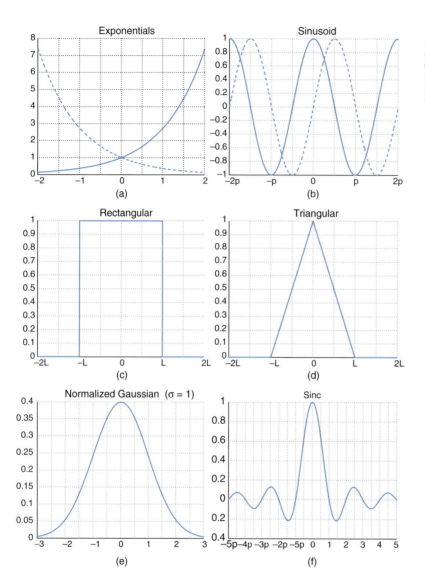

**Figure A.1** Some of the most important signals in linear system theory. **(a)** The exponentials $e^x$ (solid) and $e^{-x}$ (dashed). **(b)** $\sin(x)$ (dashed) and $\cos(x)$ (solid). **(c)** Rectangular pulse. **(d)** Triangular pulse. **(e)** Normalized Gaussian with $\mu = 0$. **(f)** $\mathrm{sinc}(x)$.

is the modulus or the amplitude and

$$\phi(x, y) = \arctan\left(\frac{v(x, y)}{u(x, y)}\right) \qquad \text{(A.11)}$$

is the argument or the phase of $s$.

A number of signals are used extensively in system theory and are important enough to have a unique name. Here are some of them (see also Figure A.1).

- *Exponential* (Figure A.1(a))

$$\exp(ax) = e^{ax}. \qquad \text{(A.12)}$$

When the constant $a > 0$, the exponential function increases continuously with increasing $x$ (solid line); when $a < 0$, it decreases toward zero with increasing $x$ (dashed line).

- *Complex exponential or sinusoid* (Figure A.1(b))

$$A\,e^{i(2\pi kx + \phi)}$$
$$= A\,(\cos(2\pi kx + \phi) + i\sin(2\pi kx + \phi)). \qquad \text{(A.13)}$$

A sinusoid is characterized by three parameters: its modulus or amplitude $A$, spatial frequency $k$, and phase $\phi$. The term i is the imaginary unit; that is

$i^2 = -1$. The real and imaginary parts of a sinusoid are, respectively, a cosine (solid line) and sine function (dashed line).

- *Unit step function (also called Heaviside's function)*

$$u(x - x_0) = \begin{cases} 0 & \text{for } x < x_0 \\ \dfrac{1}{2} & \text{for } x = x_0 \\ 1 & \text{for } x > x_0. \end{cases} \quad (A.14)$$

The constant $x_0$ denotes the location of the step. The function is discontinuous at $x_0$.

- *Rectangular function* (Figure A.1(c))

$$\Pi\left(\frac{x}{2L}\right) = \begin{cases} 1 & \text{for } |x| < L \\ \dfrac{1}{2} & \text{for } |x| = L \\ 0 & \text{for } |x| > L. \end{cases} \quad (A.15)$$

The constant $2L$ is the width of the rectangle. Because the nonzero extent of the function is finite, the function is also called a rectangular pulse.

- *Triangular function* (Figure A.1(d)):

$$\Lambda\left(\frac{x}{2L}\right) = \begin{cases} 1 - \dfrac{|x|}{L} & \text{for } |x| < L \\ 0 & \text{for } |x| \geq L. \end{cases} \quad (A.16)$$

Note that the base of the triangular pulse is equal to $2L$.

- *Normalized Gaussian* (Figure A.1(e))

$$G_{\mathrm{n}}(x) = \frac{1}{\sqrt{2\pi}\sigma} \, e^{-(x-\mu)^2/2\sigma^2}. \quad (A.17)$$

The Gaussian is normalized (i.e., its integral for all $x$ is 1). The constants $\mu$, $\sigma$, and $\sigma^2$ are the mean, the standard deviation, and the variance, respectively.

- *Sinc function* (Figure A.1(f))

$$\mathrm{sinc}(x) = \frac{\sin(x)}{x}. \quad (A.18)$$

According to L'Hôpital's rule, $\mathrm{sinc}(0) = 1$.

Note that the rectangular, the triangular, the normalized Gaussian, and the sinc function are all even and aperiodic. The step function is neither even nor odd

nor periodic. To be compatible with the theory of single-valued functions, it is common to use the mean of the value immediately left and right of the discontinuity. For example, the values at the discontinuities of the rectangular pulse equal $1/2$. For more information, we refer to [37, 38].

## The Dirac impulse

The *Dirac impulse*, also called impulse function or $\delta$-function, is a very important function in linear system theory. It is defined as

$$\delta(x - x_0) = 0 \quad \text{for } x \neq x_0,$$
$$\int_{-\infty}^{+\infty} \delta(x - x_0) \, \mathrm{d}x = 1, \quad (A.19)$$

with $x_0$ a constant. The value of a Dirac impulse is zero for all $x$ except in $x = x_0$, where it is undefined. However, the area under the impulse is finite and is by definition equal to 1. A Dirac impulse can be considered as the limit of a rectangular pulse of magnitude $1/\varepsilon$ and spatial extent $\varepsilon > 0$ such that the area of the pulse is 1:

$$\delta(x) = \lim_{\varepsilon \to 0} \frac{1}{\varepsilon} \Pi\left(\frac{x}{\varepsilon}\right). \quad (A.20)$$

When $\varepsilon$ becomes smaller, the spatial extent decreases, the amplitude increases, but the area remains the same. Clearly, the Dirac impulse is not a function in the strict mathematical sense. Its rigorous definition is given by the theory of generalized functions or distributions, which is beyond the scope of this text [40].

Using Eq. (A.20), it is clear that

$$\int_{-\infty}^{+\infty} \delta(x)s(x) \, \mathrm{d}x = \lim_{\varepsilon \to 0} \int_{-\infty}^{+\infty} \frac{1}{\varepsilon} \Pi\left(\frac{x}{\varepsilon}\right) s(x) \, \mathrm{d}x, \quad (A.21)$$

and consequently the following properties hold:

- *sifting* let $s(x)$ be continuous at $x = x_0$, then

$$\int_{-\infty}^{+\infty} s(x) \, \delta(x - x_0) \, \mathrm{d}x = s(x_0); \quad (A.22)$$

[40] R. F. Hoskins. *Generalised Functions*. New York: McGraw-Hill Book Company, 1979.

- *scaling*

$$\int_{-\infty}^{+\infty} A\,\delta(x)\,\mathrm{d}x = A, \qquad (A.23)$$

this is a special case of sifting.

The definition of the impulse function can be extended to more dimensions by replacing $x$ by $\vec{r}$. The properties are analogous; for example, the sifting property in 2D becomes

$$\iint_{-\infty}^{+\infty} s(\vec{r})\,\delta(\vec{r} - \vec{r}_0)\,\mathrm{d}\vec{r} = s(\vec{r}_0). \qquad (A.24)$$

The impulse function is crucial for a thorough understanding of *sampling*, as discussed on p. 228.

## Systems

### Definitions and examples

A system transforms an input signal (also called *excitation*) into an output signal (also called *response*). Mathematically this can be written as

$$s_o = \mathcal{L}\{s_i\}, \qquad (A.25)$$

where $s_i$ and $s_o$ are the input and output signals, respectively.* The term $\mathcal{L}$ is an operator and denotes the action of the system. A system can be complex and it can consist of many diverse parts. In system theory, however, it is often considered as a black box, and the detailed behavior of the different components is irrelevant. As a simple example, consider an amplifier. It consists of many electrical and electronic parts, but its essential action is to amplify any input signal by a certain amount, say $A$. Hence,

$$s_o(t) = \mathcal{L}\{s_i(t)\} = A\,s_i(t). \qquad (A.26)$$

The process of finding a mathematical relationship between the input and the output signal is called modeling. The simplest is an algebraic relationship, as in the example of the amplifier. More difficult are continuous dynamic relationships that involve (sets of) differential or integral equations, or both, and discrete

dynamic relationships that involve (sets of) difference equations.

With respect to their model, systems can be linear or nonlinear. A system is linear if the *superposition principle* holds, that is,

$$\mathcal{L}\{c_1 s_1 + c_2 s_2\} = c_1 \mathcal{L}\{s_1\} + c_2 \mathcal{L}\{s_2\}$$
$$\forall\, c_1, c_2 \in \mathbb{R}, \qquad (A.27)$$

with $s_1$ and $s_2$ as arbitrary signals. For example, the amplifier introduced above is linear because

$$\mathcal{L}\{c_1 s_1 + c_2 s_2\} = A(c_1 s_1 + c_2 s_2)$$
$$= c_1 A\, s_1 + c_2 A\, s_2$$
$$= c_1 \mathcal{L}\{s_1\} + c_2 \mathcal{L}\{s_2\}. \qquad (A.28)$$

A system is nonlinear if the superposition principle does not hold. For example, a system whose output is the square of the input is nonlinear because

$$\mathcal{L}\{c_1 s_1 + c_2 s_2\} = (c_1 s_1 + c_2 s_2)^2$$
$$\neq (c_1 s_1)^2 + (c_2 s_2)^2. \qquad (A.29)$$

In this text, only linear systems are dealt with.

A system is *time invariant* if its properties do not change with time. Hence, if $s_o(t)$ is the response to the excitation $s_i(t)$, $s_o(t - T)$ will be the response to $s_i(t - T)$. Analogously, a system is *shift invariant* if its properties do not change with spatial position: if $s_o(x)$ is the response to the excitation $s_i(x)$, $s_o(x - X)$ will be the response to $s_i(x - X)$. We will denote linear time-invariant systems as LTI systems and linear shift-invariant systems as LSI systems.

The response to a Dirac impulse is called the *impulse response*. From Eq. (A.22) it follows that

$$s_i(x) = \int_{-\infty}^{+\infty} s_i(\xi)\,\delta(x - \xi)\,\mathrm{d}\xi. \qquad (A.30)$$

Let $h(x)$ be the impulse response of a LSI system. Based on the superposition principle (A.27), $s_o(x)$ can then be written as

$$s_o(x) = \mathcal{L}\{s_i\} = \int_{-\infty}^{+\infty} s_i(\xi)\mathcal{L}\{\delta(x - \xi)\}\,\mathrm{d}\xi$$
$$= \int_{-\infty}^{+\infty} s_i(\xi)\,h(x - \xi)\,\mathrm{d}\xi. \qquad (A.31)$$

---

* We also use $s_o$ to represent an odd signal. However, this should cause no confusion because the exact interpretation is clear from the context.

A similar equation holds for a LTI system:

$$s_o(t) = \int_{-\infty}^{+\infty} s_i(\tau)\, h(t - \tau)\, d\tau. \qquad (A.32)$$

The integral in Eqs. (A.31) and (A.32) is a so-called *convolution* and is often represented by an asterisk:

$$s_o = s_i * h. \qquad (A.33)$$

The function $h$ is also known as the *point spread function* or PSF (see Figure 1.4). Because of its importance in this book, convolution will first be discussed in some more detail.

## Convolution

Given two signals $s_1(x)$ and $s_2(x)$, their convolution is defined as follows:

$$s_1(x) * s_2(x) = \int_{-\infty}^{+\infty} s_1(x - \xi)\, s_2(\xi)\, d\xi, \qquad (A.34)$$

or equivalently

$$s_2(x) * s_1(x) = \int_{-\infty}^{+\infty} s_1(\xi)\, s_2(x - \xi)\, d\xi. \qquad (A.35)$$

The result of both expressions is identical, as is clear when substituting $\xi$ by $x - \xi$.

A graphical interpretation of convolution is given in Figure A.2. The following steps can be discerned:

- *mirroring*, changing $\xi$ to $-\xi$,
- *translation* over a distance equal to $x$,

- *multiplication*, the product of the mirrored and shifted function $s_1(x - \xi)$ with $s_2(\xi)$ is the colored part in Figure A.2(c),
- *integration*, the area of the colored part is the convolution value in point $x$.

The convolution function is found by repeating the previous steps for each value of $x$.

Convolution can also be defined for multidimensional signals. For 2D (two-dimensional) signals, we have

$$s_1(x, y) * s_2(x, y)$$
$$= \iint_{-\infty}^{+\infty} s_1(x - \xi, y - \zeta)\, s_2(\xi, \zeta)\, d\xi\, d\zeta, \qquad (A.36)$$

or equivalently

$$s_2(x, y) * s_1(x, y)$$
$$= \iint_{-\infty}^{+\infty} s_2(x - \xi, y - \zeta)\, s_1(\xi, \zeta)\, d\xi\, d\zeta. \qquad (A.37)$$

The graphical analysis shown above can be extended to 2D. The convolution values are then represented by *volumes* rather than by areas.

The convolution integrals (A.34)–(A.37) have many properties. The most important in the context of this book include the following.

- *Commutativity*

$$s_1 * s_2 = s_2 * s_1. \qquad (A.38)$$

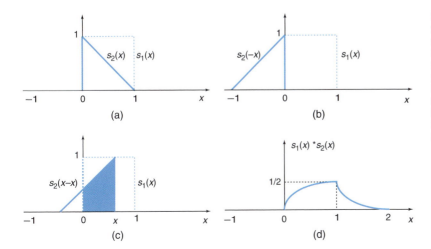

**Figure A.2** Graphical interpretation of the convolution of a rectangular pulse $s_1(x)$ with a triangle $s_2(x)$. Changing the independent variable to $\xi$ does not change the functions (**a**). After $s_2(\xi)$ is mirrored (**b**), it is translated over a distance $x$, both functions are multiplied and the result is integrated (**c**). The area of the overlapping part is the result for the chosen $x$. The convolution $s_1(x) * s_2(x)$ is shown in (**d**).

- *Associativity*

$$(s_1 * s_2) * s_3 = s_1 * (s_2 * s_3) = s_1 * s_2 * s_3. \tag{A.39}$$

- *Distributivity*

$$s_1 * (s_2 + s_3) = s_1 * s_2 + s_1 * s_3. \tag{A.40}$$

## Response of a LSI system

Let us first consider the response of a LSI system to a sinusoid. Using Eq. (A.31) with $s_i(x) = A\,e^{2\pi ikx}$ yields

$$s_o(x) = \int_{-\infty}^{+\infty} A\,e^{2\pi ik(x-\xi)}\,h(\xi)\,d\xi$$

$$= A\,e^{2\pi ikx} \int_{-\infty}^{+\infty} e^{-2\pi ik\xi}\,h(\xi)\,d\xi$$

$$= A\,e^{2\pi ikx}\,H(k), \tag{A.41}$$

with $H(k)$ the so-called *Fourier transform* of the PSF $h(x)$:

$$H(k) = \int_{-\infty}^{+\infty} e^{-2\pi ik\xi}\,h(\xi)\,d\xi. \tag{A.42}$$

The function $H(k)$ is also called the *transfer function*.

It can be shown that any input signal $s_i(x)$ can be written as an integral of weighted sinusoids with different spatial frequencies:

$$s_i(x) = \int_{-\infty}^{+\infty} S_i(k)\,e^{2\pi ikx}\,dk, \tag{A.43}$$

where $S_i(k)$ is the Fourier transform of $s_i(x)$. The signal $s_i(x)$ is the so-called *inverse Fourier transform* (because of the $+$ sign in the exponent instead of the $-$ sign in Eq. (A.42)) of $S_i(k)$.

Using Eq. (A.41) and the superposition principle, the output signal $s_o$ is then

$$s_o(x) = \int_{-\infty}^{+\infty} S_i(k)\,H(k)\,e^{2\pi ikx}\,dk. \tag{A.44}$$

Summarizing, the output function $s_o$ of a LSI system can be calculated in two ways: either by convolving the input function $s_i$ with the PSF, that is, $s_o = s_i * h$ (Eq. (A.33)), or in the $k$-space or frequency domain by multiplying the Fourier transform of $s_i$ with the

transfer function, that is, $S_o(k) = S_i(k)H(k)$, and calculating the inverse Fourier transform of $S_o(k)$.

In linear system theory, the transfer function $H(k)$ is often used instead of the PSF $h(x)$ because of its nice mathematical and interesting physical properties. The relationship between the PSF $h(x)$ and the transfer function $H(k)$ is given by the Fourier transform (A.42). Because of its importance in medical imaging, the Fourier transform is discussed in more detail in the next section. Note however that the Fourier transform is not the only possible transform. There are many others (Hilbert, Laplace, etc.), although the Fourier transform is by far the most important in the theory of medical imaging.

## The Fourier transform

### Definitions

Let $k$ and $r$ be the conjugate variables in the Fourier domain and the original domain, respectively. The *forward* Fourier transform (FT) of a signal $s(r)$ is defined as

$$S(k) = \mathcal{F}\{s(r)\} = \int_{-\infty}^{+\infty} s(r)\,e^{-2\pi irk}\,dr. \tag{A.45}$$

The operator symbol $\mathcal{F}$ (calligraphic F) is used as the notation for the transform. Uppercase letters are used for the result of the forward transform. Analogously, the *inverse* Fourier transform (IFT) is defined as

$$s(r) = \mathcal{F}^{-1}\{S(k)\} = \int_{-\infty}^{+\infty} S(k)\,e^{+2\pi irk}\,dk. \tag{A.46}$$

It can be shown that for continuous functions $s$,

$$s(r) = \mathcal{F}^{-1}\{\mathcal{F}\{s(r)\}\}. \tag{A.47}$$

From the definitions (A.45) and (A.46), it follows that for an even function $s_e(r)$,

$$\mathcal{F}\{s_e(r)\} = \mathcal{F}^{-1}\{s_e(r)\}. \tag{A.48}$$

If $r$ is time with dimension seconds, $k$ is the temporal frequency with dimension hertz. Related to the temporal frequency is the *angular frequency* $\omega = 2\pi k$ with dimension radians per second. In this case, the base function of the forward FT describes a rotation in the clockwise direction with angular velocity $\omega$. If $r$ is spatial position with dimension mm, $k$ is spatial frequency with dimension mm$^{-1}$.

In this definition, the original signal and the result of the transform are one dimensional. In medical imaging, however, the signals are often multidimensional and vectors must be used in the definitions.

Forward:

$$S(\vec{k}) = \mathcal{F}\{s(\vec{r})\} = \int_{-\infty}^{+\infty} s(\vec{r}) \, e^{-2\pi i \vec{k} \cdot \vec{r}} \, d\vec{r}.$$

Inverse:

$$s(\vec{r}) = \mathcal{F}^{-1}\{S(\vec{k})\} = \int_{-\infty}^{+\infty} S(\vec{k}) \, e^{+2\pi i \vec{k} \cdot \vec{r}} \, d\vec{k}. \quad \text{(A.49)}$$

$\vec{r}$ and $\vec{k}$ are the conjugate variables, $\vec{r}$ being spatial position and $\vec{k}$ spatial frequency. Although only one integral sign is shown, it is understood that there are as many as there are independent variables. The original signal and its transform are known as a Fourier transform pair denoted as

$$s(r) \longleftrightarrow S(k). \quad \text{(A.50)}$$

In general, the result of the forward FT of a signal is a complex function. The *amplitude spectrum* is the modulus of its FT, while the *phase spectrum* is the phase of its FT. Both spectra show how amplitude and phase vary with spatial or temporal frequencies. Often, the phase spectrum is considered irrelevant, and only the amplitude spectrum is considered. Note, however, that a signal is completely characterized if and only if *both* the amplitude and phase spectrum are specified.

# Examples
## Example 1
The FT of a rectangular pulse (Eq. (A.15)), scaled with amplitude $A$ is

$$\mathcal{F}\left\{A \, \Pi\left(\frac{x}{2L}\right)\right\} = \int_{-\infty}^{+\infty} A \, \Pi\left(\frac{x}{2L}\right) e^{-2\pi i k x} \, dx$$

$$= \int_{-L}^{+L} A \, e^{-2\pi i k x} \, dx$$

$$= -\frac{A}{2\pi i k} (e^{-2\pi i k L} - e^{+2\pi i k L}).$$
$$\text{(A.51)}$$

Using Eqs. (A.13) and (A.18), we finally obtain

$$A \, \Pi\left(\frac{x}{2L}\right) \longleftrightarrow 2AL \, \text{sinc}(2\pi k L). \quad \text{(A.52)}$$

The forward FT of a rectangular pulse is a sinc function whose maximum amplitude is equal to the area of the pulse. The first zero crossing occurs at

$$k = \frac{1}{2L}. \quad \text{(A.53)}$$

Thus, the broader the width of the rectangular pulse in the original domain, the closer the first zero-crossing lies near the origin of the Fourier domain or the more "peaked" the sinc function is (see Figure A.1(c) and (f)).

## Example 2
The forward FT of the product of a step function (Eq. (A.14)) and an exponential (Eq. (A.12)) (we assume $a > 0$) is

$$\mathcal{F}\{u(x) \, e^{-ax}\} = \int_{-\infty}^{+\infty} u(x) \, e^{-ax} \, e^{-2\pi i k x} \, dx$$

$$= \int_{0}^{+\infty} e^{-(a+2\pi i k)x} \, dx$$

$$= \frac{1}{a + 2\pi i k}$$

$$= \frac{a}{a^2 + 4\pi^2 k^2} - i\frac{2\pi k}{a^2 + 4\pi^2 k^2}.$$
$$\text{(A.54)}$$

The result is complex; according to Eqs. (A.8) and (A.9), we have the following.

$$\text{Real part:} \quad \frac{a}{a^2 + 4\pi^2 k^2}.$$

$$\text{Imaginary part:} \quad -\frac{2\pi k}{a^2 + 4\pi^2 k^2}.$$

$$\text{Modulus:} \quad \frac{1}{\sqrt{a^2 + 4\pi^2 k^2}}.$$
$$\text{(A.55)}$$

$$\text{Phase:} \quad -\arctan\left(\frac{2\pi k}{a}\right).$$

This transform pair is a mathematical model of the filter shown in Figure 4.21.

## Example 3
The forward FT of the Dirac impulse. Direct application of the sifting property (A.22) gives

$$\mathcal{F}\{\delta(x - x_0)\} = \int_{-\infty}^{+\infty} \delta(x - x_0) \, e^{-2\pi i k x} \, dx$$

$$= e^{-2\pi i k x_0}. \quad \text{(A.56)}$$

The FT of a Dirac impulse at $x_0$ is complex: in the amplitude spectrum, all spatial frequencies are present with amplitude 1. The phase varies linearly with $k$ with slope $-2\pi x_0$.

A difficulty arises when calculating the IFT:

$$s(x) = \int_{-\infty}^{+\infty} e^{-2\pi i k x_0}\, e^{+2\pi i k x}\, dk$$

$$= \int_{-\infty}^{+\infty} \cos(2\pi k(x - x_0))\, dk$$

$$+ i \int_{-\infty}^{+\infty} \sin(2\pi k(x - x_0))\, dk. \quad (A.57)$$

Because its integrand is odd, the second integral is zero. The first integral has no meaning, unless it is interpreted according to the distribution theory. In this case, it can be shown that

$$\int_{-\infty}^{+\infty} \cos(2\pi k(x - x_0))\, dk = \int_{-\infty}^{+\infty} e^{+2\pi i k(x - x_0)}\, dk$$

$$= \delta(x - x_0). \quad (A.58)$$

Hence,

$$\delta(x - x_0) \longleftrightarrow e^{-2\pi i k x_0}. \quad (A.59)$$

### Example 4

The forward FT of a cosine function is

$$\mathcal{F}\{\cos(2\pi k_0 x)\}$$

$$= \int_{-\infty}^{+\infty} \cos(2\pi k_0 x)\, e^{-2\pi i k x}\, dx$$

$$= \int_{-\infty}^{+\infty} \left( \frac{e^{+2\pi i k_0 x} + e^{-2\pi i k_0 x}}{2} \right) e^{-2\pi i k x}\, dx$$

$$= \frac{1}{2} \int_{-\infty}^{+\infty} e^{-2\pi i (k - k_0) x}\, dx$$

$$+ \frac{1}{2} \int_{-\infty}^{+\infty} e^{-2\pi i (k + k_0) x}\, dx$$

$$= \frac{1}{2} \delta(k - k_0) + \frac{1}{2} \delta(k + k_0). \quad (A.60)$$

The spectrum of a cosine function consists of two impulses at spatial frequencies $k_0$ and $-k_0$. In general it can be shown that a periodic function has a discrete spectrum (i.e., not all spatial frequencies are present), whereas an aperiodic function has a continuous spectrum. Table A.1 shows a list of FT pairs used in this book.

**Table A.1** Important Fourier transform pairs in linear system theory

| Image space | Fourier space |
|---|---|
| 1 | $\delta(k)$ |
| $\delta(x)$ | 1 |
| $\cos(2\pi k_0 x)$ | $\frac{1}{2}(\delta(k + k_0) + \delta(k - k_0))$ |
| $\sin(2\pi k_0 x)$ | $\frac{i}{2}(\delta(k + k_0) - \delta(k - k_0))$ |
| $\Pi(\frac{x}{2L})$ | $2L\,\mathrm{sinc}(2\pi L k)$ |
| $\Lambda(\frac{x}{2L})$ | $L\,\mathrm{sinc}^2(\pi L k)$ |
| $G_n(x)$ | $e^{-2\pi^2 k^2 \sigma^2}$ |

## Properties

- **Linearity** If $s_1 \longleftrightarrow S_1$ and $s_2 \longleftrightarrow S_2$, then

$$c_1 s_1 + c_2 s_2 \longleftrightarrow c_1 S_1 + c_2 S_2 \qquad \forall c_1, c_2 \in \mathbb{C}. \quad (A.61)$$

This can easily be extended to more than two signals.

- **Scaling** If $s(x) \longleftrightarrow S(k)$, then

$$s(ax) \longleftrightarrow \frac{1}{|a|} S\left(\frac{k}{a}\right) \qquad a \in \mathbb{R}_0. \quad (A.62)$$

- **Translation** If $s(x) \longleftrightarrow S(k)$, then

$$s(x - x_0) \longleftrightarrow e^{-2\pi i x_0 k} S(k) \qquad x_0 \in \mathbb{R}. \quad (A.63)$$

Thus, translating a signal over a distance $x_0$ only modifies its *phase* spectrum.

- Transfer function and impulse response (or PSF) are a FT pair. Indeed, Eq. (A.42) shows that

$$h(x) \longleftrightarrow H(k). \quad (A.64)$$

In imaging, the FT of the PSF is known as the *optical transfer function* (OTF). The modulus of the OTF is the *modulation transfer function* (MTF). As mentioned in Chapter 1, the PSF and OTF characterize the resolution of the system. If the PSF is expressed in mm, the OTF is expressed in mm$^{-1}$. Often, line pairs per millimeter (lp/mm) is used instead of mm$^{-1}$. The origin of this unit can easily be understood if an image with sinusoidal intensity lines at a frequency of 1 period per millimeter or 1 lp/mm, that is, one dark and one bright line per millimeter, is observed (Figure A.3). This line pattern can be written as $\sin(2\pi x)$, $x$ expressed in

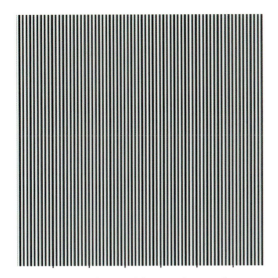

**Figure A.3** Image with sinusoidal intensity lines at a frequency of 1 lp/mm.

mm. The Fourier transform of this function consists of two impulses at spatial frequency 1 mm$^{-1}$ and $-1$ mm$^{-1}$. This then explains why the frequency units mm$^{-1}$ and lp/mm can be used as synonyms.

The resolution of an imaging system is sometimes characterized by the distinguishable number of line pairs per millimeter. It is clear now that this is a limited and subjective measure, and that it is preferable to show the complete OTF curve when talking about the resolution. Nevertheless, it is common practice in the technical documents of medical imaging equipment and in the medical literature simply to list an indication of the resolution in lp/mm at a specified small amplitude (in %) of the OTF.

- *Convolution* On p. 224 it was concluded that an output function $s_o$ of a LSI system can be calculated in two ways: (1) $s_o = s_i * h$ in the image domain or (2) $\mathcal{F}^{-1}\{S_o(k) = S_i(k)H(k)\}$ in the Fourier domain. In general, if $s_1 \longleftrightarrow S_1$ and $s_2 \longleftrightarrow S_2$, then

$$
\begin{aligned}
s_1 * s_2 &\longleftrightarrow S_1 \cdot S_2 \\
s_1 \cdot s_2 &\longleftrightarrow S_1 * S_2.
\end{aligned}
\tag{A.65}
$$

This is a very important property. The convolution of two signals can be calculated via the Fourier transform by calculating the forward–inverse FT of both signals, multiplying the FT results, and calculating the inverse–forward FT of the product.

- *The FT of a real signal is Hermitian*

$$
S(-\vec{k}) = \bar{S}(\vec{k}) \quad \text{if } s(x) \in \mathbb{R},
\tag{A.66}
$$

where $\bar{S}$ denotes the complex conjugate of $S$ (i.e., the real part is even and the imaginary part is odd). From Eqs. (A.6), (A.13), and (A.45), we obtain

$$
\begin{aligned}
S(k) &= \int_{-\infty}^{+\infty} s(x)\, e^{-2\pi i k x}\, dx \\
&= \int_{-\infty}^{+\infty} [s_e(x) + s_o(x)] \\
&\quad \cdot [\cos(2\pi\, kx) - i \sin(2\pi\, kx)]\, dx \\
&= \int_{-\infty}^{+\infty} s_e(x) \cos(2\pi\, kx)\, dx \\
&\quad - i \int_{-\infty}^{+\infty} s_o(x) \sin(2\pi\, kx)\, dx.
\end{aligned}
\tag{A.67}
$$

The first integral is the real even part of $S(k)$, and the second is the imaginary odd part of $S(k)$. Hence, to compute the FT of a real signal, it suffices to know one half-plane. The other half-plane can then be computed using Eq. (A.66).

Equation (A.67) further shows that if a function is even (odd), its FT is even (odd). Consequently, if a function is real and even, its FT is real and even, whereas if a function is real and odd, its FT is imaginary and odd.

- *Parseval's theorem*

$$
\int_{-\infty}^{+\infty} |s(x)|^2\, dx = \int_{-\infty}^{+\infty} |S(k)|^2\, dk.
\tag{A.68}
$$

- *Separability* In many cases, a 2D FT can be calculated as two subsequent 1D FTs. The transform is then called separable. For example,

$$
\begin{aligned}
&\mathcal{F}\{\operatorname{sinc}(x)\operatorname{sinc}(y)\} \\
&= \iint_{-\infty}^{+\infty} \frac{\sin(x)}{x}\frac{\sin(y)}{y} e^{-2\pi i(k_x x + k_y y)}\, dx\, dy \\
&= \int_{-\infty}^{+\infty} \frac{\sin(x)}{x} e^{-2\pi i k_x x}\, dx \\
&\quad \cdot \int_{-\infty}^{+\infty} \frac{\sin(y)}{y} e^{-2\pi i k_y y}\, dy \\
&= \mathcal{F}\{\operatorname{sinc}(x)\}\,\mathcal{F}\{\operatorname{sinc}(y)\}.
\end{aligned}
\tag{A.69}
$$

- Another important property of a 2D FT is the projection theorem or central-slice theorem. It is discussed in Chapter 3 on X-ray computed tomography.

## Polar form of the Fourier transform

Using polar coordinates

$$x = r \cos \theta$$
$$y = r \sin \theta, \tag{A.70}$$

Eq. (A.49)

$$S(k_x, k_y) = \int\int_{-\infty}^{+\infty} s(x, y)\, e^{-2\pi i(k_x x + k_y y)}\, dx\, dy \tag{A.71}$$

can be rewritten as

$$S(k_x, k_y)$$
$$= \int_0^{2\pi} \int_0^{+\infty} s(r, \theta)\, e^{-2\pi i(k_x r \cos\theta + k_y r \sin\theta)}\, r\, dr\, d\theta$$
$$= \int_0^{\pi} \int_{-\infty}^{+\infty} s(r, \theta)\, e^{-2\pi i(k_x r \cos\theta + k_y r \sin\theta)}\, |r|\, dr\, d\theta. \tag{A.72}$$

The factor $r$ in the integrand is the Jacobian of the transformation:

$$J \triangleq \begin{vmatrix} \dfrac{\partial x}{\partial r} & \dfrac{\partial x}{\partial \theta} \\[2mm] \dfrac{\partial y}{\partial r} & \dfrac{\partial y}{\partial \theta} \end{vmatrix} = \begin{vmatrix} \cos\theta & -r\sin\theta \\ \sin\theta & r\cos\theta \end{vmatrix}$$
$$= r\,(\cos^2\theta + \sin^2\theta) = r. \tag{A.73}$$

The polar form of the inverse FT is obtained analogously. Let

$$k_x = k \cos\phi$$
$$k_y = k \sin\phi, \tag{A.74}$$

then

$$s(x, y)$$
$$= \int_0^{\pi} \int_{-\infty}^{+\infty} S(k, \phi)\, e^{+2\pi i(xk \cos\phi + yk \sin\phi)}\, |k|\, dk\, d\phi. \tag{A.75}$$

## Sampling

Equation (A.1) represents an analog continuous signal, which is defined for all spatial positions and can have any (real or complex) value:

$$s(x)\ \forall\, x \in \mathbb{R}. \tag{A.76}$$

In practice, the signal is often *sampled*, that is, only discrete values at regular intervals are measured:

$$s_s(x) = s(n\Delta x)\ n \in \mathbb{Z}. \tag{A.77}$$

The constant $\Delta x$ is the sampling distance. Information may be lost by sampling. However, *under certain conditions*, a continuous signal can be completely recovered from its samples. These conditions are specified by the *sampling theorem*, which is also known as the *Nyquist criterion*. If the Fourier transform of a given signal is band limited and if the sampling frequency is *larger than twice the maximum spatial frequency* present in the signal, then the samples *uniquely* define the given signal. Hence,

$$\text{if}\quad \begin{cases} S(k) = 0 & \forall\, |k| > k_{max} \quad \text{and} \\[2mm] \dfrac{1}{\Delta x} > 2k_{max} \end{cases}$$
$$\text{then}\quad s_s(x) = s(n\Delta x) \quad \text{uniquely defines } s(x). \tag{A.78}$$

To prove this theorem, sampling is defined as a multiplication with an impulse train (see Figure A.4):

$$s_s(x) = s(x) \cdot \text{Ш}(x), \tag{A.79}$$

where $\text{Ш}(x)$ is the comb function or impulse train:

$$\text{Ш}(x) = \sum_{n=-\infty}^{+\infty} \delta(x - n\Delta x). \tag{A.80}$$

The sampling distance $\Delta x$ is the distance between any two consecutive Dirac impulses. Note that this formula is a *formal* notation because the product is only valid as an integrand.

Based on Eq. (A.80) and using the convolution theorem, the Fourier transform $S_s(k)$ can be written as follows:

$$S_s(k) = S(k) * \mathcal{F}\{\text{Ш}(x)\}. \tag{A.81}$$

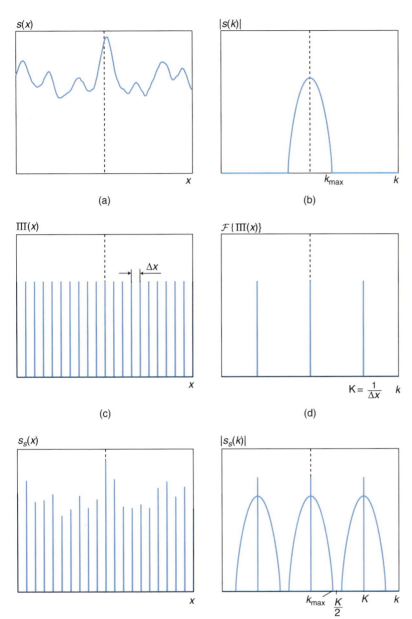

**Figure A.4** A signal with an infinite spatial extent **(a)** and its band-limited Fourier transform **(b)**. The sampled signal **(e)** is obtained by multiplying **(a)** with the impulse train **(c)**. The spectrum **(f)** of the sampled signal is found by convolving the original spectrum **(b)** with the Fourier transform of the impulse train **(d)**. This results in a periodic repetition of the original spectrum.

It can be shown that

$$\mathcal{F}\{\text{III}(x)\} = K \sum_{l=-\infty}^{+\infty} \delta(k - lK), \quad \text{(A.82)}$$

which is again an impulse train with consecutive impulses separated by the sampling frequency

$$K = \frac{1}{\Delta x}. \quad \text{(A.83)}$$

Hence,

$$S_s(k) = K(S(k) + S(k - K) + S(k + K) \\ + S(k - 2K) + S(k + 2K) + \cdots). \quad \text{(A.84)}$$

Because

$$S(k) = 0 \; \forall \; |k| \geq \frac{K}{2}$$

**229**

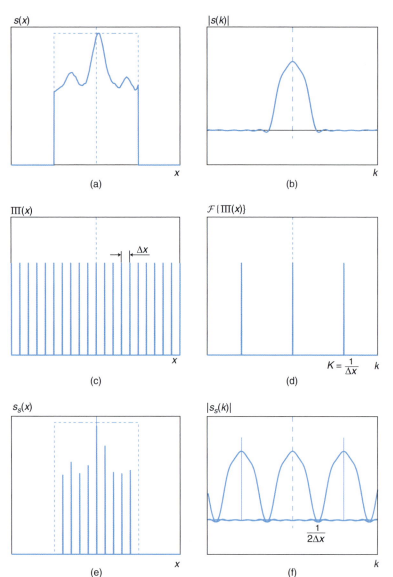

**Figure A.5** A signal with a finite spatial extent **(a)** is not band limited **(b)**. The sampled signal **(e)** is obtained by multiplying **(a)** with the impulse train **(c)**. The spectrum **(f)** of the sampled signal is found by convolving the original spectrum **(b)** with the Fourier transform of the impulse train **(d)**. This results in a periodic repetition of the original spectrum. Because of the overlap, aliasing cannot be avoided.

it follows that

$$K\,S(k) = S_{\mathrm{s}}(k)\,\Pi\!\left(\frac{x}{K}\right), \qquad (A.85)$$

and consequently $s(x)$ can be recovered from $S_{\mathrm{s}}(k)$.

If the signal $s(x)$ is not band limited or if it is band limited but $1/\Delta x \leq 2k_{\mathrm{max}}$, the shifted replicas of $S(k)$ in Eq. (A.84) will overlap (see Figure A.5). In that case, the spectrum of $s(x)$ cannot be recovered by multiplication with a rectangular pulse. This phenomenon is known as *aliasing* and is unavoidable if the original signal $s(x)$ is not band limited. As an important

example, note that a patient *always* has a limited spatial extent, which implies that the FT of an image of the body is never band limited and, consequently, aliasing is unavoidable. Several practical examples of aliasing are given in this textbook.

Numerical methods calculate the Fourier transform for a limited number of discrete points in the frequency band $(-k_N, +k_N)$. This means that not only the signal but also its Fourier transform is sampled. Sampling the Fourier data implies that it yields shifted replicas in the signal $s$, which may overlap. To avoid such overlap or aliasing of the signal, the sampling distance $\Delta k$ must also be chosen small enough. It can easily be shown that this condition can be satisfied if the number of samples in the Fourier domain is at least equal to the number of samples in the signal domain. In practice they are chosen equal.

Based on the preceding considerations, the *discrete Fourier transform* (DFT) for 2D signals can be written as (more details can be found in [38]):

$$S(m\Delta k_x, n\Delta k_y) = \sum_{q=0}^{N-1}\sum_{p=0}^{M-1} s(p\Delta x, q\Delta y)\, e^{-2\pi i\left(\frac{mp}{M}+\frac{nq}{N}\right)}.$$

$$s(p\Delta x, q\Delta y) = \sum_{n=0}^{N-1}\sum_{m=0}^{M-1} S(m\Delta k_x, n\Delta k_y)\, e^{2\pi i\left(\frac{mp}{M}+\frac{nq}{N}\right)}.$$

(A.86)

In both cases, $m, p = 0, 1, \ldots, M-1$ and $n, q = 0, 1, \ldots, N-1$. Here, $M$ and $N$ need not be equal because both directions can be sampled differently. However, for a particular direction, the number of samples in the spatial and the Fourier domain is the same.

Direct computation of the DFT is a time-consuming process. However, when the number of samples is a power of two, a computationally very fast algorithm can be employed: the *fast Fourier transform* or FFT. The FFT algorithm has become very important in signal and image processing, and hardware versions are frequently used in today's medical equipment. The properties and applications of the FFT are the subject of [38].

# Appendix

# B Exercises

## Basic image operations

1. Edge detection and edge enhancement.

    (a) Specify a differential operator (high-pass filter) to detect the horizontal edges in an image. Do the same for vertical edge detection.

    (b) How can edges of arbitrary direction be detected using the above two operators?

    (c) How can these operators be exploited for edge enhancement?

2. What is the effect of a convolution with the following $3 \times 3$ masks?

| 1 | 2 | 1 |
|---|---|---|
| 2 | 4 | 2 |
| 1 | 2 | 1 |

| −1 | 0 | 1 |
|----|---|---|
| −2 | 0 | 2 |
| −1 | 0 | 1 |

| 0 | −1 | 0 |
|---|----|---|
| −1 | 4 | −1 |
| 0 | −1 | 0 |

| 0 | −1 | 0 |
|---|----|---|
| −1 | 5 | −1 |
| 0 | −1 | 0 |

Are these operators used in clinical practice? Explain.

3. What is the effect of the following convolution operators on an image?

    * The Laplacian of a Gaussian: $\nabla^2 g\,(\vec{r})$.

    * The difference of two Gaussians:

$$g_1(\vec{r}) - g_2(\vec{r}) \text{ with different } \sigma.$$

    * The $3 \times 3$ convolution mask

| 1 | 1 | 1 |
|---|---|---|
| 1 | −8 | 1 |
| 1 | 1 | 1 |

4. Unsharp masking is defined as

$$(1 + \alpha)\, I\,(x, y) - \alpha\, g * I\,(x, y),$$

with $I\,(x, y)$ the image, $g$ a Gaussian, and $\alpha$ a parameter. The following convolution mask is an approximation of unsharp masking:

| −1/8 | −2/8 | −1/8 |
|------|------|------|
| −2/8 | ? | −2/8 |
| −1/8 | −2/8 | −1/8 |

Calculate the missing central value.

## Radiography

1. X-rays.

    (a) What is the physical difference between X-rays, $\gamma$-rays, light and radio waves? How do they interact with tissue (in the absence of a magnetic field)?

    (b) Draw the X-ray tube spectrum, i.e., the intensity distribution of X-rays as a function of the frequency of emitted X-ray photons (1) at the exit of the X-ray tube before any filtering takes place, and (2) after the filter but before the X-rays have reached the patient.

    (c) How does the tube voltage influence the wavelength of the X-rays?

    (d) Draw the linear attenuation coefficient (for an arbitrary tissue type) as a function of the energy.

2. What is the effect of the kV and mA s of an X-ray tube on

    (a) the patient dose, and

    (b) the image quality?

3. A radiograph of a structure consisting of bone and soft tissue (see Figure B.1) is acquired by a screen–film detector.

    The exposure time is 1 ms. The radiographic film has a sensitometric curve $D = 2 \log E$. The

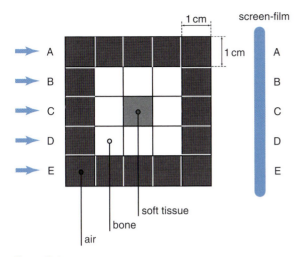

Figure B.1

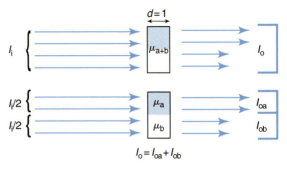

Figure B.2

film–screen system has an absorption efficiency of 25%. Assume that the X-rays are monochromatic and the linear attenuation coefficients of bone, soft tissue and air are respectively $0.50\ \mathrm{cm}^{-1}$, $0.20\ \mathrm{cm}^{-1}$, $0.00\ \mathrm{cm}^{-1}$.

(a) Calculate the optical density $D$ in positions A through E of the image.

(b) Calculate the contrast, i.e., the difference in density, between positions B and C. How can this contrast be improved?

4. In mammography the breasts are compressed with a paddle. Explain why.

# X-ray computed tomography

1. Linear absorption coefficient.

(a) Although the linear absorption coefficient $\mu$ depends on the energy, this dependence is not taken into account in filtered backprojection. Explain.

(b) What is the effect of this approximation on the image quality?

2. Given are two different tissues a and b. Two different detector sizes are used (Figure B.2).

In the first case the detector is twice as large as in the second case.

(a) Calculate the linear attenuation coefficients $\mu_a$, $\mu_b$, and $\mu_{a+b}$ from the input intensity $I_i$ and the output intensities $I_{oa}$ and $I_{ob}$.

(b) Show that $\mu_{a+b}$ is always an underestimate of the mean linear attenuation $(\mu_a + \mu_b)/2$.

(c) What is the influence of this underestimate on a reconstructed CT image? Explain.

3. Cardiac CT. The following conditions are given.

• A CT scanner with 128 detector rows.

• The detector width in the center of the FOV is 0.5 mm.

• A full rotation (360°) of the X-ray tube takes 0.33 s.

• A full data set for reconstruction requires projection values for a range of 210°.

• Maximum $1/4$ of the heart cycle can be used for acquiring projection data.

• The heart rhythm is 72 bpm.

• The scan length is 20 cm.

(a) Calculate the duration of $1/4$ heart cycle (in seconds).

(b) Calculate (in seconds) the time needed to obtain projection values for a range of 210°.

(c) What can you conclude from (a) and (b)?

(d) Assume that the table shift per heart beat is equal to the total width of the detector rows (i.e., the total $z$-collimation). Calculate the acquisition time.

(e) The assumption under (d) is approximate. Explain why? How does this approximation influence the acquisition time?

4. CT of the lungs on a 64-row scanner with detector width 0.60 mm. Given are $\mathrm{CTDI_{vol}} = 10$ mGy, 120 kV, 90 mA s, pitch 1 360° rotation time 0.33 s, slice thickness 1 mm, scan length 38.4 cm.

(a) Calculate the scan time.

233

(b) Calculate the estimated effective dose. Certain organs are only partially and/or indirectly (scatter) irradiated. The following table gives for each of the irradiated organs (1) the percentage of irradiated tissue, and (2) the tissue weighting factor $w_T$.

|  | Irradiated tissues (%) | $w_T$ |
|---|---|---|
| colon | 0.5 | 0.12 |
| lungs | 100 | 0.12 |
| breast | 100 | 0.12 |
| stomach | 50 | 0.12 |
| bone marrow | 25 | 0.12 |
| thyroid gland | 15 | 0.04 |
| liver | 50 | 0.04 |
| esophagus | 100 | 0.04 |
| bladder | 1 | 0.04 |
| skin | 25 | 0.01 |
| bone surface | 30 | 0.01 |
| remainder | 30 | 0.12 |

## Magnetic resonance imaging

1. Assume an MRI spin-echo (SE) sequence with $B_0 = 0.5$ T (see Figure B.3).
   The following conditions are given.

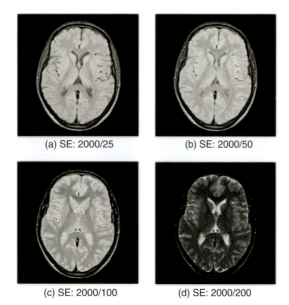

(a) SE: 2000/25    (b) SE: 2000/50

(c) SE: 2000/100    (d) SE: 2000/200

**234**

- In all the images TR = 2000ms. From (a) to (d) TE = 25ms, TE = 50ms, TE = 100ms, and TE = 200ms respectively.
- $T_1$ (white brain matter) $\sim$500 ms and $T_1$ (gray brain matter) $\sim$650 ms.
- $T_2$ (white brain matter) $\sim$90 ms and $T_2$ (gray brain matter) $\sim$100 ms.
- $T_1$ (CSF) $>$3000 ms and $T_2$ (CSF) $>$2000 ms.
- The proton density of gray matter is 14% higher than that of white matter.

The relative signal intensity can be (approximately) expressed by

$$s(t) = \rho\, e^{-TE/T_2}[1 - e^{-TR/T_1}].$$

(a) First, draw (schematically) the longitudinal magnetization ($M_z$) as a function of time after a 90° pulse for white and gray matter and for CSF.

(b) Next, draw (schematically) the transverse magnetization ($M_{xy}$) as a function of time after a 90° pulse for white and gray matter and for CSF (note that TR is 2000 ms).

(c) Explain now on this last diagram why the contrast between CSF (cerebrospinal fluid) and surrounding white brain and brain matter varies from (a) to (d).

2. The MR images in Figure B.4 were acquired with a spin-echo (SE) sequence (90° pulse) at 1.5 T. For the lower right image a so-called STIR (short tau inversion recovery) pulse sequence was used. STIR is an excellent sequence for suppressing the MR signals coming from fatty tissues. STIR is thus a fat saturation or fat suppression sequence. It is characterized by a spin preparation module containing an initial 180° RF pulse, which inverts the magnetization $M_z$, followed after a time TI by the standard RF pulse to tilt the $z$-magnetization into the $xy$-plane.
   $T_1$ (CSF) $>$3000 ms and $T_2$ (CSF) $>$2000 ms; $T_1$ (fat) $= 200$ ms and $T_2$ (fat) $= 100$ ms.

(a) Draw the magnetization $|M_z|$ as a function of time for cerebrospinal fluid (CSF) and for fat for a SE sequence without and with an inversion pulse respectively.

(b) Calculate the inversion time TI.

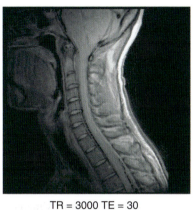

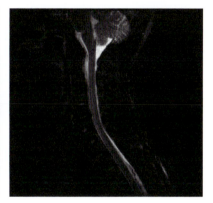

Figure B.4

TR = 3000 TE = 30          TR = 3000 TE = 150

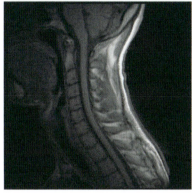

TR = 300 TE = 30          TR = 3000 TE = 150 TI = ?

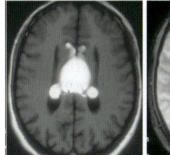

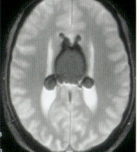

Figure B.5

(c) Draw the magnetization $|M_{xy}|$ as a function of time for CSF and for fat for each of the images (i.e., for TR = 3000 with and without saturation, and for TR = 300). Note that in practice the magnitude of the complex signal is calculated. Hence, negative signals are inverted.

(d) Explain the contrast between CSF and fat in each of the four images.

3. Suggest one or more categories for the lesion in the images of Figure B.5.

4. Assume that the magnetic field $B_0$ of an MRI magnet lies along the $z$-axis. In vector notation, this is written as $\mathbf{B} = (0, 0, B_0)$. The MRI system has three orthogonal gradient systems. We know that for protons $\gamma/2\pi = 42.57$ MHz/T.

(a) What is the precession frequency of protons in a main magnetic field $B_0 = 1.5$ T? Give the result in Hz, not in rad/s.

(b) The strengths of the gradients at a certain moment are $G_x$, $G_y$, $G_z$. What is the *magnitude* and the *direction* of the total external magnetic field in an arbitrary point $(x, y, z)$ inside the imaging volume?

5. A 2 mm slice perpendicular to the $z$-axis at position $z = 0.1$ m is excited with a radiofrequency pulse at frequency $f$. Assume $B_0 = 1.5$ T and

**235**

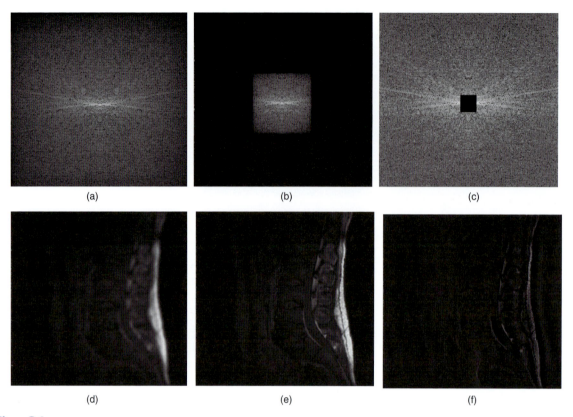

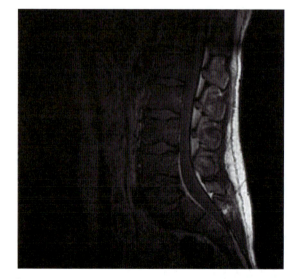

**Figure B.6**

$G_z = 10$ mT/m. What is the frequency $f$ (in Hz) of the RF pulse to excite this slice? And what is the bandwidth (in Hz)?

6. Figure B.6 shows three MR images of the lumbar spine and their $\vec{k}$-space in arbitrary order.

   (a) Which $\vec{k}$-space accompanies each of the three MR images? Explain.

   (b) The bottom left image and the bottom right image were combined using unsharp masking to obtain the image shown in Figure B.7. Explain.

7. In order to reduce the acquisition time, multiple lines in the $\vec{k}$-space can be measured per excitation.

   (a) Assume that four lines per excitation are measured. Draw these lines in the $\vec{k}$-space.

   (b) What is the effect on the image quality (as compared to measuring only one line per excitation)

**Figure B.7**

- if the lowest frequencies are measured first,
- if the highest frequencies are measured first?

8. Image reconstruction in CT and in MRI is based on Fourier theory. In both cases assumptions are made to be able to apply this theory. In CT the X-ray beam is assumed to be monochromatic. In MRI the relaxation effect during the short reading interval is neglected in the case of multiple echoes per excitations. What is the influence of these assumptions on the image quality in CT and MRI respectively?

9. Consider the pulse sequence in Figure B.8 (surface 2 equals two times surface 1). Draw the trajectory of $\vec{k}$ in the $\vec{k}$-space.

10. Draw the pulse scheme (i.e., RF pulses and magnetic gradient pulses) for the $\vec{k}$-space sampling shown in Figure B.9.

11. Given

$$k_x(t) = \frac{y}{2\pi} \, at \cos(bt)$$
$$k_y(t) = \frac{y}{2\pi} \, at \sin(bt)$$

$a, b > 0$.

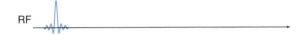

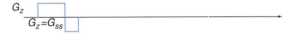

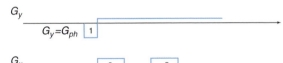

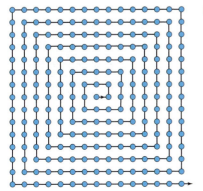

**Figure B.8**

**Figure B.9**

(a) Draw the trajectory in the $\vec{k}$-space.

(b) Calculate the necessary gradients $G_x(t)$ and $G_y(t)$.

(c) Draw the corresponding magnetic gradient pulse sequence.

12. CT is based on the projection theorem stating that the one-dimensional Fourier transform of the projections equals the two-dimensional Fourier transform of the image along a line in the 2D Fourier space, i.e.,

$$P(k, \theta) = F_1\{p_\theta(r)\} \leftrightarrow F(k_x, k_y) = F_2\{f(x, y)\}.$$

Hence an image $f(x, y)$ can be reconstructed by calculating the inverse 2D Fourier transform.

(a) In MRI it is possible to sample along radial lines in the $\vec{k}$-space (see Figure B.10(a)). Draw a suitable pulse sequence in the diagram of Figure B.10(b) to acquire samples from radial lines.

(b) Can filtered backprojection be employed for MRI reconstruction as well?

13. In molecular imaging research gene expressions in vivo can be visualized by means of the marker ferritin, which has the property of capturing iron. Which imaging technique is used to visualize this process? Explain.

14. A patient with thickness $L$ is scanned using a coil with bandwidth BW (in Hz). Note that the different frequencies that are received by this coil are defined by the range of precession frequencies of the spins.

(a) What are the conditions necessary to avoid aliasing artifacts in the readout direction?

(b) What is the maximal gradient amplitude as a function of BW and $L$ necessary to avoid aliasing?

(c) What is the relationship between BW and $\Delta t$?

15. An image is acquired with FOV $= 8$ cm and 256 phase encoding gradient steps. The phase encoding gradient equals 10 mT/m. The radiologist prefers an image with the highest resolution and without artifacts. Calculate the pulse duration of the phase

**237**

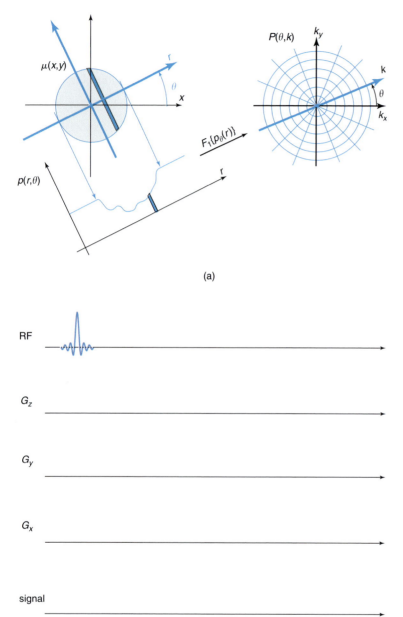

(a)

(b)

encoding gradient. You may assume that the pulse has a rectangular shape.

16. The MR images in Figure B.11 were acquired with a spin-echo (SE) sequence (90° pulse) at 1.5 T.
    Explain the origin of the artifact in the right image.

17. Most imaging modalities are very sensitive to motion.

(a) Which artifact is caused by an abrupt patient movement in CT?

(b) Which artifact is caused by breathing in MRI?

(c) How can artifacts due to respectively breathing and the beating heart be avoided in CT?

(d) How can the additional phase shift in MRI due to flowing blood be overcome?

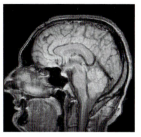
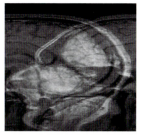

(a) TR = 3000, TE = 10
without artifact

(b) TR = 3000, TE = 10
with artifact

**Figure B.11**

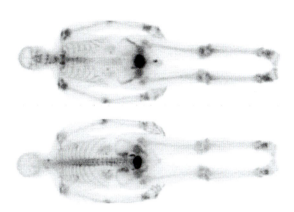

**Figure B.12**

(e) Dephasing in MRI is exploited as a means to obtain images of diffusion and perfusion. Explain.

18. Given are a turboSE sequence with 10 echoes, TR = 500 ms, TE (first echo) = 20 ms; image size 240 × 160 pixels (hence, $N_{ph}$ = 160); slice thickness 5 mm; the heart rate of the patient is 60 bpm.

(a) What is the acquisition time for one slice of the liver?

(b) What is the acquisition time for one slice of the heart? The measurements are synchronized with the ECG.

## Nuclear medicine imaging

1. Radioactivity.

(a) How can the half-life of a radioactive isotope be calculated?

(b) Give a realistic value of the half-life for some radioactive tracers.

(c) Which recommendations would you give to the patient and his/her environment?

2. What is the problem when using filtered backprojection in nuclear imaging?

3. Explain how the two images in Figure B.12 were acquired. What is the difference between them and why?

4. A colleague in a PET center would like to know whether they should put on a lead apron to protect themselves against the irradiation from the positron emitters. We know that the mass density of lead is 11.35 g/cm³ and that its linear attenuation coefficient for this kind of $\gamma$-rays is 1.75 cm$^{-1}$.

(a) An apron that absorbs $3/4$ of the irradiation would be satisfactory protection. What is the thickness of lead (in cm) required to obtain a transmission of 25% (i.e., $3/4$ is absorbed)? Assume a perpendicular incidence of the radiation with the apron.

(b) What is the weight of this lead apron with a transmission of 25% if about 1.5 m² (flexible, but lead containing) material is needed? Neglect the other material components in the apron.

(c) What is your advice with respect to the question of putting on a lead apron? Assume that 10 kg is the maximum bearable weight for an apron.

5. Given is a positron emitting point source at position $x = x^*$ in a homogeneously attenuating medium (center $x = 0$, $-L \leq x \leq L$) with attenuation coefficient $\mu$ (Figure B.13). Detector 1 has radius $R_1$ and detector 2 has radius $R_2 = R_1/2$. The detectors count all the incoming photons (i.e., the absorption efficiency is 100%). Counter A counts all photons independent of the detector, while counter B counts only the coincidences. Because $D \gg L$, $D + L \approx D$. If $\mu = 0$ detector 1 would count $N$ photons per time unit.

(a) Calculate the average number of photons per time unit measured by counter A as function of $\mu$, $x$ and $N$. Calculate the standard deviation for repeated measurements.

(b) Repeat these calculations for counter B.

6. How does a gamma camera react on a simultaneous (i.e., within a time window $\Delta T$) hit of two

**239**

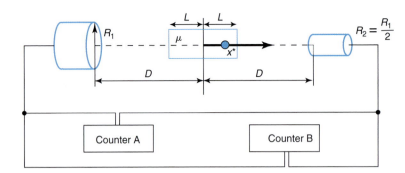

**Figure B.13**

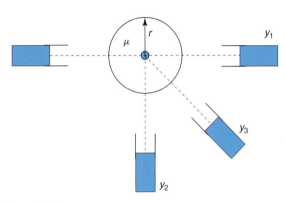

**Figure B.14**

photons of 140 keV each if the energy window is [260 keV, 300 keV]?

What is the probability of a simultaneous (i.e., within a time window $\Delta T$) hit of two photons as function of the activity $A$ (i.e., average number of photons per time unit) and the time resolution $\Delta T$?

7. A positron emitting point source is positioned in the center of a homogeneous attenuating cylinder with radius $r$ and attenuation coefficient $\mu$ (Figure B.14). Two opposing detectors, connected by an electronic coincidence circuit, measure $y_1$ photon pairs and two other single-photon detectors measure $y_2$ and $y_3$ photons respectively. The thickness of the detectors is sufficiently large to

**Figure B.15**

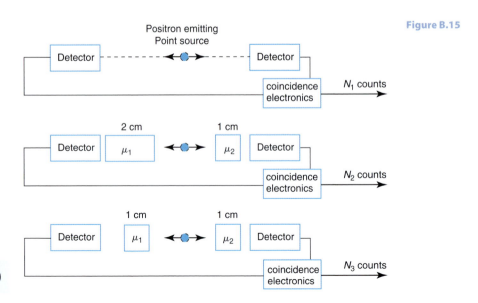

detect all the incoming photons (i.e., the absorption efficiency is 100%). All the detectors have the same size and distance to the point source.

Calculate the activity in the center of the cylinder from the measurements $y_1$, $y_2$ and $y_3$ using maximum likelihood reconstruction.

8. How does Compton scatter influence the spatial resolution in SPECT and PET respectively?

9. Two opposing detectors, connected by an electronic coincidence circuit, perform three subsequent measurements (Figure B.15). The only difference between the measurements is that the attenuation is modified by adding homogeneous blocks between the positron emitting point source and the detectors. The measurements $N_1$, $N_2$ and $N_3$ and the attenuation depths are given.

Calculate the linear absorption coefficients $\mu_1$ and $\mu_2$.

10. A radioactive point source is positioned in front of two detectors (Figure B.16). After a measurement time of one hour, two photons per second have been captured by each of the detectors.

Next, an attenuating block with attenuation depth 1 cm and an attenuation coefficient of $\ln 2$ cm$^{-1}$ is added and a new measurement is performed, this time during only one second.

What is the probability that during this measurement of one second exactly one photon is captured by detector 1 and four photons by detector 2?

11. Given are a square detector with collimator with known geometry, and a point source at distance $x$ (Figure B.17).

   (a) Calculate the sensitivity of the point source at distance $x$.

   (b) Calculate the FWHM of the point spread function at distance $x$.

   Perform the calculations for both $x \leq T$ and $x \geq T$.

12. Given are a point source and two detectors (Figure B.18). The efficiency of both detectors is known and takes both the absorption efficiency and the influence of the geometry (only limited photons travel in the direction of a detector) into account. During a short measurement exactly one photon is absorbed by each detector. What is the maximum likelihood of the total

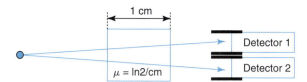

Figure B.16

Figure B.17

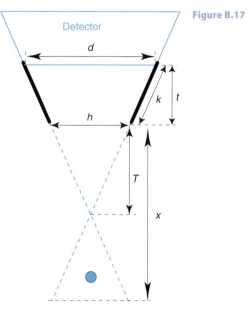

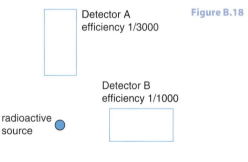

Figure B.18

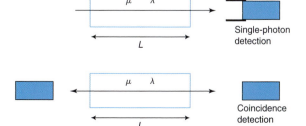

Figure B.19

number of photons that were emitted during this measurement?

13. Given a phantom with homogeneous attenuation coefficient $\mu$ and homogeneous positron activity $\lambda$ per length unit (Figure B.19). A measurement is performed with a single-photon detector and another with a pair of opposing detectors connected by an electronic coincidence circuit. The efficiency of all the detectors is constant ($S$).

    Calculate the expected number of measured photons for both cases.

14. Given is a positron emitting point source in the center of a detector pair connected by an electronic coincidence circuit (Figure B.20). The distance $R$ from the point source to the detectors is much larger than the detector size $a$. The detectors consist of different materials. The absorption efficiency of detector 1 is $\frac{3}{4}$ and that of detector 2 is $\frac{2}{3}$.

    (a) Calculate the fraction of emitted photon pairs that yields a true coincidence event.

    (b) Calculate the fraction of emitted photon pairs that yields a single event.

15. Given are two photon detectors (S and P), a point source that emits $A$ photons, and three blocks with attenuation coefficients $\mu_1 = 1/L$, $\mu_2 = 1/2L$ and $\mu_3 = 1/L$ respectively (Figure B.21). The efficiency of the detectors is known ($\varepsilon_1$ and $\varepsilon_2$ respectively) and takes both the absorption efficiency and the influence of the geometry (only limited photons travel in the direction of the detector) into account.

    (a) Calculate the expected number of detected photons in S.

    (b) Calculate the expected number of detected photon pairs if S and P are connected by an electronic coincidence circuit.

16. A positron emitting ($^{18}$F) point source is positioned in front of a detector. 3600 photons are counted during a first measurement of one hour. Next, a second measurement is performed, this time of only one second.

    (a) Calculate the probability that exactly zero photons are detected.

    (b) Calculate the probability that exactly two photons are detected.

17. Given is a point source with activity $P = 1$ mCi at a distance $L = 30$ cm from a cube with size $h = 5$ cm and attenuation coefficient $\mu = 0.1$ cm$^{-1}$ (Figure B.22). The density of the cube is 1 kg/l, and the half-life of the tracer is $T_{1/2} = 2$ h.

    Calculate the absorbed dose (in mGy) of the cube after several days. Note that 1 eV $= 1.602 \times 10^{-19}$ J and 1 mCi $= 3.7 \times 10^7$ Bq.

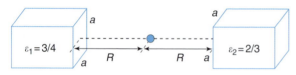

**Figure B.20**

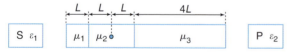

**Figure B.21**

# Ultrasound imaging

1. Ultrasonic waves.

    (a) What are reflection, refraction, scatter and absorption? What is their effect on an ultrasound image?

    (b) What is the effect of the acoustic impedance on the reflection?

    (c) What is the physical reason to avoid an air gap between the transducer and the patient? How can it be avoided?

    (d) What is constructive interference? How is this used to focus the ultrasonic beam? And how is it used to sweep the ultrasonic beam?

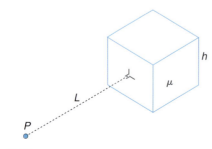

**Figure B.22**

2. What methods do you know to measure the velocity of blood?

3. Given is an ultrasound scanner with the following characteristics:

   - 5 MHz phased array transducer;
   - 16-bit, 20 MHz AD converter;
   - 256 Mb image memory (RAM).
   - operating mode: B-mode acquisition; 3000 transmitted ultrasonic pulses per second; image depth 10 cm; number of scan lines 60; sector angle 60°.

   Given an ultrasound velocity of 1530 m/s.

   (a) What is the image frequency (frame rate)?

   (b) How long does it take to fill the complete image memory with data?

   (c) How many images can maximally be stored in memory?

4. Using PW Doppler, samples $s_j$, $j = 1, 2, \ldots$ are taken of the following signal of a blood vessel:

   $$s_j = 18 \sin(\tfrac{2}{5}\pi j + 0.35) \text{ mV}.$$

   The pulse repetition frequency is 12 kHz. The frequency of the transmitted pulse is 2.5 MHz. The velocity of the ultrasonic signal in soft tissue is 1530 m/s.

   (a) What is the velocity of blood (in the direction of the transducer)?

   (b) What is the maximal velocity $v_{max}$ that can be measured without artifacts?

   (c) What is the maximal distance from the transducer required to measure this maximal velocity $v_{max}$ without artifacts?

   (d) What is the measured velocity of blood if its real velocity equals $v_{max} + 1$ m/s?

5. A radiologist would like to distinguish small details in the vessel wall. Assume that the distance between these small details is 0.5 mm, and that the blood vessel runs parallel to the surface of the tissue at a depth of 5 cm. The attenuation of the ultrasonic beam is 1 dB/(MHz cm). The maximum attenuation to guarantee that the image is practically useful is 100 dB. The ultrasonic pulse duration is 2 periods. Assume that the ultrasound velocity in tissue is 1580 m/s.

   (a) What is the minimal frequency required to distinguish the small details along the vessel wall?

   (b) Given the maximum attenuation of 100 dB, what is the maximum frequency that can be used?

   (c) Which ultrasonic frequency would you recommend to obtain the best image quality (i.e., high resolution and high SNR)?

6. Aliasing in CT, MRI and Doppler respectively.

   (a) Explain the origin of aliasing.

   (b) How does aliasing appear in an image?

   (c) How can aliasing be reduced or avoided?

7. Which methods do you know to obtain images of (a) blood vessels, (b) flow and (c) perfusion? Explain.

8. Assume that the point spread function (PSF) in the lateral direction is a $\text{sinc}^2$ function.

   (a) What is the physical principle behind this pattern?

   (b) What is the modulation transfer function (MTF)?

   (c) What is the maximal distance required between two neighboring scan lines to avoid aliasing?

   (d) What is the minimal distance in the lateral direction between two distinguishable small calcifications?

## Medical image analysis

1. Search, using the principle of dynamic programming, the best edge from left to right in the following gradient image:

   | 1 | 1 | 1 | 1 | 0 | 0 | 0 | 1 | 3 | 3 |
   |---|---|---|---|---|---|---|---|---|---|
   | 3 | 3 | 5 | 4 | 3 | 2 | 3 | 3 | 5 | 4 |
   | 4 | 5 | 4 | 4 | 5 | 4 | 5 | 5 | 2 | 2 |
   | 3 | 3 | 2 | 2 | 5 | 5 | 3 | 3 | 0 | 0 |
   | 1 | 2 | 1 | 3 | 1 | 2 | 4 | 1 | 4 | 4 |

   The cost $C(i)$ of connecting pixel $(x, y_1)$ with pixel $(x + 1, y_2)$ is defined as follows:

   $$C(i) = (5 - \text{grad}(x + 1, y_2) + |y_2 - y_1|)$$

**243**

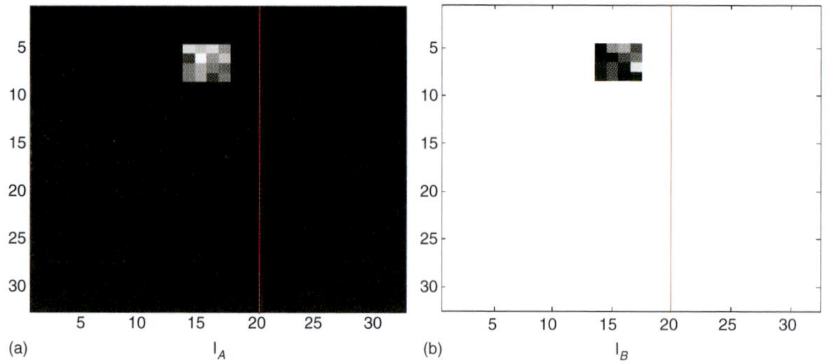

**Figure B.23**

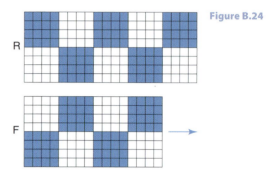

grad() is the gradient in the $y$-direction (these values are shown in the image matrix above), $x$ is the column number, $y$ is the row number, $y_1$ and $y_2$ are arbitrary $y$ values.

2. In images $I_A$ and $I_B$ in Figure B.23 two regions of interests (ROI) A and B are shown. $I_A$ and $I_B$ are geometrically aligned.

(a) Calculate the sum of squared differences (SSD) and the mutual information (MI) of the regions of interest.

(b) Do the same when image $I_B$ is translated one pixel to the right. Use matrix $B_t$ instead of $B$ this time. What can you conclude?

$$A = \begin{bmatrix} 0 & 0 & 8 & 7 & 8 & 5 & 0 & 0 \\ 0 & 0 & 2 & 9 & 5 & 7 & 0 & 0 \\ 0 & 0 & 4 & 6 & 4 & 3 & 0 & 0 \\ 0 & 0 & 4 & 6 & 2 & 4 & 0 & 0 \end{bmatrix}$$

$$B = \begin{bmatrix} 9 & 9 & 1 & 5 & 6 & 3 & 9 & 9 \\ 9 & 9 & 1 & 1 & 3 & 4 & 9 & 9 \\ 9 & 9 & 2 & 3 & 2 & 8 & 9 & 9 \\ 9 & 9 & 2 & 3 & 1 & 2 & 9 & 9 \end{bmatrix}$$

$$B_t = \begin{bmatrix} 9 & 9 & 9 & 1 & 5 & 6 & 3 & 9 \\ 9 & 9 & 9 & 1 & 1 & 3 & 4 & 9 \\ 9 & 9 & 9 & 2 & 3 & 2 & 8 & 9 \\ 9 & 9 & 9 & 2 & 3 & 1 & 2 & 9 \end{bmatrix}$$

3. Calculate the mutual information (MI) of the following arrays:

9 0 4 9          0 8 3 0
9 7 4 0          0 5 2 8
1 8 0 9          9 1 8 0
1 0 3 8          7 8 7 2

**Figure B.24**

R

F

4. To perform a pixel classification of a $T_1$-weighted brain scan, a digital atlas can be used as prior knowledge. The atlas consists of a $T_2$-weighted brain image and an image in which each voxel value expresses the probability that this voxel belongs to white brain matter, gray brain matter or cerebrospinal fluid (CSF). Explain the segmentation method.

5. Consider the binary 20 × 8 image R and 16 × 8 image F in Figure B.24. Calculate their joint histogram and mutual information (MI), given that the upper left corner of the images coincides. Repeat these calculations when image F shifts to the right about 1, 2, 3 and 4 pixels respectively.

## Visualization for diagnosis and therapy

1. Augmented reality. A preoperative 3D CT or MR image has to be registered with 2D endoscopic video images. Assume that the endoscopic camera was calibrated.

How can the video coordinates $(u, v)$ of a point $(x, y, z)$ in the preoperative images be calculated

(a) in the simple case of a static endoscope, and

(b) when the endoscope is in motion? Assume that the endoscope is a rigid instrument.

2. Image guided surgery. To perform a biopsy two on-site radiographs of the lesion are taken from two different directions. The positions of both the X-ray tube and the detector are unknown. A navigation system is used to localize the biopsy needle geometrically in real time. A number of markers, visible in both radiographs, are attached to the skin and their 3D coordinates $(x, y, z)$ can be measured by the navigation system.

   (a) Calculate the 3D coordinates $(x_l, y_l, z_l)$ of the lesion based on its projection in both radiographs. Note that these coordinates cannot simply be measured with the navigation system like the 3D marker coordinates $(x, y, z)$.

   (b) How many markers are minimally needed?

3. Preoperative maxillofacial CT images of a patient were acquired together with one or more 2D photographs taken with a digital camera. By projecting the 2D photographs onto the 3D skin surface, derived from the CT images, a textured 3D surface of the head can be obtained.

   (a) How can a 3D surface of the face be obtained from CT images?

   (b) How can the texture of a 2D photograph be projected onto this 3D surface?

# Bibliography

A. Abragam. *The Principles of Nuclear Magnetism*. Oxford: Clarendon Press, first edition, 1961.

M. Abramowitz and I. Stegun. *Handbook of Mathematical Functions*. New York: Dover Publications, ninth edition, 1970.

M. Alonso and E. J. Finn. *Physics*. Addison-Wesley, 1992.

J. Ball and J. D. Moore. *Essential Physics for Radiographers*. Oxford: Blackwell Science, 1998.

P. G. J. Barten. *Contrast Sensitivity of the Human Eye and Its Effects on Image Quality*. Washington: SPIE Optical Engineering Press, 1999.

J. Beutel, H. L. Kundel, and R. L. Van Metter. *Handbook of Medical Imaging*, Volume 1, *Physics and Psychophysics*. Washington: SPIE Press, 2000.

A. Bovik. *Handbook of Image & Video Processing*. San Diego, CA: Academic Press, 2000.

R. N. Bracewell. *The Fourier Transform and its Applications*. New York: McGraw-Hill, second edition, 1986.

E. Oran Brigham. *The Fast Fourier Transform and its Applications*. Englewood Cliffs, NJ: Prentice-Hall International, first edition, 1988.

B. H. Brown, R. H. Smallwood, D. C. Barber, P. V. Lawford, and D. R. Hose. *Medical Physics and Biomedical Engineering*. Bristol: Institute of Physics Publishing, 1999.

J. T. Bushberg, J. A. Seibert, Jr. E. M. Leidholt, and J. M. Boone. *The Essential Physics of Medical Imaging*. Philadelphia, PA: Lippincott Williams & Wilkins, second edition, 2002.

P. Carter. *Imaging Science*. Oxford: Blackwell Publishing, 2006.

C.-H. Chen. *Statistical Pattern Recognition*. Rochelle Park, NJ: Spartan Books, Hayden Book Company, 1973.

Z. H. Cho, J. P. Jones, and M. Singh. *Foundations of Medical Imaging*. New York: John Wiley & Sons, first edition, 1993.

Z. H. Cho and R. S. Ledley. *Computers in Biology and Medicine: Advances in Picture Reconstruction – Theory and Applications*, Volume 6. Oxford: Pergamon Press, 1976.

T. M. Cover and J. A. Thomas. *Elements of Information Theory*. New York: John Wiley & Sons, 1991.

R. Crane. *A Simplified Approach to Image Processing*. Englewood Cliffs, NJ: Prentice Hall, 1997.

T. S. Curry, J. E. Dowdey, and R. C. Murry. *Christensen's Physics of Diagnostic Radiology*. Philadelphia, PA: Lea and Febiger, fourth edition, 1990.

P. P. Denby and B. Heaton. *Physics for Diagnostic Radiology*. Bristol: Institute of Physics Publishing, second edition, 1999.

E. R. Dougherty and J. T. Astola. *Nonlinear Filters for Image Processing*. Washington, DC: SPIE Optical Engineering Press, 1999.

R. O. Duda and P. E. Hart. *Pattern Classification and Scene Analysis*. New York: John Wiley & Sons, 1973.

R. L. Eisenberg. *Radiology: An Illustrated History*. St. Louis, MN: Mosby Year Book, 1991.

R. F. Farr and P. J. Allisy-Roberts. *Physics for Medical Imaging*. London: WB Saunders, Harcourt Publishers, third edition, 1999.

J. D. Foley, A. van Dam, S. Feiner, and J. Hughes. *Computer Graphics: Principles and Practice*. Reading, MA: Addison-Wesley Publishing Company, second edition, 1990.

J. D. Foley, A. van Dam, S. K. Feiner, J. F. Hughes, and R. L. Phillips. *Introduction to Computer Graphics*. Reading, MA: Addison-Wesley Publishing Company, second edition, 1997.

D. A. Forsyth and J. Ponce. *Computer Vision a Modern Approach*. Englewood Cliffs, NJ: Prentice-Hall International, 2003.

G. Liney. *MRI from A to Z, A Definitive Guide for Medical Professionals*. Cambridge: Cambridge University Press, 2005.

S. Gasiorowicz. *Quantum Physics*. New York: John Wiley & Sons, first edition, 1974.

P. L. Gildenberg and R. R. Tasker. *Textbook of Stereotactic and Functional Neurosurgery*. New York: McGraw-Hill, 1998.

C. Guy and D. Ffytche. *An Introduction to the Principles of Medical Imaging*. London: Imperial College Press, revised edition, 2005.

E. M. Haacke, R. W. Brown, M. R. Thompson, and R. Venkatesan. *Magnetic Resonance Imaging, Physical Principles and Sequence Design*. New York: John Wiley & Sons, first edition, 1999.

W. R. Hendee and E. R. Ritenour. *Medical Imaging Physics*. New York: Wiley-Liss, fourth edition, 2002.

G. T. Herman. *Image Reconstruction from Projections.* Boston, MA: Academic Press, 1980.

F. S. Hill. *Computer Graphics Using OpenGL.* Englewood Cliffs, NJ: Prentice-Hall International, second edition, 2001.

J. Hsieh. *Computed Tomography: Principles, Design, Artifacts, and Recent Advances.* Cambridge: Cambridge University Press, SPIE Publications, SPIE Press Monograph, Volume PM114, 2003.

J. A. Jensen. *Estimation of Blood Velocities Using Ultrasound: a Signal Processing Approach.* Cambridge: Cambridge University Press, 1996.

H. E. Johns and J. R. Cunningham. *The Physics of Radiology.* Springfield, IL: Charles C. Thomas, third edition, 1971.

A. C. Kak and M. Slaney. *Principles of Computerized Tomographic Imaging.* New York: IEEE Press, 1987.

W. A. Kalender. *Computed Tomography: Fundamentals, System Technology, Image Quality, Applications.* Cambridge: Cambridge University Press, Wiley-VCH, SPIE Press Monograph Volume PM114, second edition, 2006.

Y. Kim and S. C. Horii. *Handbook of Medical Imaging,* Volume 3, *Display and PACS.* Washington: SPIE Press, 2000.

A. Low. *Introductory Computer Vision and Image Processing.* London: McGraw-Hill Book Company, 1991.

F. Natterer. *The Mathematics of Computerized Tomography.* New York: John Wiley & Sons, 1986.

A. Oppenheim, A. Willsky, and H. Nawab. *Signals and Systems.* Upper Saddle River, NJ: Prentice-Hall International, second edition, 1997.

W. K. Pratt. *Digital Image Processing.* New York: John Wiley & Sons, 1991.

R. A. Robb. *Three-Dimensional Biomedical Imaging.* Boca Raton, FL: CRC Press, 1985.

K. K. Shung, M. B. Smith, and B. Tsui. *Principles of Medical Imaging.* San Diego, CA: Academic Press, 1992.

M. Sonka and J. M. Fitzpatrick. *Handbook of Medical Imaging,* Volume 2, *Medical Image Processing and Analysis.* Washington, DC: SPIE Press, 2000.

R. H. Taylor, S. Lavallée, G. C. Burdea, and R. Mösges. *Computed-Integrated Surgery: Technology and Clinical Applications.* Cambridge, MA: MIT Press, 1996.

M. M. Ter-Pogossian. *Reconstruction Tomography in Diagnostic Radiology and Nuclear Medicine.* Baltimore, MD: University Park Press, 1977.

M. M. Ter-Pogossian. Instrumentation for cardiac positron emission tomography: background and historical perspective. In S. Bergmann and B. Sobel, editors, *Positron Emission Tomography of the Heart.* New York: Futura Publishing Company, 1992.

J. K. Udupa and G. T. Herman *3D Imaging in Medicine.* Boca Raton, FL: CRC Press, second edition, 2000.

M. T. Vlaardingerbroek and J. A. Den Boer. *Magnetic Resonance Imaging: Theory and Practice.* Berlin: Springer-Verlag, second edition, 1999.

# Index